ANOMALIES AND CURIOSITIES
Of
MEDICINE

Volume I

ANOMALIES AND CURIOSITIES
Of
MEDICINE

Volume I

GEORGE M. GOULD, A.M., M.D.
WALTER L. PYLE, A.M., M.D.

ANOMALIES AND CURIOSITIES OF MEDICINE
VOLUME I

Published in the United States by IndyPublish.com
Boston, Massachusetts

ISBN 1-58827-607-4 (paperback)

ANOMALIES AND CURIOSITIES OF MEDICINE

Being an encyclopedic collection of rare and extraordinary cases, and of the ost striking instances of abnormality in all branches of medicine and surgery, erived from an exhaustive research of medical literature from its origin to the present day, abstracted, classified, annotated, and indexed.

PREFATORY AND INTRODUCTORY

Since the time when man's mind first busied itself with subjects beyond his own self-preservation and the satisfaction of his bodily appetites, the anomalous and curious have been of exceptional and persistent fascination to him; and especially is this true of the construction and functions of the human body. Possibly, indeed, it was the anomalous that was largely instrumental in arousing in the savage the attention, thought, and investigation that were finally to develop into the body of organized truth which we now call Science. As by the aid of collected experience and careful inference we to-day endeavor to pass our vision into the dim twilight whence has emerged our civilization, we find abundant hint and even evidence of this truth. To the highest type of philosophic minds it is the usual and the ordinary that demand investigation and explanation. But even to such, no less than to the most naive-minded, the strange and exceptional is of absorbing interest, and it is often through the extraordinary that the philosopher gets the most searching glimpses into the heart of the mystery of the ordinary. Truly it has been said, facts are stranger than fiction. In monstrosities and dermoid cysts, for example, we seem to catch forbidden sight of the secret workroom of Nature, and drag out into the light the evidences of her clumsiness, and proofs of her lapses of skill,—evidences and proofs, moreover, that tell us much of the methods and means used by the vital artisan of Life,—the loom, and even the silent weaver at work upon the mysterious garment of corporeality.

"La premiere chose qui s'offre a l' Homme quand il se regarde, c'est son corps," says Pascal, and looking at the matter more closely we find that it was the strange and mysterious things of his body that occupied man's earliest as well as much of his later attention. In the beginning, the organs and functions of generation, the mysteries of sex, not the routine of digestion or of locomotion, stimulated his curiosity, and in them he recognized, as it were, an unseen hand reaching down into the world of matter and the workings of bodily organization, and reining them to impersonal service and far-off ends. All ethnologists and students of primitive religion well know the role that has been played in primitive society by the genetic instincts. Among the older naturalists, such as Pliny and Aristotle, and even in the older historians, whose scope included natural as well as civil and political history, the atypic and bizarre, and especially the aberrations of form or function of the generative organs, caught the eye most quickly. Judging from the records of early writers, when Medicine began to struggle toward self-consciousness, it was again the same order of facts that was singled out by the attention. The very names applied by the early anatomists to many structures so widely separated from the organs of generation as were those of the brain, give testimony of the state of mind that led to and dominated the practice of dissection.

In the literature of the past centuries the predominance of the interest in the curious is exemplified in the almost ludicrously monotonous iteration of titles, in which the conspicuous words are curiosa, rara, monstruosa, memorabilia, prodigiosa, selecta, exotica, miraculi, lusibus naturae, occultis naturae, etc., etc. Even when medical science became more strict, it was largely the curious and rare that were thought worthy of chronicling, and not the establishment or illustration of the common, or of general principles. With all his sovereign sound sense, Ambrose Pare has loaded his book with references to impossibly strange, and even mythologic cases.

In our day the taste seems to be insatiable, and hardly any medical journal is without its rare or "unique" case, or one noteworthy chiefly by reason of its anomalous features. A curious case is invariably reported, and the insertion of such a report is generally productive of correspondence and discussion with the object of finding a parallel for it.

In view of all this it seems itself a curious fact that there has never been any systematic gathering of medical curiosities. It would have been most natural that numerous encyclopedias should spring into existence in response to such a persistently dominant interest. The forelying volume appears to be the first thorough attempt to classify and epitomize the literature of this nature. It has been our purpose to briefly summarize and to arrange in order the records of the most curious, bizarre, and abnormal cases that are found in medical literature of all ages and all languages—a thaumatographia medica. It will be readily seen that such a collection must have a function far beyond the satisfaction of mere curiosity, even if that be stigmatized with the word "idle." If, as we believe, reference may here be found to all such cases in the literature of Medicine (including Anatomy, Physiology, Surgery, Obstetrics, etc.) as show the most extreme and exceptional departures from the ordinary, it follows that the future clinician and investigator must have use for a handbook that decides whether his own strange case has already been paralleled or excelled. He will thus be aided in determining the truth of his statements and the accuracy of his diagnoses. Moreover, to know extremes gives directly some knowledge of means, and by implication and inference it frequently does more. Remarkable injuries illustrate to what extent tissues and organs may be damaged without resultant death, and thus the surgeon is encouraged to proceed to his operation with greater confidence and more definite knowledge as to the issue. If a mad cow may blindly play the part of a successful obstetrician with her horns, certainly a skilled surgeon may hazard entering the womb with his knife. If large portions of an organ,—the lung, a kidney, parts of the liver, or the brain itself,—may be lost by accident, and the patient still live, the physician is taught the lesson of nil desperandum, and that if possible to arrest disease of these organs before their total destruction, the prognosis and treatment thereby acquire new and more hopeful phases.

Directly or indirectly many similar examples have also clear medicolegal bearings or suggestions; in fact, it must be acknowledged that much of the importance of medical jurisprudence lies in a thorough comprehension of the anomalous and rare cases in Medicine. Expert medical testimony has its chief value in showing the possibilities of the occurrence of alleged extreme cases, and extraordinary deviations from the natural. Every expert witness should be able to maintain his argument by a full citation of parallels to any remarkable theory or hypothesis advanced by his clients; and it is only by an exhaustive knowledge of extremes and anomalies that an authority on medical jurisprudence can hope to substantiate his testimony beyond question. In every poisoning case he is closely questioned as to the largest dose of the drug in question that has been taken with impunity, and the smallest dose that has killed, and he is expected to have the cases of reported idiosyncrasies and tolerance at his immediate command. A widow with a child of ten months' gestation may be saved the loss of reputation by mention of the authentic cases in which pregnancy has exceeded nine months' duration; the proof of the viability of a seven months' child may alter the disposition of an estate; the proof of death by a blow on the epigastrium without external marks of violence may convict a murderer; and so it is with many other cases of a medicolegal nature.

It is noteworthy that in old-time medical literature—sadly and unjustly neglected in our rage for the new—should so often be found parallels of our most wonderful and peculiar modern cases. We wish, also, to enter a mild protest against the modern egotism that would set aside with a sneer as myth and fancy the testimonies and reports of philosophers and physicians, only because they lived hundreds of years ago. We are keenly appreciative of the power exercised by the myth-making faculty in the past, but as applied to early physicians, we suggest that the suspicion may easily be too active. When Pare, for example, pictures a monster, we may distrust his art, his artist, or his engraver, and make all due allowance for his primitive knowledge of teratology, coupled with the exaggerations and inventions of the wonder-lover; but when he describes in his own writing what he or his confreres have seen on the battle-field or in the dissecting room, we think, within moderate limits, we owe him credence. For the rest, we doubt not that the modern reporter is, to be mild, quite as much of a myth-maker as his elder brother, especially if we find modern instances that are essentially like the older cases reported in reputable journals or books, and by men presumably honest. In our collection we have endeavored, so far as possible, to cite similar cases from the older and from the more recent literature.

This connection suggests the question of credibility in general. It need hardly be said that the lay-journalist and newspaper reporter have usually been ignored by us, simply because experience and investigation have many times proved that a scientific fact, by presentation in most lay-journals, becomes in some mysterious manner, ipso facto, a scientific caricature (or worse !), and if it is so with facts, what must be the effect upon reports based upon no fact whatsoever? It is manifestly impossible for us to guarantee the credibility of chronicles given. If we have been reasonably certain of unreliability, we may not even have mentioned the marvelous statement. Obviously, we could do no more with apparently credible cases, reported by reputable medical men, than to cite author and source and leave the matter there, where our responsibility must end.

But where our proper responsibility seemed likely never to end was in carrying out the enormous labor requisite for a reasonable certainty that we had omitted no searching that might lead to undiscovered facts, ancient or modern. Choice in selection is always, of course, an affair de gustibus, and especially when, like the present, there is considerable embarrassment of riches, coupled with the purpose of compressing our results in one handy volume. In brief, it may be said that several years of exhaustive research have been spent by us in the great medical libraries of the United States and Europe in collecting the material herewith presented. If, despite of this, omissions and errors are to be found, we shall be grateful to have them pointed out. It must be remembered that limits of space have forbidden satisfactory discussion of the cases, and the prime object of the whole work has been to carefully collect and group the anomalies and curiosities, and allow the reader to form his own conclusions and make his own deductions.

As the entire labor in the preparation of the forelying volume, from the inception of the idea to the completion of the index, has been exclusively the personal work of the authors, it is with full confidence of the authenticity of the reports quoted that the material is presented.

Complete references are given to those facts that are comparatively unknown or unique, or that are worthy of particular interest or further investigation. To prevent unnecessary loading of the book with foot-notes, in those instances in which there are a number of cases of the same nature, and a description has not been thought necessary, mere citation being sufficient, references are but briefly given or omitted altogether. For the same reason a bibliographic index has been added at the end of the text. This contains the most important sources of information used, and each journal or book therein has its own number, which is used in its stead all through the book (thus, 476 signifies The Lancet, London; 597, the New York Medical Journal; etc.). These bibliographic numbers begin at 100.

Notwithstanding that every effort has been made to conveniently and satisfactorily group the thousands of cases contained in the book (a labor of no small proportions in itself), a complete general index is a practical necessity for the full success of what is essentially a reference-volume, and consequently one has been added, in which may be found not only the subjects under consideration and numerous cross-references, but also the names of the authors of the most important reports. A table of contents follows this preface.

We assume the responsibility for innovations in orthography, certain abbreviations, and the occasional substitution of figures for large numerals, fractions, and decimals, made necessary by limited space, and in some cases to more lucidly show tables and statistics. From the variety of the reports, uniformity of nomenclature and numeration is almost impossible.

As we contemplate constantly increasing our data, we shall be glad to receive information of any unpublished anomalous or curious cases, either of the past or in the future.

For many courtesies most generously extended in aiding our research-work we wish, among others, to acknowledge our especial gratitude and indebtedness to the officers and assistants of the Surgeon-General's Library at Washington, D.C., the Library of the Royal College of Surgeons of London, the Library of the British Museum, the Library of the British Medical Association, the Bibliotheque de Faculte de Medecine de Paris, the Bibliotheque Nationale, and the Library of the College of Physicians of Philadelphia.

GEORGE M. GOULD.
PHILADELPHIA, October, 1896.   WALTER L. PYLE.

TABLE OF CONTENTS

CHAPTER   PAGES

I. GENETIC ANOMALIES 1

II. PRENATAL ANOMALIES 32

III. OBSTETRIC ANOMALIES 87

IV. PROLIFICITY 116

V. MAJOR TERATA 134

VI. MINOR TERATA 175

VII. ANOMALIES OF STATURE, SIZE, AND DEVELOPMENT. 271

VIII. LONGEVITY 305

IX. PHYSIOLOGIC AND FUNCTIONAL ANOMALIES 325

CHAPTER I

GENETIC ANOMALIES.

Menstruation has always been of interest, not only to the student of medicine, but to the lay-observer as well. In olden times there were many opinions concerning its causation, all of which, until the era of physiologic investigation, were of superstitious derivation. Believing menstruation to be the natural means of exit of the feminine bodily impurities, the ancients always thought a menstruating woman was to be shunned; her very presence was deleterious to the whole animal economy, as, for instance, among the older writers we find that Pliny remarks: "On the approach of a woman in this state, must will become sour, seeds which are touched by her become sterile, grass withers away, garden plants are parched up, and the fruit will fall from the tree beneath which she sits." He also says that the menstruating women in Cappadocia were perambulated about the fields to preserve the vegetation from worms and caterpillars. According to Flemming, menstrual blood was believed to be so powerful that the mere touch of a menstruating woman would render vines and all kinds of fruit-trees sterile. Among the indigenous Australians, menstrual superstition was so intense that one of the native blacks, who discovered his wife lying on his blanket during her menstrual period, killed her, and died of terror himself in a fortnight. Hence, Australian women during this season are forbidden to touch anything that men use. Aristotle said that the very look of a menstruating woman would take the polish out of a mirror, and the next person looking in it would be bewitched. Frommann mentions a man who said he saw a tree in Goa which withered because a catamenial napkin was hung on it. Bourke remarks that the dread felt by the American Indians in this respect corresponds with the particulars recited by Pliny. Squaws at the time of menstrual purgation are obliged to seclude themselves, and in most instances to occupy isolated lodges, and in all tribes are forbidden to prepare food for anyone save themselves. It was believed that, were a menstruating woman to step astride a rifle, a bow, or a lance, the weapon would have no utility. Medicine men are in the habit of making a "protective" clause whenever they concoct a "medicine," which is to the effect that the "medicine" will be effective provided that no woman in this condition is allowed to approach the tent of the official in charge.

Empiricism had doubtless taught the ancient husbands the dangers of sexual intercourse during this period, and the after-results of many such connections were looked upon as manifestations of the contagiousness of the evil excretions issuing at this period. Hence at one time menstruation was held in much awe and abhorrence.

On the other hand, in some of the eastern countries menstruation was regarded as sacred, and the first menstrual discharge was considered so valuable that premenstrual marriages were inaugurated in order that the first ovum might not be wasted, but fertilized, because it was supposed to be the purest and best for the purpose. Such customs are extant at the present day in some parts of India, despite the efforts of the British Government to suppress them, and descriptions of child-marriages and their evil results have often been given by missionaries.

As the advances of physiology enlightened the mind as to the true nature of the menstrual period, and the age of superstition gradually disappeared, the intense interest in menstruation vanished, and now, rather than being held in fear and awe, the physicians of to-day constantly see the results of copulation during this period. The uncontrollable desire of the husband and the mercenary aims of the prostitute furnish examples of modern disregard.

The anomalies of menstruation must naturally have attracted much attention, and we find medical literature of all times replete with examples. While some are simply examples of vicarious or compensatory menstruation, and were so explained even by the older writers, there are many that are physiologic curiosities of considerable interest. Lheritier furnishes the oft-quoted history of the case of a young girl who suffered from suppression of menses, which, instead of flowing through the natural channels, issued periodically from vesicles on the leg for a period of six months, when the seat of the discharge changed to an eruption on the left arm, and continued in this location for one year; then the discharge shifted to a sore on the thumb, and at the end of another six months again changed, the next location being on the upper eyelid; here it continued for a period of two years. Brierre de Boismont and Meisner describe a case apparently identical with the foregoing, though not quoting the source.

Haller, in a collection of physiologic curiosities covering a period of a century and a half, cites 18 instances of menstruation from the skin. Parrot has also mentioned several cases of this nature. Chambers speaks of bloody sweat occurring periodically in a woman of twenty-seven; the intervals, however, were occasionally but a week or a fortnight, and the exudation was not confined to any one locality. Van Swieten quotes the history of a case of suppression of the menstrual function in which there were convulsive contractions of the body, followed by paralysis of the right arm. Later on, the patient received a blow on the left eye causing amaurosis; swelling of this organ followed, and one month later blood issued from it, and subsequently blood oozed from the skin of the nose, and ran in jets from the skin of the fingers and from the nails.

D'Andrade cites an account of a healthy Parsee lady, eighteen years of age, who menstruated regularly from thirteen to fifteen and a half years; the catamenia then became irregular and she suffered occasional hemorrhages from the gums and nose, together with attacks of hematemesis. The menstruation returned, but she never became pregnant, and, later, blood issued from the healthy skin of the left breast and right forearm, recurring every month or two, and finally additional dermal hemorrhage developed on the forehead. Microscopic examination of the exuded blood showed usual constituents present. There are two somewhat similar cases spoken of in French literature. The first was that of a young lady, who, after ten years' suppression of the menstrual discharge, exhibited the flow from a vesicular eruption on the finger. The other case was quite peculiar, the woman being a prostitute, who menstruated from time to time through spots, the size of a five-franc piece, developing on the breasts, buttocks, back, axilla, and epigastrium. Barham records a case similar to the foregoing, in which the menstruation assumed the character of periodic purpura. Duchesne mentions an instance of complete amenorrhea, in which the ordinary flow was replaced by periodic sweats.

Parrot speaks of a woman who, when seven months old, suffered from strumous ulcers, which left cicatrices on the right hand, from whence, at the age of six years, issued a sanguineous discharge with associate convulsions. One day, while in violent grief, she shed bloody tears. She menstruated at the age of eleven, and was temporarily improved in her condition; but after any strong emotion the hemorrhages returned. The subsidence of the bleeding followed her first pregnancy, but subsequently on one occasion, when the menses were a few days in arrears, she exhibited a blood-like exudation from the forehead, eyelids, and scalp. As in the case under D'Andrade's observation, the exudation was found by microscopic examination to consist of the true constituents of blood. An additional element of complication in this case was the occurrence of occasional attacks of hematemesis.

Menstruation from the Breasts.—Being in close sympathy with the generative function, we would naturally expect to find the female mammae involved in cases of anomalous menstruation, and the truth of this supposition is substantiated in the abundance of such cases on record. Schenck reports instances of menstruation from the nipple; and Richter, de Fontechia, Laurentius, Marcellus Donatus, Amatus Lusitanus, and Bierling are some of the older writers who have observed this anomaly. Pare says the wife of Pierre de Feure, an iron merchant, living at Chasteaudun, menstruated such quantities from the breasts each month that several serviettes were necessary to receive the discharge. Cazenave details the history of a case in which the mammary menstruation was associated with a similar exudation from the face, and Wolff saw an example associated with hemorrhage from the fauces. In the Lancet (1840-1841) is an instance of monthly discharge from beneath the left mamma. Finley also writes of an example of mammary hemorrhage simulating menstruation. Barnes saw a case in St. George's Hospital, London, 1876, in which the young girl menstruated vicariously from the nipple and stomach. In a London discussion there was mentioned the case of a healthy woman of fifty who never was pregnant, and whose menstruation had ceased two years previously, but who for twelve months had menstruated regularly from the nipples, the hemorrhage being so profuse as to require constant change of napkins. The mammae were large and painful, and the accompanying symptoms were those of ordinary menstruation. Boulger mentions an instance of periodic menstrual discharge from beneath the left mamma. Jacobson speaks of habitual menstruation by both breasts. Rouxeau describes amenorrhea in a girl of seventeen, who menstruated from the breast; and Teufard reports a case in which there was reestablishment of menstruation by the mammae at the age of fifty-six. Baker details in full the description of a case of vicarious menstruation from an ulcer on the right mamma of a woman of twenty. At the time he was called to see her she was suffering with what was called "green-sickness." The girl had never menstruated regularly or freely. The right mamma was quite well developed, flaccid, the nipple prominent, and the superficial veins larger and more tortuous than usual. The patient stated that the right mamma had always been larger than the left. The areola was large and well marked, and 1/4 inch from its outer edge, immediately under the nipple, there was an ulcer with slightly elevated edges measuring about 1 1/4 inches across the base, and having an opening in its center 1/4 inch in diameter, covered with a thin scab. By removing the scab and making pressure at the base of the ulcer, drops of thick, mucopurulent matter were made to exude. This discharge, however, was not offensive to the smell. On March 17, 1846, the breast became much enlarged and congested, as portrayed in Plate 1. The ulcer was much inflamed and painful, the veins corded and deep colored, and there was a free discharge of sanguineous yellowish matter. When the girl's general health improved and menstruation became more natural, the vicarious discharge diminished in proportion, and the ulcer healed shortly afterward. Every month this breast had enlarged, the ulcer became inflamed and discharged vicariously, continuing in this manner for a few days, with all the accompanying menstrual symptoms, and then dried up gradually. It was stated that the ulcer was the result of the girl's stooping over some bushes to take an egg from a hen's nest, when the point of a palmetto stuck in her breast and broke off. The ulcer subsequently formed, and ultimately discharged a piece of palmetto. This happened just at the time of the beginning of the menstrual epoch. The accompanying figures, Plate 1, show the breast in the ordinary state and at the time of the anomalous discharge.

Hancock relates an instance of menstruation from the left breast in a large, otherwise healthy, Englishwoman of thirty-one, who one and a half years after the birth of the youngest child (now ten years old) commenced to have a discharge of fluid from the left breast three days before the time of the regular period. As the fluid escaped from the nipple it became changed in character, passing from a whitish to a bloody and to a yellowish color respectively, and suddenly terminating at the beginning of the real flow from the uterus, to reappear again at the breast at the close of the flow, and then lasting two or three days longer. Some pain of a lancinating type occurred in the breast at this time. The patient first discovered her peculiar condition by a stain of blood upon the night-gown on awakening in the morning, and this she traced to the breast. From an examination it appeared that a neglected lacerated cervix during the birth of the last child had given rise to endometritis, and for a year the patient had suffered from severe menorrhagia, for which she was subsequently treated. At this time the menses became scanty, and then supervened the discharge of bloody fluid from the left breast, as heretofore mentioned. The right breast remained always entirely passive. A remarkable feature of the case was that some escape of fluid occurred from the left breast during coitus. As a possible means of throwing light on this subject it may be added that the patient was unusually vigorous, and during the nursing of her two children she had more than the ordinary amount of milk (galactorrhea), which poured from the breast constantly. Since this time the breasts had been quite normal, except for the tendency manifested in the left one under the conditions given.

Cases of menstruation through the eyes are frequently mentioned by the older writers. Bellini, Hellwig, and Dodonaeus all speak of menstruation from the eye. Jonston quotes an example of ocular menstruation in a young Saxon girl, and

Bartholinus an instance associated with bloody discharge of the foot. Guepin has an example in a case of a girl of eighteen, who commenced to menstruate when three years old. The menstruation was tolerably regular, occurring every thirty-two or thirty-three days, and lasting from one to six days. At the cessation of the menstrual flow, she generally had a supplementary epistaxis, and on one occasion, when this was omitted, she suffered a sudden effusion into the anterior chamber of the eye. The discharge had only lasted two hours on this occasion. He also relates an example of hemorrhage into the vitreous humor in a case of amenorrhea. Conjunctival hemorrhage has been noticed as a manifestation of vicarious menstruation by several American observers. Liebreich found examples of retinal hemorrhage in suppressed menstruation, and Sir James Paget says that he has seen a young girl at Moorfields who had a small effusion of blood into the anterior chamber of the eye at the menstrual period, which became absorbed during the intervals of menstruation. Blair relates the history of a case of vicarious menstruation attended with conjunctivitis and opacity of the cornea. Law speaks of a plethoric woman of thirty who bled freely from the eyes, though menstruating regularly.

Relative to menstruation from the ear, Spindler, Paullini, and Alibert furnish examples. In Paullini's case the discharge is spoken of as very foul, which makes it quite possible that this was a case of middle-ear disease associated with some menstrual disturbance, and not one of true vicarious menstruation. Alibert's case was consequent upon suppression of the menses. Law cites an instance in a woman of twenty-three, in whom the menstrual discharge was suspended several months. She experienced fulness of the head and bleeding (largely from the ears), which subsequently occurred periodically, being preceded by much throbbing; but the patient finally made a good recovery. Barnes, Stepanoff, and Field adduce examples of this anomaly. Jouilleton relates an instance of menstruation from the right ear for five years, following a miscarriage.

Hemorrhage from the mouth of a vicarious nature has been frequently observed associated with menstrual disorders. The Ephemerides, Meibomius, and Rhodius mention instances. The case of Meibomius was that of an infant, and the case mentioned by Rhodius was associated with hemorrhages from the lungs, umbilicus, thigh, and tooth-cavity. Allport reports the history of a case in which there was recession of the gingival margins and alveolar processes, the consequence of amenorrhea. Caso has an instance of menstruation from the gums, and there is on record the description of a woman, aged thirty-two, who had bleeding from the throat preceding menstruation; later the menstruation ceased to be regular, and four years previously, after an unfortunate and violent connection, the menses ceased, and the woman soon developed hemorrhoids and hemoptysis. Henry speaks of a woman who menstruated from the mouth; at the necropsy 207 stones were found in the gall-bladder. Krishaber speaks of a case of lingual menstruation at the epoch of menstruation.

Descriptions of menstruation from the extremities are quite numerous. Pechlin offers an example from the foot; Boerhaave from the skin of the hand; Ephemerides from the knee; Albertus from the foot; Zacutus Lusitanus from the left thumb; Bartholinus a curious instance from the hand; and the Ephemerides another during pregnancy from the ankle.

Post speaks of a very peculiar case of edema of the arm alternating with the menstrual discharge. Sennert writes of menstruation from the groin associated with hemorrhage from the umbilicus and gums. Moses offers an example of hemorrhage from the umbilicus, doubtless vicarious. Verduc details the history of two cases from the top of the head, and Kerokring cites three similar instances, one of which was associated with hemorrhage from the hand.

A peculiar mode is vicarious menstrual hemorrhage through old ulcers, wounds, or cicatrices, and many examples are on record, a few of which will be described. Calder gives an excellent account of menstruation at an ankle-ulcer, and Brincken says he has seen periodical bleeding from the cicatrix of a leprous ulcer. In the Lancet is an account of a case in the Vienna Hospital of simulated stigmata; the scar opened each month and a menstrual flow proceeded therefrom; but by placing a plaster-of-Paris bandage about the wound, sealing it so that tampering with the wound could be easily detected, healing soon ensued, and the imposture was thus exposed. Such would likely be the result of the investigation of most cases of "bleeding wounds" which are exhibited to the ignorant and superstitious for religious purposes.

Hogg publishes a report describing a young lady who injured her leg with the broken steel of her crinoline. The wound healed nicely, but always burst out afresh the day preceding the regular period. Forster speaks of a menstrual ulcer of the face, and Moses two of the head. White, quoted by Barnes, cites an instance of vicarious hemorrhage from five deep fissures of the lips in a girl of fourteen; the hemorrhage was periodical and could not be checked. At the advent of each menstrual period the lips became much congested, and the recently-healed menstrual scars burst open anew.

Knaggs relates an interesting account of a sequel to an operation for ovarian disease. Following the operation, there was a regular, painless menstruation every month, at which time the lower part of the wound re-opened, and blood issued forth during the three days of the catamenia. McGraw illustrates vicarious menstruation by an example, the discharge issuing from an ovariotomy-scar, and Hooper cites an instance in which the vicarious function was performed by a sloughing ulcer. Buchanan and Simpson describe "amenorrheal ulcers." Dupuytren speaks of denudation of the skin from a burn, with the subsequent development of vicarious catamenia from the seat of the injury.

There are cases on record in which the menstruation occurs by the rectum or the urinary tract. Barbee illustrates this by a case in which cholera morbus occurred monthly in lieu of the regular menstrual discharge. Barrett speaks of a case of vicarious menstruation by the rectum. Astbury says he has seen a case of menstruation by the hemorrhoidal vessels, and instances of relief from plethora by vicarious menstruation in this manner are quite common. Rosenbladt cites an instance of menstruation by the bladder, and Salmuth speaks of a pregnant woman who had her monthly flow by the urinary tract. Ford illustrates this anomaly by the case of a woman of thirty-two, who began normal menstruation at fourteen; for quite a period she had vicarious menstruation from the urinary tract, which ceased after the birth of her last child. The coexistence of a floating kidney in this case may have been responsible for this hemorrhage, and in reading reports of so-called menstruation due consideration must be given to the existence of any other than menstrual derangement before we can accept the cases as true vicarious hemorrhage. Tarnier cites an instance of a girl without a uterus, in whom menstruation proceeded from the vagina. Zacutus Lusitanus relates the history of a case of uterine occlusion, with the flow from the lips of the cervix. There is mentioned an instance of menstruation from the labia.

The occurrence of menstruation after removal of the uterus or ovaries is frequently reported. Storer, Clay, Tait, and the British and Foreign Medico-Chirurgical Review report cases in which menstruation took place with neither uterus nor ovary. Doubtless many authentic instances like the preceding could be found to-day. Menstruation after hysterectomy and ovariotomy has been attributed to the incomplete removal of the organs in question, yet upon postmortem examination of some cases no vestige of the functional organs in question has been found.

Hematemesis is a means of anomalous menstruation, and several instances are recorded. Marcellus Donatus and Benivenius exemplify this with cases. Instances of vicarious and compensatory epistaxis and hemoptysis are so common that any examples would be superfluous. There is recorded an inexplicable case of menstruation from the region of the sternum, and among the curious anomalies of menstruation must be mentioned that reported by Parvin seen in a woman, who, at the menstrual epoch, suffered hemoptysis and oozing of blood from the lips and tongue. Occasionally there was a substitution of a great swelling of the tongue, rendering mastication and articulation very difficult for four or five days. Parvin gives portraits showing the venous congestion and discoloration of the lips.

Instances of migratory menstruation, the flow moving periodically from the ordinary passage to the breasts and mammae, are found in the older writers. Salmuth speaks of a woman on whose hands appeared spots immediately before the establishment of the menses. Cases of semimonthly menstruation and many similar anomalies of periodicity are spoken of.

The Ephemerides contains an instance of the simulation of menstruation after death, and Testa speaks of menstruation lasting through a long sleep. Instances of black menstruation are to be found, described in full, in the Ephemerides, by Paullini and by Schurig, and in some of the later works; it is possible that an excess of iron, administered for some menstrual disorder, may cause such an alteration in the color of the menstrual fluid.

Suppression of menstruation is brought about in many peculiar ways, and sometimes by the slightest of causes, some authentic instances being so strange as to seem mythical. Through the Ephemerides we constantly read of such causes as contact with a corpse, the sight of a serpent or mouse, the sight of monsters, etc. Lightning stroke and curious neuroses have been reported as causes. Many of the older books on obstetric subjects are full of such instances, and modern illustrations are constantly reported.

Menstruation in Man.—Periodic discharges of blood in man, constituting what is called "male menstruation," have been frequently noticed and are particularly interesting when the discharge is from the penis or urethra, furnishing a striking analogy to the female function of menstruation. The older authors quoted several such instances, and Mehliss says that in the ancient days certain writers remarked that catamenial lustration from the penis was inflicted on the Jews as a divine punishment. Bartholinus mentions a case in a youth; the Ephemerides several instances; Zacutus Lusitanus, Salmuth, Hngedorn, Fabricius Hildanus, Vesalius, Mead, and Acta Eruditorum all mention instances. Forel saw menstruation in a man. Gloninger tells of a man of thirty-six, who, since the age of seventeen years and five months, had had lunar manifestations of menstruation. Each attack was accompanied by pains in the back and hypogastric region, febrile disturbance, and a sanguineous discharge from the urethra, which resembled in color, consistency, etc., the menstrual flux. King relates that while attending a course of medical lectures at the University of Louisiana he formed the acquaintance of a young student who possessed the normal male generative organs, but in whom the simulated function of menstruation was periodically performed. The cause was inexplicable, and the unfortunate victim was the subject of deep chagrin, and was afflicted with melancholia. He had menstruated for three years in this manner: a fluid exuded from the sebaceous glands of the deep fossa behind the corona glandis; this fluid was of the same appearance as the menstrual flux. The quantity was from one to two ounces, and the discharge lasted from three to six days. At this time the student was twenty-two years of age, of a lymphatic temperament, not particularly lustful, and was never the victim of any venereal disease. The author gives no account of the after-life of this man, his whereabouts being, unfortunately, unknown or omitted.

Vicarious Menstruation in the Male.—This simulation of menstruation by the male assumes a vicarious nature as well as in the female. Van Swieten, quoting from Benivenius, relates a case of a man who once a month sweated great quantities of blood from his right flank. Pinel mentions a case of a captain in the army (M. Regis), who was wounded by a bullet in the body and who afterward had a monthly discharge from the urethra. Pinel calls attention particularly to the analogy in this case by mentioning that if the captain were exposed to fatigue, privation, cold, etc., he exhibited the ordinary symptoms of amenorrhea or suppression. Fournier speaks of a man over thirty years old, who had been the subject of a menstrual evacuation since puberty, or shortly after his first sexual intercourse. He would experience pains of the premenstrual type, about twenty-four hours before the appearance of the flow, which subsided when the menstruation began. He was of an intensely voluptuous nature, and constantly gave himself up to sexual excesses. The flow was abundant on the first day, diminished on the second, and ceased on the third. Halliburton, Jouilleton, and Rayman also record male menstruation.

Cases of menstruation during pregnancy and lactation are not rare. It is not uncommon to find pregnancy, lactation, and menstruation coexisting. No careful obstetrician will deny pregnancy solely on the regular occurrence of the menstrual periods, any more than he would make the diagnosis of pregnancy from the fact of the suppression of menses. Blake reports an instance of catamenia and mammary secretion during pregnancy. Denaux de Breyne mentions a similar case. The child was born by a face-presentation. De Saint-Moulin cites an instance of the persistence of menstruation during pregnancy in a woman of twenty-four, who had never been regular; the child was born at term. Gelly speaks of a case in which menstruation continued until the third month of pregnancy, when abortion occurred. Post, in describing the birth of a two-pound child, mentions that menstruation had persisted during the mother's pregnancy. Rousset reports a peculiar case in which menstruation appeared during the last four months of pregnancy.

There are some cases on record of child-bearing after the menopause, as, for instance, that of Pearson, of a woman who had given birth to nine children up to September, 1836; after this the menses appeared only slightly until July, 1838, when they ceased entirely. A year and a half after this she was delivered of her tenth child. Other cases, somewhat similar, will be found under the discussion of late conception.

Precocious menstruation is seen from birth to nine or ten years. Of course, menstruation before the third or fourth year is extremely rare, most of the cases reported before this age being merely accidental sanguineous discharges from the genitals, not regularly periodical, and not true catamenia. However, there are many authentic cases of infantile menstruation on record, which were generally associated with precocious development in other parts as well. Billard says that the source of infantile menstruation is the lining membrane of the uterus; but Camerer explains it as due to ligature of the umbilical cord before the circulation in the pulmonary vessels is thoroughly established. In the consideration of this subject, we must bear in mind the influence of climate and locality on the time of the appearance of menstruation. In the southern countries, girls arrive at maturity at an earlier age than their sisters of the north. Medical reports from India show early puberty of the females of that country. Campbell remarks that girls attain the age of puberty at twelve in Siam, while, on the contrary, some observers report the fact that menstruation does not appear in the Esquimaux women until the age of twenty-three, and then is very scanty, and is only present in the summer months.

Cases of menstruation commencing within a few days after birth and exhibiting periodical recurrence are spoken of by Penada, Neues Hannoverisehes Magazin, Drummond, Buxtorf, Arnold, The Lancet, and the British Medical Journal.

Cecil relates an instance of menstruation on the sixth day, continuing for five days, in which six or eight drams of blood were lost. Peeples cites an instance in Texas in an infant at the age of five days, which was associated with a remarkable development of the genital organs and breasts. Van Swieten offers an example at the first month; the British Medical Journal at the second month; Conarmond at the third month. Ysabel, a young slave girl belonging to Don Carlos Pedro of Havana, began to menstruate soon after birth, and at the first year was regular in this function. At birth her mamma were well developed and her axillae were slightly covered with hair. At the age of thirty-two months she was three feet ten inches tall, and her genitals and mammae resembled those of a girl of thirteen. Her voice was grave and sonorous; her moral inclinations were not known.

Deever records an instance of a child two years and seven months old who, with the exception of three months only, had menstruated regularly since the fourth month. Harle speaks of a child, the youngest of three girls, who had a bloody discharge at the age of five months which lasted three days and recurred every month until the child was weaned at the tenth month. At the eleventh month it returned and continued periodically until death, occasioned by diarrhea at the fourteenth month. The necropsy showed a uterus 1 5/8 inches long, the lips of which were congested; the left ovary was twice the size of the right, but displayed nothing strikingly abnormal. Baillot and the British Medical Journal cite instances of menstruation at the fourth month. A case is on record of an infant who menstruated at the age of six months, and whose menses returned on the twenty-eighth day exactly. Clark, Wall, and the Lancet give descriptions of cases at the ninth month. Naegele has seen a case at the eighteenth month, and Schmidt and Colly in the second year. Another case is that of a child, nineteen months old, whose breasts and external genitals were fully developed, although the child had shown no sexual desire, and did not exceed other children of the same age in intellectual development. This prodigy was symmetrically formed and of pleasant appearance. Warner speaks of Sophie Gantz, of Jewish parentage, born in Cincinnati, July 27, 1865, whose menses began at the twenty-third month and had continued regularly up to the time of reporting. At the age of three years and six months she was 38 inches tall, 38 pounds in weight, and her girth at the hip was 33 1/2 inches. The pelvis was broad and well shaped, and measured 10 1/2 inches from the anterior surface of the spinous process of one ilium to that of the other, being a little more than the standard pelvis of Churchill, and, in consequence of this pelvic development, her legs were bowed. The mammae and labia had all the appearance of established puberty, and the pubes and axillae were covered with hair. She was lady-like and maidenly in her demeanor, without unnatural constraint or effrontery. A case somewhat similar, though the patient had the appearance of a little old woman, was a child of three whose breasts were as well developed as in a girl of twenty, and whose sexual organs resembled those of a girl at puberty. She had menstruated regularly since the age of two years. Woodruff describes a child who began to menstruate at two years of age and continued regularly thereafter. At the age of six years she was still menstruating, and exhibited beginning signs of puberty. She was 118 cm. tall, her breasts were developed, and she had hair on the mons veneris. Van der Veer mentions an infant who began menstruating at the early age of four months and had continued regularly for over two years. She had the features and development of a child ten or twelve years old. The external labia and the vulva in all its parts were well formed, and the mons veneris was covered with a full growth of hair. Sir Astley Cooper, Mandelshof, the Ephemerides, Rause, Geoffroy-Saint-Hilaire, and several others a report instances of menstruation occurring at three years of age. Le Beau describes an infant prodigy who was born with the mammae well formed and as much hair on the mons veneris as a girl of thirteen or fourteen. She menstruated at three and continued to do so regularly, the flow lasting four days and being copious. At the age of four years and five months she was 42 1/2 inches tall; her features were regular, the complexion rosy, the hair chestnut, the eyes blue-gray, her mamma the size of a large orange, and indications that she would be able to bear children at the age of eight. Prideaux cites a case at five, and Gaugirau Casals, a doctor of Agde, has seen a girl of six years who suffered abdominal colic, hemorrhage from the nose, migraine, and neuralgia, all periodically, which, with the association of pruritus of the genitals and engorged mammae, led him to suspect amenorrhea. He ordered baths, and shortly the menstruation appeared and became regular thereafter. Brierre de Boismont records cases of catamenia at five, seven, and eight years; and Skene mentions a girl who menstruated at ten years and five months. She was in the lowest grade of society, living with a drunken father in a tenement house, and was of wretched physical constitution, quite ignorant, and of low moral character, as evinced by her specific vaginitis. Occurring from nine years to the ordinary time of puberty, many cases are recorded.

Instances of protracted menstruation are, as a rule, reliable, the individuals themselves being cognizant of the nature of true menstruation, and themselves furnishing the requisite information as to the nature and periodicity of the discharge in question. Such cases range even past the century-mark. Many elaborate statistics on this subject have been gathered by men of ability. Dr. Meyer of Berlin quotes the following:—

> 28 at 50 years of age,
> 3 at 57 years of age,
> 18 " 51 " " "
> 3 " 58 " " "
> 18 " 52 " " "
> 1 " 59 " " "
> 11 " 53 " " "
> 4 " 60 " " "
> 13 " 54 " " "
> 4 " 62 " " "
> 5 " 55 " " "
> 3 " 63 " " "
> 4 " 56 " " "

These statistics were from examination of 6000 cases of menstruating women. The last seven were found to be in women in the highest class of society.

Mehliss has made the following collection of statistics of a somewhat similar nature—

	Late Dentition. Male.	Late Dentition. Female.	Late Lactation.	Late Menstruation.
Between 40 and 50	0	4	0	0
" 50 " 60	1	4	2	1
" 60 " 70	3	2	1	0
" 70 " 80	3	2	0	7
" 80 " 90	6	2	0	0
" 90 " 100	1	1	0	1
Above 100	6	1	0	1
	20	16	3	10

These statistics seem to have been made with the idea of illustrating the marvelous rather than to give the usual prolongation of these functions. It hardly seems possible that ordinary investigation would show no cases of menstruation between sixty and seventy, and seven cases between seventy and eighty; however, in searching literature for such a collection, we must bear in mind that the more extraordinary the instance, the more likely it is that it would be spoken of, as the natural tendency of medical men is to overlook the important ordinary and report the nonimportant extraordinary. Dewees mentions an example of menstruation at sixty-five, and others at fifty-four and fifty-five years. Motte speaks of a case at sixty-one; Ryan and others, at fifty-five, sixty, and sixty-five; Parry, from sixty-six to seventy seven; Desormeux, from sixty to seventy-five; Semple, at seventy and eighty seven; Higgins, at seventy-six; Whitehead, at seventy-seven; Bernstein, at seventy-eight; Beyrat, at eighty-seven; Haller, at one hundred; and highest of all is Blancardi's case, in which menstruation was present at one hundred and six years. In the London Medical and Surgical Journal, 1831, are reported cases at eighty and ninety-five years. In Good's System of Nosology there are instances occurring at seventy-one, eighty, and ninety years. There was a woman in Italy whose menstrual function continued from twenty-four to ninety years. Emmet cites an instance of menstruation at seventy, and Brierre de Boismont one of a woman who menstruated regularly from her twenty-fourth year to the time of her death at ninety-two.

Strasberger of Beeskow describes a woman who ceased menstruating at forty-two, who remained in good health up to eighty, suffering slight attacks of rheumatism only, and at this late age was seized with abdominal pains, followed by menstruation, which continued for three years; the woman died the next year. This late menstruation had all the sensible characters of the early one. Kennard mentions a negress, aged ninety-one, who menstruated at fourteen, ceased at forty-nine, and at eighty-two commenced again, and was regular for four years, but had had no return since. On the return of her menstruation, believing that her procreative powers were returning, she married a vigorous negro of thirty-five and experienced little difficulty in satisfying his desires. Du Peyrou de Cheyssiole and Bonhoure speak of an aged peasant woman, past ninety-one years of age, who menstruated regularly.

Petersen describes a woman of seventy-nine, who on March 26th was seized with uterine pains lasting a few days and terminating with hemorrhagic discharge. On April 23d she was seized again, and a discharge commenced on the 25th, continuing four days. Up to the time of the report, one year after, this menstruation had been regular. There is an instance on record of a female who menstruated every three months during the period from her fiftieth to her seventy-fourth year, the discharge, however, being very slight. Thomas cites an instance of a woman of sixty-nine who had had no menstruation since her forty-ninth year, but who commenced again the year he saw her. Her mother and sister were similarly affected at the age of sixty, in the first case attributable to grief over the death of a son, in the second ascribed to fright. It seemed to be a peculiar family idiosyncrasy. Velasquez of Tarentum says that the Abbess of Monvicaro at the very advanced age of one hundred had a recurrence of catamenia after a severe illness, and subsequently a new set of teeth and a new growth of hair.

Late Establishment of Menstruation.—In some cases menstruation never appears until late in life, presenting the same phenomena as normal menstruation. Perfect relates the history of a woman who had been married many years, and whose menstruation did not appear until her forty-seventh year. She was a widow at the time, and had never been pregnant. Up to the time of her death, which was occasioned by a convulsive colic, in her fifty-seventh year, she had the usual prodromes of menstruation followed by the usual discharge. Rodsewitch speaks of a widow of a peasant who menstruated for the first time at the age of thirty-six. Her first coitus took place at the age of fifteen, before any signs of menstruation had appeared, and from this time all through her married life she was either pregnant or suckling. Her husband died when thirty-six years old, and ever since the catamenial flow had shown itself with great regularity. She had borne twins in her second, fourth, and eighth confinement, and altogether had 16 children. Holdefrund in 1836 mentions a case in which menstruation did not commence until the seventieth year, and Hoyer mentions one delayed to the seventy-sixth year. Marx of Krakau speaks of a woman, aged forty-eight, who had never menstruated; until forty-two years old she had felt no symptoms, but at this time pain began, and at forty-eight regular menstruation ensued. At the time of report, four years after, she was free from pain and amenorrhea, and her flow was regular, though scant. She had been married since she was twenty-eight years of age. A somewhat similar case is mentioned by Gregory of a mother of 7 children who had never had her menstrual flow. There are two instances of delayed menstruation quoted: the first, a woman of thirty, well formed, healthy, of good social position, and with all the signs of puberty except menstruation, which had never appeared; the second, a married woman of forty-two, who throughout a healthy connubial life had never menstruated. An instance is known to the authors of a woman of forty who has never menstruated, though she is of exceptional vigor and development. She has been married many years without pregnancy.

The medical literature relative to precocious impregnation is full of marvelous instances. Individually, many of the cases would be beyond credibility, but when instance after instance is reported by reliable authorities we must accept the possibility of their occurrence, even if we doubt the statements of some of the authorities. No less a medical celebrity than the illustrious Sir Astley Cooper remarks that on one occasion he saw a girl in Scotland, seven years old, whose pelvis was so fully developed that he was sure she could easily give birth to a child; and Warner's case of the Jewish girl three and a half years old, with a pelvis of normal width, more than substantiates this supposition. Similar examples of precocious pelvic and sexual development are on record in abundance, and nearly every medical man of experience has seen cases of infantile masturbation.

The ordinary period of female maturity is astonishingly late when compared with the lower animals of the same size, particularly when viewed with cases of animal precocity on record. Berthold speaks of a kid fourteen days old which was impregnated by an adult goat, and at the usual period of gestation bore a kid, which was mature but weak, to which it gave milk in abundance, and both the mother and kid grew up strong. Compared with the above, child-bearing by women of eight is not extraordinary.

The earliest case of conception that has come to the authors' notice is a quotation in one of the last century books from von Mandelslo of impregnation at six; but a careful search in the British Museum failed to confirm this statement, and, for the present, we must accept the statement as hearsay and without authority available for reference-purposes.

Molitor gives an instance of precocious pregnancy in a child of eight. It was probably the same case spoken of by Lefebvre and reported to the Belgium Academy:

A girl, born in Luxemborg, well developed sexually, having hair on the pubis at birth, who menstruated at four, and at the age of eight was impregnated by a cousin of thirty-seven, who was sentenced to five years' imprisonment for seduction. The pregnancy terminated by the expulsion of a mole containing a well-characterized human embryo. Schmidt's case in 1779 was in a child who had menstruated at two, and bore a dead fetus when she was but eight years and ten months old. She had all the appearance and development of a girl of seventeen. Kussmaul gives an example of conception at eight. Dodd speaks of a child who menstruated early and continued up to the time of impregnation. She was a hard worker and did all her mother's washing. Her labor pains did not continue over six hours, from first to the last. The child was a large one, weighing 7 pounds, and afterward died in convulsions. The infant's left foot had but 3 toes. The young mother at the time of delivery was only nine years and eight months old, and consequently must have been impregnated before the age of nine. Meyer gives an astonishing instance of birth in a Swiss girl at nine. Carn describes a case of a child who menstruated at two, became pregnant at eight, and lived to an advanced age. Ruttel reports conception in a girl of nine, and as far north as St. Petersburg a girl has become a mother before nine years. The Journal de Scavans, 1684, contains the report of the case of a boy, who survived, being born to a mother of nine years.

Beck has reported an instance of delivery in a girl a little over ten years of age. There are instances of fecundity at nine years recorded by Ephemerides, Wolffius, Savonarola, and others. Gleaves reports from Wytheville, Va., the history of what he calls the case of the youngest mother in Virginia —Annie H.—who was born in Bland County, July 15, 1885, and, on September 10, 1895, was delivered of a well-formed child weighing 5 pounds. The girl had not the development of a woman, although she had menstruated regularly since her fifth year. The labor was short and uneventful, and, two hours afterward, the child-mother wanted to arise and dress and would have done so had she been permitted. There were no developments of the mammae nor secretion of milk. The baby was nourished through its short existence (as it only lived a week) by its grandmother, who had a child only a few months old. The parents of this child were prosperous, intelligent, and worthy people, and there was no doubt of the child's age. "Annie is now well and plays about with the other children as if nothing had happened." Harris refers to a Kentucky woman, a mother at ten years, one in Massachusetts a mother at ten years, eight months, and seventeen days, and one in Philadelphia at eleven years and three months. The first case was one of infantile precocity, the other belonging to a much later period, the menstrual function having been established but a few months prior to conception. All these girls had well-developed pelves, large mammae, and the general marks of womanhood, and bore living children. It has been remarked of 3 very markedly precocious cases of pregnancy that one was the daughter of very humble parents, one born in an almshouse, and the other raised by her mother in a house of prostitution. The only significance of this statement is the greater amount of vice and opportunity for precocious sexual intercourse to which they were exposed; doubtless similar cases under more favorable conditions would never be recognized as such.

The instance in the Journal decavans is reiterated in 1775, which is but such a repetition as is found all through medical literature—"new friends with old faces," as it were. Haller observed a case of impregnation in a girl of nine, who had menstruated several years, and others who had become pregnant at nine, ten, and twelve years respectively. Rowlett, whose case is mentioned by Harris, saw a child who had menstruated the first year and regularly thereafter, and gave birth to a child weighing 7 3/4 pounds when she was only ten years and thirteen days old. At the time of delivery she measured 4 feet 7 inches in height and weighed 100 pounds. Curtis, who is also quoted by Harris, relates the history of Elizabeth Drayton, who became pregnant before she was ten, and was delivered of a full-grown, living male child weighing 8 pounds. She had menstruated once or twice before conception, was fairly healthy during gestation, and had a rather lingering but natural labor. To complete the story, the father of this child was a boy of fifteen. One of the faculty of Montpellier has reported an instance at New Orleans of a young girl of eleven, who became impregnated by a youth who was not yet sixteen. Maygrier says that he knew a girl of twelve, living in the Faubourg Saint-Germain, who was confined.

Harris relates the particulars of the case of a white girl who began to menstruate at eleven years and four months, and who gave birth to an over-sized male child on January 21, 1872, when she was twelve years and nine months old. She had an abundance of milk and nursed the child; the labor was of about eighteen hours' duration, and laceration was avoided. He also speaks of a mulatto girl, born in 1848, who began to menstruate at eleven years and nine months, and gave birth to a female child before she reached thirteen, and bore a second child when fourteen years and seven months old. The child's father was a white boy of seventeen.

The following are some Indian statistics: 1 pregnancy at ten, 6 at eleven, 2 at eighteen, 1 at nineteen. Chevers speaks of a mother at ten and others at eleven and twelve; and Green, at Dacca, performed craniotomy upon the fetus of a girl of twelve. Wilson gives an account of a girl thirteen years old, who gave birth to a full-grown female child after three hours' labor. She made a speedy convalescence, but the child died four weeks afterward from bad nursing. The lad who acknowledged paternity was nineteen years old. King reports a well-verified case of confinement in a girl of eleven. Both the mother and child did well.

Robertson of Manchester describes a girl, working in a cotton factory, who was a mother at twelve; de La Motte mentions pregnancy before twelve; Kilpatrick in a negress, at eleven years and six months; Fox, at twelve; Hall, at twelve; Kinney, at twelve years, ten months, and sixteen days; Herrick, at thirteen years and nine months; Murillo, at thirteen years; Philippart, at fourteen years; Stallcup, at eleven years and nine months; Stoakley, at thirteen years; Walker, at the age of twelve years and eight months; another case, at twelve years and six months; and Williams, at eleven.

An editorial article in the Indian Medical Gazette of Sept., 1890, says:—

"The appearance of menstruation is held by the great majority of natives of India to be evidence and proof of marriageability, but among the Hindu community it is considered disgraceful that a girl should remain unmarried until this function is established. The consequence is that girls are married at the age of nine or ten years, but it is understood or professed that the consummation of the marriage is delayed until after the first menstrual period. There is, however, too much reason to believe that the earlier ceremony is very frequently, perhaps commonly, taken to warrant resort to sexual intercourse before the menstrual flux has occurred: it may be accepted as true that premenstrual copulation is largely practised under the cover of marriage in this country.

"From this practice it results that girls become mothers at the earliest possible period of their lives. A native medical witness testified that in about 20 per cent of marriages children were born by wives of from twelve to thirteen years of age. Cases of death caused by the first act of sexual intercourse are by no means rare. They are naturally concealed, but ever and anon they come to light. Dr. Chevers mentioned some 14 cases of this sort in the last edition of his 'Handbook of Medical Jurisprudence for India,' and Dr. Harvey found 5 in the medicolegal returns submitted by the Civil Surgeons of the Bengal Presidency during the years 1870-71-72.

"Reform must come from conviction and effort, as in every other case, but meantime the strong arm of the law should be put forth for the protection of female children from the degradation and hurt entailed by premature sexual intercourse. This can easily be done by raising the age of punishable intercourse, which is now fixed at the absurd limit of ten years. Menstruation very seldom appears in native girls before the completed age of twelve years, and if the 'age of consent' were raised to that limit, it would not interfere with the prejudices and customs which insist on marriage before menstruation."

In 1816 some girls were admitted to the Paris Maternite as young as thirteen, and during the Revolution several at eleven, and even younger. Smith speaks of a legal case in which a girl, eleven years old, being safely delivered of a living child, charged her uncle with rape. Allen speaks of a girl who became pregnant at twelve years and nine months, and was delivered of a healthy, 9-pound boy before the physician's arrival; the placenta came away afterward, and the mother made a speedy recovery. She was thought to have had "dropsy of the abdomen," as the parents had lost a girl of about the same age who was tapped for ascites. The father of the child was a boy only fourteen years of age.

Marvelous to relate, there are on record several cases of twins being born to a child mother. Kay reports a case of twins in a girl of thirteen; Montgomery, at fourteen; and Meigs reports the case of a young girl, of Spanish blood, at Maracaibo, who gave birth to a child before she was twelve and to twins before reaching fourteen years.

In the older works, the following authors have reported cases of pregnancy before the appearance of menstruation: Ballonius, Vogel, Morgagni, the anatomist of the kidney, Schenck, Bartholinus, Bierling, Zacchias, Charleton, Mauriceau, Ephemerides, and Fabricius Hildanus.

In some cases this precocity seems to be hereditary, being transmitted from mother to daughter, bringing about an almost incredible state of affairs, in which a girl is a grandmother about the ordinary age of maternity. Kay says that he had reported to him, on "pretty good" authority, an instance of a Damascus Jewess who became a grandmother at twenty-one years. In France they record a young grandmother of twenty-eight. Ketchum speaks of a negress, aged thirteen, who gave birth to a well-developed child which began to menstruate at ten years and nine months and at thirteen became pregnant; hence the negress was a grandmother at twenty-five years and nine months. She had a second child before she was sixteen, who began to menstruate at seven years and six months, thus proving the inheritance of this precocity, and leaving us at sea to figure what degree of grandmother she may be if she lives to an advanced age. Another interesting case of this nature is that of Mrs. C., born 1854, married in 1867, and who had a daughter ten months after. This daughter married in 1882, and in March, 1883, gave birth to a 9-pound boy. The youthful grandmother, not twenty-nine, was present at the birth. This case was remarkable, as the children were both legitimate.

Fecundity in the old seems to have attracted fully as much attention among the older observers as precocity. Pliny speaks of Cornelia, of the family of Serpios, who bore a son at sixty, who was named Volusius Saturnius; and Marsa, a physician of Venice, was deceived in a pregnancy in a woman of sixty, his diagnosis being "dropsy." Tarenta records the history of the case of a woman who menstruated and bore children when past the age of sixty. Among the older reports are those of Blanchard of a woman who bore a child at sixty years; Fielitz, one at sixty; Ephemerides, one at sixty-two; Rush, one at sixty; Bernstein, one at sixty years; Schoepfer, at seventy years; and, almost beyond belief, Debes cites an instance as taking place at the very advanced age of one hundred and three. Wallace speaks of a woman in the Isle of Orkney bearing children when past the age of sixty. We would naturally expect to find the age of child-bearing prolonged in the northern countries where the age of maturity is later. Capuron cites an example of childbirth in a woman of sixty; Haller, cases at fifty-eight, sixty-three, and seventy; Dewees, at sixty-one; and Thibaut de Chauvalon, in a woman of Martinique aged ninety years. There was a woman delivered in Germany, in 1723, at the age of fifty-five; one at fifty-one in Kentucky; and one in Russia at fifty. Depasse speaks of a woman of fifty-nine years and five months old who was delivered of a healthy male child, which she suckled, weaning it on her sixtieth birthday. She had been a widow for twenty years, and had ceased to menstruate nearly ten years before. In St. Peter's Church, in East Oxford, is a monument bearing an inscription recording the death in child-birth of a woman sixty-two years old. Cachot relates the case of a woman of fifty-three, who was delivered of a living child by means of the forceps, and a year after bore a second child without instrumental interference. She had no milk in her breasts at the time and no signs of secretion. This aged mother had been married at fifty-two, five years after the cessation of her menstruation, and her husband was a young man, only twenty-four years old.

Kennedy reports a delivery at sixty-two years, and the Cincinnati Enquirer, January, 1863, says: "Dr. W. McCarthy was in attendance on a lady of sixty-nine years, on Thursday night last, who gave birth to a fine boy. The father of the child is seventy-four years old, and the mother and child are doing well." Quite recently there died in Great Britain a Mrs. Henry of Gortree at the age of one hundred and twelve, leaving a daughter of nine years.

Mayham saw a woman seventy-three years old who recovered after delivery of a child. A most peculiar case is that of a widow, seventy years old, a native of Garches. She had been in the habit of indulging freely in wine, and, during the last six months, to decided excess. After an unusually prolonged libation she found herself unable to walk home; she sat down by the roadside waiting until she could proceed, and was so found by a young man who knew her and who proposed helping her home. By the time her house was reached night was well advanced, and she invited him to stop over night; finding her more than affable, he stopped at her house over four nights, and the result of his visits was an ensuing pregnancy for Madame.

Multiple births in the aged have been reported from authentic sources. The Lancet quotes a rather fabulous account of a lady over sixty-two years of age who gave birth to triplets, making her total number of children 13. Montgomery, Colomb, and Knehel, each, have recorded the birth of twins in women beyond the usual age of the menopause, and there is a case recorded of a woman of fifty-two who was delivered of twins.

Impregnation without completion of the copulative act by reason of some malformation, such as occlusion of the vagina or uterus, fibrous and unruptured hymen, etc., has been a subject of discussion in the works of medical jurisprudence of all ages; and cases of conception without entrance of the penis are found in abundance throughout medical literature, and may have an important medicolegal bearing. There is little doubt of the possibility of spermatozoa deposited on the genitalia making progress to the seat of fertilization, as their power of motility and tenacity of life have been well demonstrated. Percy reports an instance in which semen was found issuing from the os uteri eight and one-half days after the last intercourse; and a microscopic examination of this semen revealed the presence of living as well as dead spermatozoa. We have occasional instances of impregnation by rectal coitus, the semen finding its way into an occluded vaginal canal by a fistulous communication.

Guillemeau, the surgeon of the French king, tells of a girl of eighteen, who was brought before the French officials in Paris, in 1607, on the citation of her husband of her inability to allow him completion of the marital function. He alleged that he had made several unsuccessful attempts to enter her, and in doing so had caused paraphimosis. On examination by the surgeons she was found to have a dense membrane, of a fibrous nature, entirely occluding the vagina, which they incised. Immediately afterward the woman exhibited morning sickness and the usual signs of pregnancy, and was delivered in four months of a full-term child, the results of an impregnation occasioned by one of the unsuccessful attempts at entrance. Such instances are numerous in the older literature, and a mere citation of a few is considered sufficient here. Zacchias, Amand, Fabricius Hildanus, Graaf, the discoverer of the follicles that bear his name, Borellus, Blegny, Blanchard, Diemerbroeck, Duddell, Mauriceau, a Reyes, Riolan, Harvey, the discoverer of the circulation of the blood, Wolfius, Walther, Rongier, Ruysch, Forestus, Ephemerides, and Schurig all mention cases of conception with intact hymen, and in which there was no entrance of the penis. Tolberg has an example of hymen integrum after the birth of a fetus five months old, and there is recorded a case of tubal pregnancy in which the hymen was intact.

Gilbert gives an account of a case of pregnancy in an unmarried woman, who successfully resisted an attempt at criminal connection and yet became impregnated and gave birth to a perfectly formed female child. The hymen was not ruptured, and the impregnation could not have preceded the birth more than thirty-six weeks. Unfortunately, this poor woman was infected with gonorrhea after the attempted assault. Simmons of St. Louis gives a curious peculiarity of conception, in which there was complete closure of the vagina, subsequent conception, and delivery at term. He made the patient's acquaintance from her application to him in regard to a malcondition of her sexual apparatus, causing much domestic infelicity.

Lawson speaks of a woman of thirty-five, who had been married ten months, and whose husband could never effect an entrance; yet she became pregnant and had a normal labor, despite the fact that, in addition to a tough and unruptured hymen, she had an occluding vaginal cyst. Hickinbotham of Birmingham reports the history of two cases of labor at term in females whose hymens were immensely thickened. H. Grey Edwards has seen a case of imperforate hymen which had to be torn through in labor; yet one single act of copulation, even with this obstacle to entrance, sufficed to impregnate. Champion speaks of a woman who became pregnant although her hymen was intact. She had been in the habit of having coitus by the urethra, and all through her pregnancy continued this practice.

Houghton speaks of a girl of twenty-five into whose vagina it was impossible to pass the tip of the first finger on account of the dense cicatricial membrane in the orifice, but who gave birth, with comparative ease, to a child at full term, the only interference necessary being a few slight incisions to permit the passage of the head. Tweedie saw an Irish girl of twenty-three, with an imperforate os uteri, who had menstruated only scantily since fourteen and not since her marriage. She became pregnant and went to term, and required some operative interference. He incised at the point of usual location of the os, and one of his incisions was followed by the flow of liquor amnii, and the head fell upon the artificial opening, the diameter of which proved to be one and a half or two inches; the birth then progressed promptly, the child being born alive.

Guerard notes an instance in which the opening barely admitted a hair; yet the patient reached the third month of pregnancy, at which time she induced abortion in a manner that could not be ascertained. Roe gives a case of conception in an imperforate uterus, and Duncan relates the history of a case of pregnancy in an unruptured hymen, characterized by an extraordinary ascent of the uterus. Among many, the following modern observers have also reported instances of pregnancy with hymen integrum: Braun, 3 cases; Francis, Horton, Oakman, Brill, 2 cases; Burgess, Haig, Hay, and Smith.

Instances in which the presence of an unruptured hymen has complicated or retarded actual labor are quite common, and until the membrane is ruptured by external means the labor is often effectually obstructed. Among others reporting cases of this nature are Beale, Carey, Davis, Emond Fetherston, Leisenring, Mackinlay, Martinelli, Palmer, Rousseau, Ware, and Yale.

There are many cases of stricture or complete occlusion of the vagina, congenital or acquired from cicatricial contraction, obstructing delivery, and in some the impregnation seems more marvelous than cases in which the obstruction is only a thin membranous hymen. Often the obstruction is so dense as to require a large bistoury to divide it, and even that is not always sufficient, and the Cesarean operation only can terminate the obstructed delivery; we cannot surmise how conception could have been possible. Staples records a case of pregnancy and parturition with congenital stricture of the vagina. Maisonneuve mentions the successful practice of a Cesarean operation in a case of congenital occlusion of the vagina forming a complete obstruction to delivery. Verdile records an instance of imperforate vagina in which rectovaginal wall was divided and the delivery effected through the rectum and anus. Lombard mentions an observation of complete occlusion of the vagina in a woman, the mother of 4 living children and pregnant for the fifth time. Thus, almost incredible to relate, it is possible for a woman to become a mother of a living child and yet preserve all the vaginal evidences of virginity. Cole describes a woman of twenty-four who was delivered without the rupture of the hymen, and Meek remarks on a similar case. We can readily see that, in a case like that of Verdile, in which rectal delivery is effected, the hymen could be left intact and the product of conception be born alive.

A natural sequence to the subject of impregnation without entrance is that of artificial impregnation. From being a matter of wonder and hearsay, it has been demonstrated as a practical and useful method in those cases in which, by reason of some unfortunate anatomic malformation on either the male or the female side, the marriage is unfruitful. There are many cases constantly occurring in which the birth of an heir is a most desirable thing in a person's life. The historic instance of Queen Mary of England, whose anxiety and efforts to bear a child were the subject of public comment and prayers, is but an example of a fact that is occurring every day, and doubtless some of these cases could be righted by the pursuance of some of the methods suggested.

There have been rumors from the beginning of the century of women being impregnated in a bath, from contact with cloths containing semen, etc., and some authorities in medical jurisprudence have accepted the possibility of such an occurrence. It is not in the province of this work to speculate on what may be, but to give authoritative facts, from which the reader may draw his own deductions. Fertilization of plants has been thought to have been known in the oldest times, and there are some who believe that the library at Alexandria must have contained some information relative to it. The first authentic account that we have of artificial impregnation is that of Schwammerdam, who in 1680 attempted it without success by the fecundation of the eggs of fish. Roesel, his scholar, made an attempt in 1690, but also failed; and to Jacobi, in 1700, belongs the honor of success. In 1780, Abbe Spallanzani, following up the success of Jacobi, artificially impregnated a bitch, who brought forth in sixty-two days 3 puppies, all resembling the male. The illustrious John Hunter advised a man afflicted with hypospadias to impregnate his wife by vaginal injections of semen in water with an ordinary syringe, and, in spite of the simplicity of this method, the attempt was followed by a successful issue. Since this time, Nicholas of Nancy and Lesueur have practised the simple vaginal method; while Gigon, d'Angouleme (14 cases), Girault (10 cases), Marion Sims, Thomas, Salmon, Pajot, Gallard, Courty, Roubaud, Dehaut, and others have used the more modern uterine method with success.

A dog-breeder, by syringing the uterus of a bitch, has succeeded in impregnating her. Those who are desirous of full information on this subject, as regards the modus operandi, etc., are referred to Girault; this author reports in full several examples. One case was that of a woman, aged twenty-five, afflicted with blenorrhea, who, chagrined at not having issue, made repeated forcible injections of semen in water for two months, and finally succeeded in impregnating herself, and was delivered of a living child. Another case was that of a female, aged twenty-three, who had an extra long vaginal canal, probably accounting for the absence of pregnancy. She made injections of semen, and was finally delivered of a child. He also reports the case of a distinguished musician who, by reason of hypospadias, had never impregnated his wife, and had resorted to injections of semen with a favorable result. This latter case seems hardly warranted when we consider that men afflicted with hypospadias and epispadias have become fathers. Percy gives the instance of a gentleman whom he had known for some time, whose urethra terminated a little below the frenum, as in other persons, but whose glans bulged quite prominently beyond it, rendering urination in the forward direction impossible. Despite the fact that this man could not perform the ejaculatory function, he was the father of three children, two of them inheriting his penile formation.

The fundamental condition of fecundity being the union of a spermatozoid and an ovum, the object of artificial impregnation is to further this union by introducing semen directly to the fundus of the uterus. The operation is quite simple and as follows: The husband, having been found perfectly healthy, is directed to cohabit with his wife, using a condom. The semen ejaculated is sucked up by an intrauterine syringe which has been properly disinfected and kept warm. The os uteri is now exposed and wiped off with some cotton which has been dipped in an antiseptic fluid; introduced to the fundus of the uterus, and some drops of the fluid slowly expressed into the uterus. The woman is then kept in bed on her back. This operation is best carried out immediately before or immediately after the menstrual epoch, and if not successful at the first attempt should be repeated for several months. At the present day artificial impregnation in pisciculture is extensively used with great success.

{footnote} The following extraordinary incident of accidental impregnation, quoted from the American Medical Weekly by the Lancet, is given in brief, not because it bears any semblance of possibility, but as a curious example from the realms of imagination in medicine.

L. G. Capers of Vicksburg, Miss., relates an incident during the late Civil War, as follows: A matron and her two daughters, aged fifteen and seventeen years, filled with the enthusiasm of patriotism, stood ready to minister to the wounds of their countrymen in their fine residence near the scene of the battle of R———, May 12, 1863, between a portion of Grant's army and some Confederates. During the fray a gallant and noble young friend of the narrator staggered and fell to the earth; at the same time a piercing cry was heard in the house near by. Examination of the wounded soldier showed that a bullet had passed through the scrotum and carried away the left testicle. The same bullet had apparently penetrated the left side of the abdomen of the elder young lady, midway between the umbilicus and the anterior superior spinous process of the ilium, and had become lost in the abdomen. This daughter suffered an attack of peritonitis, but recovered in two months under the treatment administered.

Marvelous to relate, just two hundred and seventy-eight days after the reception of the minie-ball, she was delivered of a fine boy, weighing 8 pounds, to the surprise of herself and the mortification of her parents and friends. The hymen was intact, and the young mother strenuously insisted on her virginity and innocence. About three weeks after this remarkable birth Dr. Capers was called to see the infant, and the grandmother insisted that there was something wrong with the child's genitals. Examination showed a rough, swollen, and sensitive scrotum, containing some hard substance. He operated, and extracted a smashed and battered minie-ball. The doctor, after some meditation, theorized in this manner: He concluded that this was the same ball that had carried away the testicle of his young friend, that had penetrated the ovary of the young lady, and, with some spermatozoa upon it, had impregnated her. With this conviction he approached the young man and told him the circumstances; the soldier appeared skeptical at first, but consented to visit the young mother; a friendship ensued which soon ripened into a happy marriage, and the pair had three children, none resembling, in the same degree as the first, the heroic pater familias.

Interesting as are all the anomalies of conception, none are more so than those of unconscious impregnation; and some well-authenticated cases can be mentioned. Instances of violation in sleep, with subsequent pregnancy as a result, have been reported in the last century by Valentini, Genselius, and Schurig. Reports by modern authorities seem to be quite scarce, though there are several cases on record of rape during anesthesia, followed by impregnation. Capuron relates a curious instance of a woman who was raped during lethargy, and who subsequently became pregnant, though her condition was not ascertained until the fourth month, the peculiar abdominal sensation exciting suspicion of the true nature of the case, which had previously been thought impossible.

There is a record of a case of a young girl of great moral purity who became pregnant without the slightest knowledge of the source; although, it might be remarked, such cases must be taken "cum grano salis." Cases of conception without the slightest sexual desire or pleasure, either from fright, as in rape, or naturally deficient constitution, have been recorded; as well as conception during intoxication and in a hypnotic trance, which latter has recently assumed a much mooted legal aspect. As far back as 1680, Duverney speaks of conception without the slightest sense of desire or pleasure on the part of the female.

Conception with Deficient Organs.—Having spoken of conception with some obstructive interference, conception with some natural or acquired deficiency of the functional, organic, or genital apparatus must be considered. It is a well-known fact that women exhibiting rudimentary development of the uterus or vagina are still liable to become pregnant, and many such cases have been recorded; but the most peculiar cases are those in which pregnancy has appeared after removal of some of the sexual apparatus.

Pregnancy going to term with a successful delivery frequently follows the performance of ovariotomy with astonishing rapidity. Olier cites an instance of ovariotomy with a pregnancy of twins three months afterward, and accouchement at term of two well-developed boys. Polaillon speaks of a pregnancy consecutive to ovariotomy, the accouchement being normal at term. Crouch reports a case of successful parturition in a patient who had previously undergone ovariotomy by a large incision. Parsons mentions a case of twin pregnancy two years after ovariotomy attended with abnormal development of one of the children. Cutter speaks of a case in which a woman bore a child one year after the performance of ovariotomy, and Pippingskold of two cases of pregnancy after ovariotomy in which the stump as well as the remaining ovary were cauterized. Brown relates a similar instance with successful delivery. Bixby, Harding, Walker (1878-9), and Mears all report cases, and others are not at all rare. In the cases following shortly after operation, it has been suggested that they may be explained by the long retention of the ova in the uterus, deposited them prior to operation. In the presence of such facts one can but wonder if artificial fecundation of an ovum derived from another woman may ever be brought about in the uterus of a sterile woman!

Conception Soon After a Preceding Pregnancy.—Conception sometimes follows birth (or abortion) with astonishing rapidity, and some women seem for a period of their lives either always pregnant or with infants at their breasts. This prolificity is often alluded to, and is not confined to the lower classes, as often stated, but is common even among the nobility. Illustrative of this, we have examples in some of the reigning families in Europe to-day. A peculiar instance is given by Sparkman in which a woman conceived just forty hours after abortion. Rice mentions the case of a woman who was confined with her first child, a boy, on July 31, 1870, and was again delivered of another child on June 4, 1871. She had become pregnant twenty-eight days after delivery. He also mentions another case of a Mrs. C., who, at the age of twenty-three, gave birth to a child on September 13, 1880, and bore a second child on July 2, 1881. She must have become pregnant twenty-one days after the delivery of her first child.

Superfetation has been known for many centuries; the Romans had laws prescribing the laws of succession in such cases, and many medical writers have mentioned it. Hippocrates and Aristotle wrote of it, the former at some length. Pliny speaks of a slave who bore two infants, one resembling the master, the other a man with whom she had intercourse, and cites the case as one of superfetation. Schenck relates instances, and Zacchias, Velchius, and Sinibaldus mention eases. Pare seemed to be well conversant with the possibility as well as the actuality of superfetation; and Harvey reports that a certain maid, gotten with child by her master, in order to hide her knavery came to London in September, where she lay in by stealth, and being recovered, returned home. In December of the same year she was unexpectedly delivered of another child, a product of superfetation, which proclaimed the crime that she had so cunningly concealed before.

Marcellus Donatus, Goret, Schacher, and Mauriceau mention superfetation. In the Academie des Sciences, at Paris, in 1702, there was mentioned the case of a woman who was delivered of a boy; in the placenta was discovered a sort of bladder which was found to contain a female fetus of the age of from four to five months; and in 1729, before the same society, there was an instance in which two fetuses were born a day apart, one aged forty days and the other at full term. From the description, it does not seem possible that either of these were blighted twin pregnancies. Ruysch gives an account of a surgeon's wife at Amsterdam, in 1686, who was delivered of a strong child which survived, and, six hours after, of a small embryo, the funis of which was full of hydatids and the placenta as large and thick as one of three months. Ruysch accompanies his description with an illustrative figure. At Lyons, in 1782, Benoite Franquet was unexpectedly delivered of a child seven months old; three weeks later she experienced symptoms indicative of the existence of another fetus, and after five months and sixteen days she was delivered of a remarkably strong and healthy child.

Baudeloque speaks of a case of superfetation observed by Desgranges in Lyons in 1780. After the birth of the first infant the lochia failed to flow, no milk appeared in the breasts, and the belly remained large. In about three weeks after the accouchement she had connection with her husband, and in a few days felt fetal movements. A second child was born at term, sixty-eight days after the first; and in 1782 both children were living. A woman of Arles was delivered on November 11, 1796, of a child at term; she had connection with her husband four days after; the lochia stopped, and the milk did not flow after this intercourse. About one and a half months after this she felt quickening again, and naturally supposed that she had become impregnated by the first intercourse after confinement; but five months after the first accouchement she was delivered of another child at term, the result of a superfetation. Milk in abundance made its appearance, and she was amply able to nourish both children from the breasts. Lachausse speaks of a woman of thirty who bore one child on April 30, 1748, and another on September 16th in the same year. Her breasts were full enough to nourish both of the children. It might be remarked in comment on this case that, according to a French authority, the woman died in 1755, and on dissection was found to have had a double uterus.

A peculiar instance of superfetation was reported by Langmore in which there was an abortion of a fetus between the third and fourth months, apparently dead some time, and thirteen hours later a second fetus; an ovum of about four weeks and of perfect formation was found adherent near the fundus. Tyler Smith mentions a lady pregnant for the first time who miscarried at five months and some time afterward discharged a small clot containing a perfectly fresh and healthy ovum of about four weeks' formation. There was no sign of a double uterus, and the patient menstruated regularly during pregnancy, being unwell three weeks before the abortion. Harley and Tanner speak of a woman of thirty-eight who never had borne twins, and who aborted a fetus of four months' gestation; serious hemorrhage accompanied the removal of the placenta, and on placing the hand in the uterine cavity an embryo of five or six weeks was found inclosed in a sac and floating in clear liquor amnii. The patient was the mother of nine children, the youngest of which was three years old.

Young speaks of a woman who three months previously had aborted a three months' fetus, but a tumor still remained in the abdomen, the auscultation of which gave evidence of a fetal heart-beat. Vaginal examination revealed a dilatation of the os uteri of at least one inch and a fetal head pressing out; subsequently a living fetus of about six months of age was delivered. Severe hemorrhage complicated the case, but was controlled, and convalescence speedily ensued. Huse cites an instance of a mother bearing a boy on November 4, 1834, and a girl on August 3, 1835. At birth the boy looked premature, about seven months old, which being the case, the girl must have been either a superfetation or a seven months' child also. Van Bibber of Baltimore says he met a young lady who was born five months after her sister, and who was still living.

The most curious and convincing examples of superfetation are those in which children of different colors, either twins or near the same age, are born to the same woman,—similar to that exemplified in the case of the mare who was covered first by a stallion and a quarter of an hour later by an ass, and gave birth at one parturition to a horse and a mule. Parsons speaks of a case at Charleston, S.C., in 1714, of a white woman who gave birth to twins, one a mulatto and the other white. She confessed that after her husband left her a negro servant came to her and forced her to comply with his wishes by threatening her life. Smellie mentions the case of a black woman who had twins, one child black and the other almost white. She confessed having had intercourse with a white overseer immediately after her husband left her bed. Dewees reports a similar case. Newlin of Nashville speaks of a negress who bore twins, one distinctly black with the typical African features, while the other was a pretty mulatto exhibiting the distinct characters of the Caucasian race. Both the parents were perfect types of the black African negro. The mother, on being questioned, frankly acknowledged that shortly after being with her husband she had lain a night with a white man. In this case each child had its own distinct cord and placenta.

Archer gives facts illustrating and observations showing: "that a white woman, by intercourse with a white man and negro, may conceive twins, one of which shall be white and the other a mulatto; and that, vice versa, a black woman, by intercourse with a negro and a white man, may conceive twins, one of which shall be a negro and the other a mulatto." Wight narrates that he was called to see a woman, the wife of an East Indian laborer on the Isle of Trinidad, who had been delivered of a fetus 6 inches long, about four months old, and having a cord of about 18 inches in length. He removed the placenta, and in about half an hour the woman was delivered of a full-term white female child. The first child was dark, like the mother and father, and the mother denied any possibility of its being a white man's child; but this was only natural on her part, as East Indian husbands are so intensely jealous that they would even kill an unfaithful wife. Both the mother and the mysterious white baby are doing well. Bouillon speaks of a negress in Guadeloupe who bore twins, one a negro and the other a mulatto. She had sexual congress with both a negro and a white man.

Delmas, a surgeon of Rouen, tells of a woman of thirty-six who was delivered in the hospital of his city on February 26, 1806, of two children, one black and the other a mulatto. She had been pregnant eight months, and had had intercourse with a negro twice about her fourth month of pregnancy, though living with the white man who first impregnated her. Two placentae were expelled some time after the twins, and showed a membranous junction. The children died shortly after birth.

Pregnancy often takes place in a unicorn or bicorn uterus, leading to similar anomalous conditions. Galle, Hoffman, Massen, and Sanger give interesting accounts of this occurrence, and Ross relates an instance of triple pregnancy in a double uterus. Cleveland describes a discharge of an anomalous deciduous membrane during pregnancy which was probably from the unimpregnated half of a double uterus.

CHAPTER II

PRENATAL ANOMALIES.

Extrauterine Pregnancy.—In the consideration of prenatal anomalies, the first to be discussed will be those of extrauterine pregnancy. This abnormalism has been known almost as long as there has been any real knowledge of obstetrics. In the writings of Albucasis, during the eleventh century, extrauterine pregnancy is discussed, and later the works of N. Polinus and Cordseus, about the sixteenth century, speak of it; in the case of Cordseus the fetus was converted into a lithopedion and carried in the abdomen twenty-eight years. Horstius in the sixteenth century relates the history of a woman who conceived for the third time in March, 1547, and in 1563 the remains of the fetus were still in the abdomen.

Israel Spach, in an extensive gynecologic work published in 1557, figures a lithopedion drawn in situ in the case of a woman with her belly laid open. He dedicated to this calcified fetus, which he regarded as a reversion, the following curious epigram, in allusion to the classical myth that after the flood the world was repopulated by the two survivors, Deucalion and Pyrrha, who walked over the earth and cast stones behind them, which, on striking the ground, became people. Roughly translated from the Latin, this epigram read as follows: "Deucalion cast stones behind him and thus fashioned our tender race from the hard marble. How comes it that nowadays, by a reversal of things, the tender body of a little babe has limbs nearer akin to stone?" Many of the older writers mention this form of fetation as a curiosity, but offer no explanation as to its cause. Mauriceau and de Graaf discuss in full extrauterine pregnancy, and Salmuth, Hannseus, and Bartholinus describe it. From the beginning of the eighteenth century this subject always demanded the attention and interest of medical observers. In more modern times, Campbell and Geoffroy-Saint-Hilaire, who named it "Grossesse Pathologique," have carefully defined and classified the forms, and to-day every text-book on obstetrics gives a scientific discussion and classification of the different forms of extrauterine pregnancy.

The site of the conception is generally the wall of the uterus, the Fallopian tube, or the ovary, although there are instances of pregnancy in the vagina, as for example when there is scirrhus of the uterus; and again, cases supposed to be only extrauterine have been instances simply of double uterus, with single or concurrent pregnancy. Ross speaks of a woman of thirty-three who had been married fourteen years, had borne six children, and who on July 16, 1870, miscarried with twins of about five months' development. After a week she declared that she was still pregnant with another child, but as the physician had placed his hand in the uterine cavity after the abortion, he knew the fetus must be elsewhere or that no pregnancy existed. We can readily see how this condition might lead to a diagnosis of extrauterine pregnancy, but as the patient insisted on a thorough examination, the doctor found by the stethoscope the presence of a beating fetal heart, and by vaginal examination a double uterus. On introducing a sound into the new aperture he discovered that it opened into another cavity; but as the woman was pregnant in this, he proceeded no further. On October 31st she was delivered of a female child of full growth. She had menstruated from this bipartite uterus three times during the period between the miscarriage of the twins and the birth of the child. Both the mother and child did well.

In most cases there is rupture of the fetal sac into the abdominal cavity or the uterus, and the fetus is ejected into this location, from thence to be removed or carried therein many years; but there are instances in which the conception has been found in situ, as depicted in Figure 2. A sturdy woman of thirty was executed on January 16, 1735, for the murder of her child. It was ascertained that she had passed her catamenia about the first of the month, and thereafter had sexual intercourse with one of her fellow-prisoners. On dissection both Fallopian tubes were found distended, and the left ovary, which bore signs of conception, was twice as large as the right. Campbell quotes another such case in a woman of thirty-eight who for twenty years had practised her vocation as a Cyprian, and who unexpectedly conceived. At the third month of pregnancy a hard extrauterine tumor was found, which was gradually increasing in size and extending to the left side of the hypogastrium, the associate symptoms of pregnancy, sense of pressure, pain, tormina, and dysuria, being unusually severe. There was subsequently at attack of inflammatory fever, followed by tumefaction of the abdomen, convulsions, and death on the ninth day. The fetus had been contained in the peritoneal coat of the ovary until the fourth month, when one of the feet passed through the cyst and caused the fatal result. Signs of acute peritonitis were seen postmortem, the abdominal cavity was full of blood, and the ovary much lacerated.

The termination of extrauterine pregnancy varies; in some cases the fetus is extracted by operation after rupture; in others the fetus has been delivered alive by abdominal section; it may be partially absorbed, or carried many years in the abdomen; or it may ulcerate through the confining walls, enter the bowels or bladder, and the remnants of the fetal body be discharged.

The curious cases mentioned by older writers, and called abortion by the mouth, etc., are doubtless, in many instances, remnants of extrauterine pregnancies or dermoid cysts. Maroldus speaks in full of such cases; Bartholinus, Salmuth, and a Reyes speak of women vomiting remnants of fetuses. In Germany, in the seventeenth century, there lived a woman who on three different occasions is said to have vomited a fetus. The last miscarriage in this manner was of eight months' growth and was accompanied by its placenta. The older observers thought this woman must have had two orifices to her womb, one of which had some connection with the stomach, as they had records of the dissection of a female in whom was found a conformation similar to this.

Discharge of the fetal bones or even the whole of an extrauterine fetus by the rectum is not uncommon. There are two early cases mentioned in which the bones of a fetus were discharged at stool, causing intense pain. Armstrong describes an anomalous case of pregnancy in a syphilitic patient who discharged fetal bones by the rectum. Bubendorf reports the spontaneous elimination of a fetal skeleton by the rectum after five years of retention, with recovery of the patient. Butcher speaks of delivery through the rectum at the fourth month, with recovery. Depaul mentions a similar expulsion after a pregnancy of about two months and a half. Jackson reports the dissection of an extrauterine sac which communicated freely with the large intestine. Peck has an example of spontaneous delivery of an extrauterine fetus by the rectum, with recovery of the mother. Skippon, in the early part of the last century, reports the discharge of the bones of a fetus through an "imposthume" in the groin. Other cases of anal discharge of the product of extrauterine conception are recorded by Winthrop, Woodbury, Tuttle, Atkinson, Browne, Weinlechner, Gibson, Littre, Magruder, Gilland, and many others. De Brun du Bois-Noir speaks of the expulsion of extrauterine remains by the anus after seven years, and Heyerdahl after thirteen years. Benham mentions the discharge of a fetus by the rectum; there was a stricture of the rectum associated with syphilitic patches, necessitating the performance of colotomy.

Bartholinus and Rosseus speak of fetal bones being discharged from the urinary passages. Ebersbach, in the Ephemerides of 1717, describes a necropsy in which a human fetus was found contained in the bladder. In 1878 White reported an instance of the discharge of fetal remains through the bladder.

Discharge of the Fetus through the Abdominal Walls.—Margaret Parry of Berkshire in 1668 voided the bones of a fetus through the flesh above the os pubis, and in 1684 she was alive and well, having had healthy children afterward. Brodie reports the history of a case in a negress who voided a fetus from an abscess at the navel about the seventeenth month of conception. Modern instances of the discharge of the extrauterine fetus from the walls of the abdomen are frequently reported. Algora speaks of an abdominal pregnancy in which there was spontaneous perforation of the anterior abdominal parietes, followed by death. Bouzal cites an extraordinary case of ectopic gestation in which there was natural expulsion of the fetus through abdominal walls, with subsequent intestinal strangulation. An artificial anus was established and the mother recovered. Brodie, Dunglison, Erich, Rodbard, Fox, and Wilson are among others reporting the expulsion of remnants of ectopic pregnancies through the abdominal parietes. Campbell quotes the case of a Polish woman, aged thirty-five, the mother of nine children, most of whom were stillborn, who conceived for the tenth time, the gestation being normal up to the lying-in period. She had pains followed by extraordinary effusion and some blood into the vagina. After various protracted complaints the abdominal tumor became painful and inflamed in the umbilical region. A breach in the walls soon formed, giving exit to purulent matter and all the bones of a fetus. During this process the patient received no medical treatment, and frequently no assistance in dressing the opening. She recovered, but had an artificial anus all her life. Sarah McKinna was married at sixteen and menstruated for the first time a month thereafter. Ten months after marriage she showed signs of pregnancy and was delivered at full term of a living child; the second child was born ten months after the first, and the second month after the second birth she again showed signs of pregnancy. At the close of nine months these symptoms, with the exception of the suppression of menses, subsided, and in this state she continued for six years. During the first four years she felt discomfort in the region of the umbilicus. About the seventh year she suffered tumefaction of the abdomen and thought she had conceived again. The abscess burst and an elbow of the fetus protruded from the wound. A butcher enlarged the wound and, fixing his finger under the jaw of the fetus, extracted the head. On looking into the abdomen he perceived a black object, whereupon he introduced his hand and extracted piecemeal an entire fetal skeleton and some decomposed animal-matter. The abdomen was bound up, and in six weeks the woman was enabled to superintend her domestic affairs; excepting a ventral hernia she had no bad after-results. Kimura, quoted by Whitney, speaks of a case of extrauterine pregnancy in a Japanese woman of forty-one similar to the foregoing, in which an arm protruded through the abdominal wall above the umbilicus and the remains of a fetus were removed through the aperture. The accompanying illustration shows the appearance of the arm in situ before extraction of the fetus and the location of the wound.

Bodinier and Lusk report instances of the delivery of an extrauterine fetus by the vagina; and Mathieson relates the history of the delivery of a living ectopic child by the vagina, with recovery of the mother. Gordon speaks of a curious case in a negress, six months pregnant, in which an extrauterine fetus passed down from the posterior culdesac and occluded the uterus. It was removed through the vagina, and two days later labor-pains set in, and in two hours she was delivered of a uterine child. The placenta was left behind and drainage established through the vagina, and the woman made complete recovery.

Combined Intrauterine and Extrauterine Gestation.—Many well-authenticated cases of combined pregnancy, in which one of the products of conception was intrauterine and the other of extrauterine gestation, have been recorded. Clark and Ramsbotham report instances of double conception, one fetus being born alive in the ordinary manner and the other located extrauterine. Chasser speaks of a case in which there was concurrent pregnancy in both the uterus and the Fallopian tube. Smith cites an instance of a woman of twenty-three who became pregnant in August, 1870. In the following December she passed fetal bones from the rectum, and a month later gave birth to an intrauterine fetus of six months' growth. McGee mentions the case of a woman of twenty-eight who became pregnant in July, 1872, and on October 20th and 21st passed several fetal bones by the rectum, and about four months later expelled some from the uterus. From this time she rapidly recovered her strength and health. Devergie quotes an instance of a woman of thirty who had several children, but who died suddenly, and being pregnant was opened. In the right iliac fossa was found a male child weighing 5 pounds and 5 ounces, 8 1/2 inches long, and of about five months' growth. The uterus also contained a male fetus of about three months' gestation. Figure 4 shows combined intrauterine and extrauterine gestation. Hodgen speaks of a woman of twenty-seven, who was regular until November, 1872; early in January, 1873, she had an attack of pain with peritonitis, shortly after which what was apparently an extrauterine pregnancy gradually diminished. On August 17, 1873, after a labor of eight hours, she gave birth to a healthy fetus. The hand in the uterus detected a tumor to the left, which wag reduced to about one-fourth the former size. In April, 1874, the woman still suffered pain and tenderness in the tumor. Hodgen believed this to have been originally a tubal pregnancy, which burst, causing much hemorrhage and the death of the fetus, together with a limited peritonitis. Beach has seen a twin compound pregnancy in which after connection there was a miscarriage in six weeks, and four years after delivery of an extrauterine fetus through the abdominal walls. Cooke cites an example of intrauterine and extrauterine pregnancy progressing simultaneously to full period of gestation, with resultant death. Rosset reports the case of a woman of twenty-seven, who menstruated last in November, 1878, and on August 5, 1879, was delivered of a well-developed dead female child weighing seven pounds. The uterine contractions were feeble, and the attached placenta was removed only with difficulty; there was considerable hemorrhage. The hemorrhage continued to occur at intervals of two weeks, and an extrauterine tumor remained. Two weeks later septicemia supervened and life was despaired of. On the 15th of October a portion of a fetus of five months' growth in an advanced stage of decomposition protruded from the vulva. After the escape of this putrid mass her health returned, and in four months she was again robust and healthy. Whinery speaks of a young woman who at the time of her second child-birth observed a tumor in the abdomen on her right side and felt motion in it. In about a month she was with severe pain which continued a week and then ceased. Health soon improved, and the woman afterward gave birth to a third child; subsequently she noticed that the tumor had enlarged since the first birth, and she had a recurrence of pain and a slight hemorrhage every three weeks, and distinctly felt motion in the tumor. This continued for eighteen months, when, after a most violent attack of pain, all movement ceased, and, as she expressed it, she knew the moment the child died. The tumor lost its natural consistence and felt flabby and dead. An incision was made through the linea alba, and the knife came in contact with a hard, gritty substance, three or four lines thick. The escape of several quarts of dark brown fluid followed the incision, and the operation had to be discontinued on account of the ensuing syncope. About six weeks afterward a bone presented at the orifice, which the woman extracted, and this was soon followed by a mass of bones, hair, and putrid matter. The discharge was small, and gradually grew less in quantity and offensiveness, soon ceasing altogether, and the wound closed. By December health was good and the menses had returned.

Ahlfeld, Ambrosioni, Galabin, Packard, Thiernesse, Maxson, de Belamizaran, Dibot, and Chabert are among others recording the phenomenon of coexisting extrauterine and intrauterine pregnancy. Argles mentions simultaneous extrauterine fetation and superfetation.

Sanger mentions a triple ectopic gestation, in which there was twin pregnancy in the wall of the uterus and a third ovum at the fimbriated end of the right tube. Careful examination showed this to be a case of intramural twin pregnancy at the point of entrance of the tube and the uterus, while at the abdominal end of the same tube there was another ovum,—the whole being an example of triple unilateral ectopic gestation.

The instances of delivery of an extrauterine fetus, with viability of the child, from the abdomen of the mother would attract attention from their rarity alone, but when coupled with associations of additional interest they surely deserve a place in a work of this nature. Osiander speaks of an abdominal fetus being taken out alive, and there is a similar case on record in the early part of this century. The London Medical and Physical Journal, in one of its early numbers, contained an account of an abdominal fetus penetrating the walls of the bladder and being extracted from the walls of the hypogastrium; but Sennertus gives a case which far eclipses this, both mother and fetus surviving. He says that in this case the woman, while pregnant, received a blow on the lower part of her body, in consequence of which a small tumor appeared shortly after the accident. It so happened in this case that the peritoneum was extremely dilatable, and the uterus, with the child inside, made its way into the peritoneal sac. In his presence an incision was made and the fetus taken out alive. Jessop gives an example of extrauterine gestation in a woman of twenty-six, who had previously had normal delivery. In this case an incision was made and a fetus of about eight months' growth was found lying loose in the abdominal cavity in the midst of the intestines. Both the mother and child were saved. This is a very rare result. Campbell, in his celebrated monograph, in a total of 51 operations had only seen recorded the accounts of two children saved, and one of these was too marvelous to believe. Lawson Tait reports a case in which he saved the child, but lost the mother on the fourth day. Parvin describes a case in which death occurred on the third day. Browne quotes Parry as saying that there is one twin pregnancy in 23 extrauterine conceptions. He gives 24 cases of twin conception, one of which was uterine, the other extrauterine, and says that of 7 in the third month, with no operation, the mother died in 5. Of 6 cases of from four and a half to seven months' duration, 2 lived, and in 1 case at the fifth month there was an intrauterine fetus delivered which lived. Of 11 such cases at nine months, 6 mothers lived and 6 intrauterine fetuses lived. In 6 of these cases no operation was performed. In one case the mother died, but both the uterine and the extrauterine conceptions lived. In another the mother and intrauterine fetus died, and the extrauterine fetus lived. Wilson a gives an instance of a woman delivered of a healthy female child at eight months which lived. The after-birth came away without assistance, but the woman still presented every appearance of having another child within her, although examination by the vagina revealed none. Wilson called Chatard in consultation, and from the fetal heart-sounds and other symptoms they decided that there was another pregnancy wholly extrauterine. They allowed the case to go twenty-three days, until pains similar to those of labor occurred, and then decided on celiotomy. The operation was almost bloodless, and a living child weighing eight pounds was extracted. Unfortunately, the mother succumbed after ninety hours, and in a month the intrauterine child died from inanition, but the child of extrauterine gestation thrived. Sales gives the case of a negress of twenty-two, who said that she had been "tricked by a negro," and had a large snake in the abdomen, and could distinctly feel its movements. She stoutly denied any intercourse. It was decided to open the abdominal cyst; the incision was followed by a gush of blood and a placenta came into view, which was extracted with a living child. To the astonishment of the operators the uterus was distended, and it was decided to open it, when another living child was seen and extracted. The cyst and the uterus were cleansed of all clots and the wound closed. The mother died of septicemia, but the children both lived and were doing well six weeks after the operation. A curious case was seen in 1814 of a woman who at her fifth gestation suffered abdominal uneasiness at the third month, and this became intolerable at the ninth month. The head of the fetus could be felt through the abdomen; an incision was made through the parietes; a fully developed female child was delivered, but, unfortunately, the mother died of septic infection.

The British Medical Journal quotes: "Pinard (Bull. de l'Acad. de Med., August 6, 1895) records the following, which he describes as an ideal case. The patient was aged thirty-six, had had no illness, and had been regular from the age of fourteen till July, 1894. During August of that year she had nausea and vomiting; on the 22d and 23d she lost a fluid, which was just pink. The symptoms continued during September, on the 22d and 23d of which month there was a similar loss. In October she was kept in bed for two days by abdominal pain, which reappeared in November, and was then associated with pain in micturition and defecation. From that time till February 26, 1895, when she came under Pinard's care, she was attended by several doctors, each of whom adopted a different diagnosis and treatment. One of them, thinking she had a fibroid, made her take in all about an ounce of savin powder, which did not, however, produce any ill effect. When admitted she looked ill and pinched. The left thigh and leg were painful and edematous. The abdomen looked like that of the sixth month of pregnancy. The abdominal wall was tense, smooth, and without lineae albicantes. Palpation revealed a cystic immobile tumor, extending 2 inches above the umbilicus and apparently fixed by deep adhesions. The fetal parts could only be made out with difficulty by deep palpation, but the heart-sounds were easily heard to the right of and below the umbilicus. By the right side of this tumor one could feel a small one, the size of a Tangerine orange, which hardened and softened under examination. When contracted the groove between it and the large tumor became evident. Vaginal examination showed that the cervix, which was slightly deflected forward and to the right and softened, as in uterine gestation, was continuous with the smaller tumor. Cephalic ballottement was obtained in the large tumor. No sound was passed into the uterus for fear of setting up reflex action; the diagnosis of extrauterine gestation at about six and a half months with a living child was established without requiring to be clinched by proving the uterus empty. The patient was kept absolutely at rest in bed and the edema of the left leg cured by position. On April 30th the fundus of the tumor was 35 cm. above the symphysis and the uterus 11 1/2 cm.; the cervix was soft as that of a primipara at term. Operation, May 2d: Uterus found empty, cavity 14 1/2 cm. long. Median incision in abdominal wall; cyst walls exposed; seen to be very slight and filled with enormous vessels, some greater than the little finger. On seizing the wall one of these vessels burst, and the hemorrhage was only rendered greater on attempting to secure it, so great was the friability of the walls. The cyst was therefore rapidly opened and the child extracted by the foot. Hemorrhage was restrained first by pressure of the hands, then by pressure-forceps and ligatures. The walls of the cyst were sewn to the margins of the abdominal wound, the edge of the placenta being included in the suture. A wound was thus formed 10 cm. in diameter, with the placenta for its base; it was filled with iodoform and salicylic gauze. The operation lasted an hour, and the child, a boy weighing 5 1/2 pounds, after a brief period of respiratory difficulties, was perfectly vigorous. There was at first a slight facial asymmetry and a depression on the left upper jaw caused by the point of the left shoulder, against which it had been pressed in the cyst; these soon disappeared, and on the nineteenth day the boy weighed 12 pounds. The maternal wound was not dressed till May 13th, when it was washed with biniodid, 1:4000. The placenta came away piecemeal between May 25th and June 2d. The wound healed up, and the patient got up on the forty-third day, having suckled her infant from the first day after its birth."

Quite recently Werder has investigated the question of the ultimate fate of ectopic children delivered alive. He has been able to obtain the record of 40 cases. Of these, 18 died within a week after birth; 5 within a month; 1 died at six months of bronchopneumonia; 1 at seven months of diarrhea; 2 at eleven months, 1 from croup; 1 at eighteen months from cholera infantum—making a total of 26 deaths and leaving 14 children to be accounted for. Of these, 5 were reported as living and well after operation, with no subsequent report; 1 was strong and healthy after three weeks, but there has been no report since; 1 was well at six months, then was lost sight of; 1 was well at the last report; 2 live and are well at one year; 2 are living and well at two years; 1 (Beisone's case) is well at seven years; and 1 (Tait's case) is well at fourteen and one-half years. The list given on pages 60 and 61 has been quoted by Hirst and Dorland. It contains data relative to 17 cases in which abdominal section has been successfully performed for advanced ectopic gestation with living children.

Long Retention of Extrauterine Pregnancy.—The time of the retention of an extrauterine gestation is sometimes remarkable, and it is no uncommon occurrence for several pregnancies to successfully ensue during such retention. The Ephemerides contains examples of extrauterine pregnancy remaining in the abdomen forty-six years; Hannaeus mentioned an instance remaining ten years, the mother being pregnant in the meantime; Primperosius speaks of a similar instance; de Blegny, one of twenty-five years in the abdomen; Birch, a case of eighteen years in the abdomen, the woman bearing in the meantime; Bayle, one of twenty-six years, and the Ephemerides, another. In a woman of forty-six, the labor pains intervened without expulsion of the fetus. Impregnation ensued twice afterward, each followed by the birth of a living child. The woman lived to be ninety-four, and was persuaded that the fetus was still in the abdomen, and directed a postmortem examination to be made after her decease, which was done, and a large cyst containing an ossified fetus was discovered in the left side of the cavity. In 1716 a woman of Joigny when thirty years old, having been married four years, became pregnant, and three months later felt movements and found milk in her breasts. At the ninth month she had labor-pains, but the fetus failed to present; the pains ceased, but recurred in a month, still with a negative result. She fell into a most sickly condition and remained so for eighteen months, when the pains returned again, but soon ceased. Menstruation ceased and the milk in her breasts remained for thirty years. She died at sixty-one of peripneumonia, and on postmortem examination a tumor was found occupying part of the hypogastric and umbilical regions. It weighed eight pounds and consisted of a male fetus of full term with six teeth; it had no odor and its sac contained no liquid. The bones seemed better developed than ordinarily; the skin was thick, callous, and yellowish The chorion, amnion, and placenta were ossified and the cord dried up. Walther mentions the case of an infant which remained almost petrified in the belly of its mother for twenty-three years. No trace of the placenta, cord, or enveloping membrane could be found.

Cordier publishes a paper on ectopic gestation, with particular reference to tubal pregnancy, and mentions that when there is rupture between the broad ligaments hemorrhage is greatly limited by the resistance of the surrounding structures, death rarely resulting from the primary rupture in this location. Cordier gives an instance in which he successfully removed a full-grown child, the result of an ectopic gestation which had ruptured intraligamentally and had been retained nearly two years.

Lospichlerus gives an account of a mother carrying twins, extrauterine, for six years. Mounsey of Riga, physician to the army of the Czarina, sent to the Royal Society in 1748 the bones of a fetus that had been extracted from one of the fallopian tubes after a lodgment of thirteen years. Starkey Middleton read the report of a case of a child which had been taken out of the abdomen, having lain there nearly sixteen years, during which time the mother had borne four children. It was argued at this time that boys were conceived on the right side and girls on the left, and in commenting on this Middleton remarks that in this case the woman had three boys and one girl after the right fallopian tube had lost its function. Chester cites the instance of a fetus being retained fifty-two years, the mother not dying until her eightieth year. Margaret Mathew carried a child weighing eight pounds in her abdomen for twenty-six years, and which after death was extracted. Aubrey speaks of a woman aged seventy years unconsciously carrying an extrauterine fetus for many years, which was only discovered postmortem. She had ceased to menstruate at forty and had borne a child at twenty-seven. Watkins speaks of a fetus being retained forty-three years; James, others for twenty-five, thirty, forty-six, and fifty years; Murfee, fifty-five years; Cunningham, forty years; Johnson, forty-four years; Josephi, fifteen years (in the urinary bladder); Craddock, twenty-two years, and da Costa Simoes, twenty-six years.

Long Retention of Uterine Pregnancy.—Cases of long retained intrauterine pregnancies are on record and deserve as much consideration as those that were extrauterine. Albosius speaks of a mother carrying a child in an ossified condition in the uterus for twenty-eight years. Cheselden speaks of a case in which a child was carried many years in the uterus, being converted into a clay-like substance, but preserving form and outline. Caldwell mentions the case of a woman who carried an ossified fetus in her uterus for sixty years. Camerer describes the retention of a fetus in the uterus for forty-six years; Stengel, one for ten years, and Storer and Buzzell, for twenty-two months. Hannaeus, in 1686, issued a paper on such a case under the title, "Mater, Infantis Mortui Vivum Sepulchrum," which may be found in French translation.

Buchner speaks of a fetus being retained in the uterus for six years, and Horstius relates a similar case. Schmidt's Jahrbucher contain the report of a woman of forty-nine, who had borne two children. While threshing corn she felt violent pain like that of labor, and after an illness suffered a constant fetid discharge from the vagina for eleven years, fetal bones being discharged with occasional pain. This poor creature worked along for eleven years, at the end of which time she was forced to bed, and died of symptoms of purulent peritonitis. At the necropsy the uterus was found adherent to the anterior wall of the abdomen and containing remnants of a putrid fetus with its numerous bones. There is an instance recorded of the death of a fetus occurring near term, its retention and subsequent discharge being through a spontaneous opening in the abdominal wall one or two months after.

Meigs cites the case of a woman who dated her pregnancy from March, 1848, and which proceeded normally for nine months, but no labor supervened at this time and the menses reappeared. In March, 1849, she passed a few fetal bones by the rectum, and in May, 1855, she died. At the necropsy the uterus was found to contain the remains of a fully developed fetus, minus the portions discharged through a fistulous connection between the uterine cavity and the rectum. In this case there had been retention of a fully developed fetus for nine years. Cox describes the case of a woman who was pregnant seven months, and who was seized with convulsions; the supposed labor-pains passed off, and after death the fetus was found in the womb, having lain there for five years. She had an early return of the menses, and these recurred regularly for four years. Dewees quotes two cases, in one of which the child was carried twenty months in the uterus; in the other, the mother was still living two years and five months after fecundation. Another case was in a woman of sixty, who had conceived at twenty-six, and whose fetus was found, partly ossified, in the uterus after death.

There are many narratives of the long continuation of fetal movements, and during recent years, in the Southern States, there was quite a prevalence of this kind of imposters. Many instances of the exhibition of fetal movements in the bellies of old negro women have been noticed by the lay journals, but investigation proves them to have been nothing more than an exceptional control over the abdominal muscles, with the ability to simulate at will the supposed fetal jerks. One old woman went so far as to show the fetus dancing to the music of a banjo with rhythmical movements. Such imposters flourished best in the regions given to "voodooism." We can readily believe how easy the deception might be when we recall the exact simulation of the fetal movements in instances of pseudocyesis.

The extraordinary diversity of reports concerning the duration of pregnancy has made this a much mooted question. Many opinions relative to the longest and shortest period of pregnancy, associated with viability of the issue, have been expressed by authors on medical jurisprudence. There is perhaps no information more unsatisfactory or uncertain. Mistakes are so easily made in the date of the occurrence of pregnancy, or in the date of conception, that in the remarkable cases we can hardly accept the propositions as worthy evidence unless associated with other and more convincing facts, such as the appearance and stage of development of the fetus, or circumstances making conception impossible before or after the time mentioned, etc. It will be our endeavor to cite the more seemingly reliable instances of the anomalies of the time or duration of pregnancy reported in reputable periodicals or books.

Short Pregnancies.—Hasenet speaks of the possibility of a living birth at four months; Capuron relates the instance of Fortunio Liceti, who was said to have been born at the end of four and a half months and lived to complete his twenty-fourth year. In the case of the Marechal de Richelieu, the Parliament of Paris decreed that an infant of five months possessed that capability of living the ordinary period of existence, i.e., the "viabilite," which the law of France requires for the establishment of inheritance. In his seventh book Pliny gives examples of men who were born out of time. Jonston gives instances of births at five, six, seven, and eight months. Bonnar quotes 5 living births before the one hundred and fiftieth day; 1 of one hundred and twenty-five days; 1 of one hundred and twenty days; 1 of one hundred and thirty-three days, surviving to twenty-one months; and 1 of one hundred and thirty-five days' pregnancy surviving to eighty years. Maisonneuve describes a case in which abortion took place at four and a half months; he found the fetus in its membranes two hours after delivery, and, on laying the membranes open, saw that it was living. He applied warmth, and partly succeeded in restoring it; for a few minutes respiratory movements were performed regularly, but it died in six hours. Taylor quotes Carter concerning the case of a fetus of five months which cried directly after it was born, and in the half hour it lived it tried frequently to breathe. He also quotes Davies, mentioning an instance of a fetus of five months, which lived twelve hours, weighing 2 pounds, and measuring 12 inches, and which cried vigorously. The pupillary membrane was entire, the testes had not descended, and the head was well covered with hair. Usher speaks of a woman who in 1876 was delivered of 2 male children on the one hundred and thirty-ninth day; both lived for an hour; the first weighed 10 ounces 6 drams and measured 9 3/4 inches; the other 10 ounces 7 drams, with the same length as the first. Routh speaks of a Mrs. F——, aged thirty-eight, who had borne 9 children and had had 3 miscarriages, the last conception terminating as such. Her husband was away, and returned October 9, 1869. She did not again see her husband until the 3d or 4th of January. The date of quickening was not observed, and the child was born June 8, 1870. During gestation she was much frightened by a rat. The child was weak, the testes undescended, and it lived but eighteen days, dying of symptoms of atrophy. The parents were poor, of excellent character, and although, according to the evidence, this pregnancy lasted but twenty-two weeks and two days, there was absolutely no reason to suspect infidelity.

Ruttel speaks of a child of five months who lived twenty-four hours; and he saw male twins born at the sixth month weighing 3 pounds each who were alive and healthy a year after. Barker cites the case of a female child born on the one hundred and fifty-eighth day that weighed 1 pound and was 11 inches long. It had rudimentary nails, very little hair on the head, its eyelids were closed, and the skin much shriveled; it did not suckle properly, and did not walk until nineteen months old. Three and a half years after, the child was healthy and thriving, but weighed only 29 1/2 pounds. At the time of birth it was wrapped up in a box and placed before the fire. Brouzet speaks of living births of from five to six months' pregnancy, and Kopp speaks of a six months' child which lived four days. The Ephemerides contains accounts of living premature births.

Newinton describes a pregnancy of five months terminating with the birth of twins, one of whom lived twenty minutes and the other fifteen. The first was 11 1/2 inches long, and weighed 1 pound 3 1/2 ounces, and the other was 11 inches long, and weighed 1 pound. There is a recent instance of premature birth following a pregnancy of between five and a half and six months, the infant weighing 955 grams. One month after birth, through the good offices of the wet-nurse and M. Villemin, who attended the child and who invented a "couveuse" for the occasion, it measured 38 cm. long.

Moore is accredited with the trustworthy report of the case of a woman who bore a child at the end of the fifth month weighing 1 1/2 pounds and measuring 9 inches. It was first nourished by dropping liquid food into its mouth; and at the age of fifteen months it was healthy and weighed 18 pounds. Eikam saw a case of abortion at the fifth month in which the fetus was 6 inches in length and weighed about 8 ounces. The head was sufficiently developed and the cranial bones considerably advanced in ossification. He tied the cord and placed the fetus in warm water. It drew up its feet and arms and turned its head from one side to the other, opening its mouth and trying to breathe. It continued in this wise for an hour, the action of the heart being visible ten minutes after the movements ceased. From its imperfectly developed genitals it was supposed to have been a female. Professor J. Muller, to whom it was shown, said that it was not more than four months old, and this coincided with the mother's calculation.

Villemin before the Societe Obstetricale et Gynecologique reported the case of a two-year-old child, born in the sixth month of pregnancy. That the child had not had six months of intrauterine life he could vouch, the statement being borne out by the last menstrual period of the mother, the date of the first fetal movements, the child's weight, which was 30 1/2 ounces, and its appearance. Budin had had this infant under observation from the beginning and corroborated Villemin's statements. He had examined infants of six or seven months that had cried and lived a few days, and had found the alveolar cavities filled with epithelial cells, the lung sinking when placed in a vessel of water. Charpentier reported a case of premature birth in his practice, the child being not more than six and a half months and weighing 33 1/2 ounces. So sure was he that it would not live that he placed it in a basin while he attended to the mother. After this had been done, the child being still alive, he wrapped it in cotton and was surprised next day to find it alive. It was then placed in a small, well-heated room and fed with a spoon on human milk; on the twelfth day it could take the breast, since which time it thrived and grew.

There is a case on record of a child viable at six months and twenty days. The mother had a miscarriage at the beginning of 1877, after which menstruation became regular, appearing last from July 3 to 9, 1877. On January 28, 1878, she gave birth to a male infant, which was wrapped in wadding and kept at an artificial temperature. Being unable to suckle, it was fed first on diluted cow's milk. It was so small at birth that the father passed his ring over the foot almost to the knee. On the thirteenth day it weighed 1250 grams, and at the end of a week it was taking the breast. In December, 1879, it had 16 teeth, weighed 10 kilograms, walked with agility, could pronounce some words, and was especially intelligent. Capuron relates an instance of a child born after a pregnancy of six and a half months and in excellent health at two years, and another living at ten years of the same age at birth. Tait speaks of a living female child, born on the one hundred and seventy-ninth day, with no nails on its fingers or toes, no hair, the extremities imperfectly developed, and the skin florid and thin. It was too feeble to grasp its mother's nipple, and was fed for three weeks by milk from the breast through a quill. At forty days it weighed 3 pounds and measured 13 inches. Before the expiration of three months it died of measles. Dodd describes a case in which the catamenia were on the 24th of June, 1838, and continued a week; the woman bore twins on January 11, 1839, one of which survived, the other dying a few minutes after birth. She was never irregular, prompt to the hour, and this fact, coupled with the diminutive size of the children, seemed to verify the duration of the pregnancy. In 1825, Baber of Buxur, India, spoke of a child born at six and a half months, who at the age of fifty days weighed 1 pound and 13 ounces and was 14 inches long. The longest circumference of the head was 10 inches and the shortest 9.1 inches. The child suckled freely and readily. In Spaeth's clinic there was a viable infant at six and a half months weighing 900 grams. Spaeth says that he has known a child of six months to surpass in eventual development its brothers born at full term.

In some cases there seems to be a peculiarity in women which manifests itself by regular premature births. La Motte, van Swieten, and Fordere mention females who always brought forth their conceptions at the seventh month.

The incubator seems destined to be the future means of preserving these premature births. Several successful cases have been noticed, and by means of an incubator Tarnier succeeded in raising infants which at the age of six months were above the average. A full description of the incubator may be found. The modified Auvard incubator is easily made; the accompanying illustrations (Figs. 5, 6, and 7) explain its mechanism. Several improved incubators have been described in recent years, but the Auvard appears to be the most satisfactory.

The question of retardation of labor, like that of premature birth, is open to much discussion, and authorities differ as to the limit of protraction with viability. Aulus Gellius says that, after a long conversation with the physicians and wise men, the Emperor Adrian decided in a case before him, that of a woman of chaste manners and irreproachable character, the child born eleven months after her husband's death was legitimate. Under the Roman law the Decenviri established that a woman may bear a viable child at the tenth month of pregnancy. Paulus Zacchias, physician to Pope Innocent X, declared that birth may be retarded to the tenth month, and sometimes to a longer period. A case was decided in the Supreme Court of Friesland, a province in the northern part of the Netherlands, October, 1634, in which a child born three hundred and thirty-three days after the death of the husband was pronounced legitimate. The Parliament of Paris was gallant enough to come to the rescue of a widow and save her reputation by declaring that a child born after a fourteen months' gestation was legitimate. Bartholinus speaks of an unmarried woman of Leipzig who was delivered after a pregnancy of sixteen months. The civil code of France provides that three hundred days shall constitute the longest period of the legitimacy of an infant; the Scottish law, three hundred days; and the Prussian law, three hundred and one days.

There are numerous cases recorded by the older writers. Amman has one of twelve months' duration; Enguin, one of twelve months'; Buchner, a case of twelve months'; Benedictus, one of fourteen months'; de Blegny, one of nineteen months'; Marteau, Osiander, and others of forty-two and forty-four weeks'; and Stark's Archives, one of forty-five weeks', living, and also another case of forty-four weeks'. An incredible case is recorded of an infant which lived after a three years' gestation. Instances of twelve months' duration are also recorded. Jonston quotes Paschal in relating an instance of birth after pregnancy of twenty-three months; Aventium, one after two years; and Mercurialis, a birth after a four years' gestation—which is, of course, beyond belief.

Thormeau writes from Tours, 1580, of a case of gestation prolonged to the twenty-third month, and Santorini, at Venice, in 1721, describes a similar case, the child reaching adult life. Elvert records a case of late pregnancy, and Henschel one of forty-six weeks, but the fetus was dead. Schneider cites an instance of three hundred and eight days' duration. Campbell says that Simpson had cases of three hundred and nineteen, three hundred and thirty-two, and three hundred and thirty-six days'; Meigs had one of four hundred and twenty. James Reid, in a table of 500 mature births, gives 14 as being from three hundred and two to three hundred and fifteen days'.

Not so long ago a jury rendered a verdict of guilty of fornication and bastardy when it was alleged that the child was born three hundred and seventeen days after intercourse. Taylor relates a case of pregnancy in which the wife of a laborer went to America three hundred and twenty-two days before the birth. Jaffe describes an instance of the prolongation of pregnancy for three hundred and sixty-five days, in which the developments and measurements corresponded to the length of protraction. Bryan speaks of a woman of twenty-five who became pregnant on February 10, 1876, and on June 17th felt motion. On July 28th she was threatened with miscarriage, and by his advice the woman weaned the child at the breast. She expected to be confined the middle of November, 1876, but the expected event did not occur until April 26, 1877, nine months after the quickening and four hundred and forty days from the time of conception. The boy was active and weighed nine pounds. The author cites Meigs' case, and also one of Atlee's, at three hundred and fifty-six days.

Talcott, Superintendent of the State Homeopathic Asylum for the Insane, explained the pregnancy of an inmate who had been confined for four years in this institution as one of protracted labor. He said that many such cases have been reported, and that something less than two years before he had charge of a case in which the child was born. He made the report to the New York Senate Commission on Asylums for the Insane as one of three years' protraction. Tidd speaks of a woman who was delivered of a male child at term, and again in ten months delivered of a well-developed male child weighing 7 1/4 pounds; he relates the history of another case, in Clifton, W. Va., of a woman expecting confinement on June 1st going over to September 16th, the fetus being in the uterus over twelve months, and nine months after quickening was felt.

Two extraordinary cases are mentioned, one in a woman of thirty-five, who expected to be confined April 24, 1883. In May she had a few labor-pains that passed away, and during the next six months she remained about as large as usual, and was several times thought to be in the early stages of labor. In September the os dilated until the first and second fingers could be passed directly to the head. This condition lasted about a month, but passed away. At times during the last nine months of pregnancy she was almost unable to endure the movements of the child. Finally, on the morning of November 6th, after a pregnancy of four hundred and seventy-six days, she was delivered of a male child weighing 13 pounds.

Both the mother and child did well despite the use of chloroform and forceps. The other case was one lasting sixteen months and twenty days.

In a rather loose argument, Carey reckons a case of three hundred and fifty days. Menzie gives an instance in a woman aged twenty-eight, the mother of one child, in whom a gestation was prolonged to the seventeenth month. The pregnancy was complicated by carcinoma of the uterus. Ballard describes the case of a girl of sixteen years and six months, whose pregnancy, the result of a single intercourse, lasted three hundred and sixty days. Her labor was short and easy for a primipara, and the child was of the average size. Mackenzie cites the instance of a woman aged thirty-two, a primipara, who had been married ten years and who always had been regular in menstruation. The menses ceased on April 28, 1888, and she felt the child for the first time in September. She had false pains in January, 1889, and labor did not begin until March 8th, lasting sixty-six hours. If all these statements are correct, the probable duration of this pregnancy was eleven months and ten days.

Lundie relates an example of protracted gestation of eleven months, in which an anencephalous fetus was born; and Martin of Birmingham describes a similar case of ten and a half months' duration. Raux-Tripier has seen protraction to the thirteenth month. Enguin reports an observation of an accouchement of twins after a pregnancy that had been prolonged for eleven months. Resnikoff mentions a pregnancy of eleven months' duration in an anemic secundipara. The case had been under his observation from the beginning of pregnancy; the patient would not submit to artificial termination at term, which he advised. After a painful labor of twenty-four hours a macerated and decomposed child was born, together with a closely-adherent placenta. Tarnier reports an instance of partus serotinus in which the product of conception was carried in the uterus forty days after term. The fetus was macerated but not putrid, and the placenta had undergone fatty degeneration. At a recent meeting of the Chicago Gynecological Society, Dr. F. A. Stahl reported the case of a German-Bohemian woman in which the fifth pregnancy terminated three hundred and two days after the last menstruation. Twenty days before there had occurred pains similar to those of labor, but they gradually ceased. The sacral promontory was exaggerated, and the anteroposterior pelvic diameter of the inlet in consequence diminished. The fetus was large and occupied the first position. Version was with difficulty effected and the passage of the after-coming head through the superior strait required expression and traction, during which the child died. The mother suffered a deep laceration of the perineum involving an inch of the wall of the rectum.

Among others reporting instances of protracted pregnancy are Collins, eleven months; Desbrest, eighteen months; Henderson, fifteen months; Jefferies, three hundred and fifty-eight days, and De la Vergne gives the history of a woman who carried an infant in her womb for twenty-nine months; this case may possibly belong under the head of fetus long retained in the uterus.

Unconscious Pregnancy.—There are numerous instances of women who have had experience in pregnancy unconsciously going almost to the moment of delivery, yet experiencing none of the usual accompanying symptoms of this condition. Crowell speaks of a woman of good social position who had been married seven years, and who had made extensive preparations for a long journey, when she was seized with a "bilious colic," and, to her dismay and surprise, a child was born before the arrival of the doctor summoned on account of her sudden colic and her inability to retain her water. A peculiar feature of this case was the fact that mental disturbance set in immediately afterward, and the mother became morbid and had to be removed to an asylum, but recovered in a few months. Tanner saw a woman of forty-two who had been suffering with abdominal pains. She had been married three years and had never been pregnant. Her catamenia were very scant, but this was attributed to her change of life. She had conceived, had gone to the full term of gestation, and was in labor ten hours without any suspicion of pregnancy. She was successfully delivered of a girl, which occasioned much rejoicing in the household.

Tasker of Kendall's Mills, Me., reports the case of a young married woman calling him for bilious colic. He found the stomach slightly distended and questioned her about the possibility of pregnancy. Both she and her husband informed him that such could not be the case, as her courses had been regular and her waist not enlarged, as she had worn a certain corset all the time. There were no signs of quickening, no change in the breasts, and, in fact, none of the usual signs of pregnancy present. He gave her an opiate, and to her surprise, in about six hours she was the mother of a boy weighing five pounds. Both the mother and child made a good recovery. Duke cites the instance of a woman who supposed that she was not pregnant up to the night of her miscarriage. She had menstruated and was suckling a child sixteen months old. During the night she was attacked with pains resembling those of labor and a fetus slipped into the vagina without any hemorrhage; the placenta came away directly afterward. In this peculiar case the woman was menstruating regularly, suckling a child, and at the same time was unconsciously pregnant.

Isham speaks of a case of unconscious pregnancy in which extremely small twins were delivered at the eighth month. Fox cites an instance of a woman who had borne eight children, and yet unconscious of pregnancy. Merriman speaks of a woman forty years of age who had not borne a child for nine years, but who suddenly gave birth to a stout, healthy boy without being cognizant of pregnancy. Dayral tells of a woman who carried a child all through pregnancy, unconscious of her condition, and who was greatly surprised at its birth. Among the French observers speaking of pregnancy remaining unrecognized by the mother until the period of accouchement, Lozes and Rhades record peculiar cases; and Mouronval relates an instance in which a woman who had borne three children completely ignored the presence of pregnancy until the pains of labor were felt. Fleishman and Munzenthaler also record examples of unconscious pregnancy.

Pseudocyesis.—On the other hand, instances of pregnancy with imaginary symptoms and preparations for birth are sometimes noticed, and many cases are on record. In fact, nearly every text-book on obstetrics gives some space to the subject of pseudocyesis. Suppression of the menses, enlargement of the abdomen, engorgement of the breasts, together with the symptoms produced by the imagination, such as nausea, spasmodic contraction of the abdomen, etc., are for the most part the origin of the cases of pseudocyesis. Of course, many of the cases are not examples of true pseudocyesis, with its interesting phenomena, but instances of malingering for mercenary or other purposes, and some are calculated to deceive the most expert obstetricians by their tricks. Weir Mitchell delineates an interesting case of pseudocyesis as follows: "A woman, young, or else, it may be, at or past the climacteric, eagerly desires a child or is horribly afraid of becoming pregnant. The menses become slight in amount, irregular, and at last cease or not. Meanwhile the abdomen and breasts enlarge, owing to a rapid taking on of fat, and this is far less visible elsewhere. There comes with this excess of fat the most profound conviction of the fact of pregnancy. By and by the child is felt, the physician takes it for granted, and this goes on until the great diagnostician, Time, corrects the delusion. Then the fat disappears with remarkable speed, and the reign of this singular simulation is at an end." In the same article, Dr. Mitchell cites the two following cases under his personal observation: "I was consulted by a lady in regard to a woman of thirty years of age, a nurse in whom she was interested. This person had been married some three years to a very old man possessed of a considerable estate. He died, leaving his wife her legal share and the rest to distant cousins, unless the wife had a child. For two months before he died the woman, who was very anemic, ceased to menstruate. She became sure that she was pregnant, and thereupon took on flesh at a rate and in a way which seemed to justify her belief. Her breasts and abdomen were the chief seats of this overgrowth. The menses did not return, her pallor increased; the child was felt, and every preparation made for delivery. At the eighth month a physician made an examination and assured her of the absence of pregnancy. A second medical opinion confirmed the first, and the tenth month found her of immense size and still positive as to her condition. At the twelfth month her menstrual flow returned, and she became sure it was the early sign of labor. When it passed over she became convinced of her error, and at once dropped weight at the rate of half a pound a day despite every effort to limit the rate of this remarkable loss. At the end of two months she had parted with fifty pounds and was, on the whole, less anemic. At this stage I was consulted by letter, as the woman had become exceedingly hysteric. This briefly stated case, which occurred many years ago, is a fair illustration of my thesis.

"Another instance I saw when in general practice. A lady who had several children and suffered much in her pregnancies passed five years without becoming impregnated. Then she missed a period, and had, as usual, vomiting. She made some wild efforts to end her supposed pregnancy, and failing, acquiesced in her fate. The menses returned at the ninth month and were presumed to mean labor. Meanwhile she vomited, up to the eighth month, and ate little. Nevertheless, she took on fat so as to make the abdomen and breasts immense and to excite unusual attention. No physician examined her until the supposed labor began, when, of course, the truth came out. She was pleased not to have another child, and in her case, as in all the others known to me, the fat lessened as soon as the mind was satisfied as to the non-existence of pregnancy. As I now recall the facts, this woman was not more than two months in getting rid of the excess of adipose tissue. Dr. Hirst tells me he has met with cases of women taking on fat with cessation of the menses, and in which there was also a steady belief in the existence of pregnancy. He has not so followed up these cases as to know if in them the fat fell away with speed when once the patient was assured that no child existed within her."

Hirst, in an article on the difficulties in the diagnosis of pregnancy, gives several excellent photographs showing the close resemblance between several pathologic conditions and the normal distention of the abdomen in pregnancy. A woman who had several children fell sick with a chest-affection, followed by an edema. For fifteen months she was confined to her bed, and had never had connection with her husband during that time. Her menses ceased; her mammae became engorged and discharged a serous lactescent fluid; her belly enlarged, and both she and her physician felt fetal movements in her abdomen. As in her previous pregnancies, she suffered nausea. Naturally, a suspicion as to her virtue came into her husband's mind, but when he considered that she had never left her bed for fifteen months he thought the pregnancy impossible. Still the wife insisted that she was pregnant and was confirmed in the belief by a midwife. The belly continued to increase, and about eleven months after the cessation of the menses she had the pains of labor. Three doctors and an accoucheur were present, and when they claimed that the fetal head presented the husband gave up in despair; but the supposed fetus was born shortly after, and proved to be only a mass of hydatids, with not the sign of a true pregnancy. Girard of Lyons speaks of a female who had been pregnant several times, but again experienced the signs of pregnancy. Her mammae were engorged with a lactescent fluid, and she felt belly-movements like those of a child; but during all this time she had regular menstruation. Her abdomen progressively increased in size, and between the tenth and eleventh months she suffered what she thought to be labor-pains. These false pains ceased upon taking a bath, and with the disappearance of the other signs was dissipated the fallacious idea of pregnancy.

There is mentioned an instance of medicolegal interest of a young girl who showed all the signs of pregnancy and confessed to her parents that she had had commerce with a man. The parents immediately prosecuted the seducer by strenuous legal methods, but when her ninth month came, and after the use of six baths, all the signs of pregnancy vanished. Harvey cites several instances of pseudocyesis, and says we must not rashly determine of the the inordinate birth before the seventh or after the eleventh month. In 1646 a woman, after having laughed heartily at the jests of an ill-bred, covetous clown, was seized with various movements and motions in her belly like those of a child, and these continued for over a month, when the courses appeared again and the movements ceased. The woman was certain that she was pregnant.

The most noteworthy historic case of pseudocyesis is that of Queen Mary of England, or "Bloody Mary," as she was called. To insure the succession of a Catholic heir, she was most desirous of having a son by her consort,

Philip, and she constantly prayed and wished for pregnancy. Finally her menses stopped; the breasts began to enlarge and became discolored around the nipples. She had morning-sickness of a violent nature and her abdomen enlarged. On consultation with the ladies of her court, her opinion of pregnancy was strongly confirmed. Her favorite amusement then was to make baby-clothes and count on her fingers the months of pregnancy. When the end of the ninth month approached, the people were awakened one night by the joyous peals of the bells of London announcing the new heir. An ambassador had been sent to tell the Pope that Mary could feel the new life within her, and the people rushed to St. Paul's Cathedral to listen to the venerable Archbishop of Canterbury describe the baby-prince and give thanks for his deliverance. The spurious labor pains passed away, and after being assured that no real pregnancy existed in her case, Mary went into violent hysterics, and Philip, disgusted with the whole affair, deserted her; then commenced the persecution of the Protestants, which blighted the reign.

Putnam cites the case of a healthy brunet, aged forty, the mother of three children. She had abrupt vertical abdominal movements, so strong as to cause her to plunge and sway from side to side. Her breasts were enlarged, the areolae dark, and the uterus contained an elastic tumor, heavy and rolling under the hand. Her abdomen progressively enlarged to the regular size of matured gestation; but the extrauterine pregnancy, which was supposed to have existed, was not seen at the autopsy, nothing more than an enlarged liver being found. The movement was due to spasmodic movements of the abdominal muscles, the causes being unknown. Madden gives the history of a primipara of twenty-eight, married one year, to whom he was called. On entering the room he was greeted by the midwife, who said she expected the child about 8 P.M. The woman was lying in the usual obstetric position, on the left side, groaning, crying loudly, and pulling hard at a strap fastened to the bed-post. She had a partial cessation of menses, and had complained of tumultuous movements of the child and overflow of milk from the breasts. Examination showed the cervix low down, the os small and circular, and no signs of pregnancy in the uterus. The abdomen was distended with tympanites and the rectum much dilated with accumulated feces. Dr. Madden left her, telling her that she was not pregnant, and when she reappeared at his office in a few days, he reassured her of the nonexistence of pregnancy; she became very indignant, triumphantly squeezed lactescent fluid from her breasts, and, insisting that she could feel fetal movements, left to seek a more sympathetic accoucheur. Underhill, in the words of Hamilton, describes a woman as "having acquired the most accurate description of the breeding symptoms, and with wonderful facility imagined that she had felt every one of them." He found the woman on a bed complaining of great labor-pains, biting a handkerchief, and pulling on a cloth attached to her bed. The finger on the abdomen or vulva elicited symptoms of great sensitiveness. He told her she was not pregnant, and the next day she was sitting up, though the discharge continued, but the simulated throes of labor, which she had so graphically pictured, had ceased.

Haultain gives three examples of pseudocyesis, the first with no apparent cause, the second due to carcinoma of the uterus, while in the third there was a small fibroid in the anterior wall of the uterus. Some cases are of purely nervous origin, associated with a purely muscular distention of the abdomen. Clay reported a case due to ascites. Cases of pseudocyesis in women convicted of murder are not uncommon, though most of them are imposters hoping for an extra lease of life.

Croon speaks of a child seven years old on whom he performed ovariotomy for a round-celled sarcoma. She had been well up to May, but since then she had several times been raped by a boy, in consequence of which she had constant uterine hemorrhage. Shortly after the first coitus her abdomen began to enlarge, the breasts to develop, and the areolae to darken. In seven months the abdomen presented the signs of pregnancy, but the cervix was soft and patulous; the sound entered three inches and was followed by some hemorrhage. The child was well developed, the mons was covered with hair, and all the associate symptoms tended to increase the deception.

Sympathetic Male Nausea of Pregnancy.—Associated with pregnancy there are often present morning-nausea and vomiting as prominent and reliable symptoms. Vomiting is often so excessive as to be provocative of most serious issue and even warranting the induction of abortion. This fact is well known and has been thoroughly discussed, but with it is associated an interesting point, the occasional association of the same symptoms sympathetically in the husband. The belief has long been a superstition in parts of Great Britain, descending to America, and even exists at the present day. Sir Francis Bacon has written on this subject, the substance of his argument being that certain loving husbands so sympathize with their pregnant wives that they suffer morning-sickness in their own person. No less an authority than S. Weir Mitchell called attention to the interesting subject of sympathetic vomiting in the husband in his lectures on nervous maladies some years ago. He also quotes the following case associated with pseudocyesis:—

"A woman had given birth to two female children. Some years passed and her desire for a boy was ungratified. Then she missed her flow once, and had thrice after this, as always took place with her when pregnant, a very small but regular loss. At the second month morning-vomiting came on as usual with her. Meanwhile she became very fat, and as the growth was largely, in fact excessively, abdominal, she became easily sure of her condition. She was not my patient, but her husband consulted me as to his own morning-sickness, which came on with the first occurrence of this sign in his wife, as had been the case twice before in her former pregnancies. I advised him to leave home, and this proved effectual. I learned later that the woman continued to gain flesh and be sick every morning until the seventh month. Then menstruation returned, an examination was made, and when sure that there was no possibility of her being pregnant she began to lose flesh, and within a few months regained her usual size."

Hamill reports an instance of morning-sickness in a husband two weeks after the appearance of menstruation in the wife for the last time. He had daily attacks, and it was not until the failure of the next menses that the woman had any other sign of pregnancy than her husband's nausea. His nausea continued for two months, and was the same as that which he had suffered during his wife's former pregnancies, although not until both he and his wife became aware of the existence of pregnancy. The Lancet describes a case in which the husband's nausea and vomiting, as well as that of the wife, began and ended simultaneously. Judkins cites an instance of a man who was sick in the morning while his wife was carrying a child. This occurred during every pregnancy, and the man related that his own father was similarly affected while his mother was in the early months of pregnancy with him, showing an hereditary predisposition.

The perverted appetites and peculiar longings of pregnant women furnish curious matter for discussion. From the earliest times there are many such records. Borellus cites an instance, and there are many others, of pregnant women eating excrement with apparent relish. Tulpius, Sennert, Langius, van Swieten, a Castro, and several others report depraved appetites. Several writers have seen avidity for human flesh in such females. Fournier knew a woman with an appetite for the blood of her husband. She gently cut him while he lay asleep by her side and sucked blood from the wounds—a modern "Succubus." Pare mentions the perverted appetites of pregnant women, and says that they have been known to eat plaster, ashes, dirt, charcoal, flour, salt, spices, to drink pure vinegar, and to indulge in all forms of debauchery. Plot gives the case of a woman who would gnaw and eat all the linen off her bed. Hufeland's Journal records the history of a case of a woman of thirty-two, who had been married ten years, who acquired a strong taste for charcoal, and was ravenous for it. It seemed to cheer her and to cure a supposed dyspepsia. She devoured enormous quantities, preferring hardwood charcoal. Bruyesinus speaks of a woman who had a most perverted appetite for her own milk, and constantly drained her breasts; Krafft-Ebing cites a similar case. Another case is that of a pregnant woman who had a desire for hot and pungent articles of food, and who in a short time devoured a pound of pepper. Scheidemantel cites a case in which the perverted appetite, originating in pregnancy, became permanent, but this is not the experience of most observers. The pregnant wife of a farmer in Hassfort-on-the-Main ate the excrement of her husband.

Many instances could be quoted, some in which extreme cases of polydipsia and bulimia developed; these can be readily attributed to the increased call for liquids and food. Other cases of diverse new emotions can be recalled, such as lasciviousness, dirty habits, perverted thoughts, and, on the other hand, extreme piety, chastity, and purity of the mind. Some of the best-natured women are when pregnant extremely cross and irritable and many perversions of disposition are commonly noticed in pregnancy. There is often a longing for a particular kind of food or dish for which no noticeable desire had been displayed before.

Maternal Impressions.—Another curious fact associated with pregnancy is the apparent influence of the emotions of the mother on the child in utero. Every one knows of the popular explanation of many birth-marks, their supposed resemblance to some animal or object seen by the mother during pregnancy, etc. The truth of maternal impressions, however, seems to be more firmly established by facts of a substantial nature. There is a natural desire to explain any abnormality or anomaly of the child as due to some incident during the period of the mother's pregnancy, and the truth is often distorted and the imagination heavily drawn upon to furnish the satisfactory explanation. It is the customary speech of the dime-museum lecturer to attribute the existence of some "freak" to an episode in the mother's pregnancy. The poor "Elephant-man" firmly believed his peculiarity was due to the fact that his mother while carrying him in utero was knocked down at the circus by an elephant. In some countries the exhibition of monstrosities is forbidden because of the supposed danger of maternal impression. The celebrated "Siamese Twins" for this reason were forbidden to exhibit themselves for quite a period in France.

We shall cite only a few of the most interesting cases from medical literature. Hippocrates saved the honor of a princess, accused of adultery with a negro because she bore a black child, by citing it as a case of maternal impression, the husband of the princess having placed in her room a painting of a negro, to the view of which she was subjected during the whole of her pregnancy. Then, again, in the treatise "De Superfoetatione" there occurs the following distinct statement: "If a pregnant woman has a longing to eat earth or coals, and eats of them, the infant which is born carries on its head the mark of these things." This statement, however, occurs in a work which is not mentioned by any of the ancient authorities, and is rejected by practically all the modern ones; according to Ballantyne, there is, therefore, no absolute proof that Hippocrates was a believer in one of the most popular and long-persisting beliefs concerning fetal deformities.

In the explanation of heredity, Hippocrates states "that the body of the male as well as that of the female furnishes the semen. That which is weak (unhealthy) is derived from weak (unhealthy) parts, that which is strong (healthy) from strong (healthy) parts, and the fetus will correspond to the quality of the semen. If the semen of one part come in greater quantity from the male than from the female, this part will resemble more closely the father; if, however, it comes more from the female, the part will rather resemble the mother. If it be true that the semen comes from both parents, then it is impossible for the whole body to resemble either the mother or the father, or neither the one nor the other in anything, but necessarily the child will resemble both the one and the other in something. The child will most resemble the one who contributes most to the formation of the parts." Such was the Hippocratic theory of generation and heredity, and it was ingeniously used to explain the hereditary nature of certain diseases and malformations. For instance, in speaking of the sacred disease (epilepsy), Hippocrates says: "Its origin is hereditary, like that of other diseases; for if a phlegmatic person be born of a phlegmatic, and a bilious of a bilious, and a phthisical of a phthisical, and one having spleen disease of another having disease of the spleen, what is to hinder it from happening that where the father and mother were subject to this disease certain of their offspring should be so affected also? As the semen comes from all parts of the body, healthy particles will come from healthy parts, and unhealthy from unhealthy parts."

According to Pare, Damascene saw a girl with long hair like a bear, whose mother had constantly before her a picture of the hairy St. John. Pare also appends an illustration showing the supposed resemblance to a bear. Jonston quotes a case of Heliodorus; it was an Ethiopian, who by the effect of the imagination produced a white child. Pare describes this case more fully: "Heliodorus says that Persina, Queen of Ethiopia, being impregnated by Hydustes, also an Ethiopian, bore a daughter with a white skin, and the anomaly was ascribed to the admiration that a picture of Andromeda excited in Persina throughout the whole of the pregnancy." Van Helmont cites the case of a tailor's wife at Mechlin, who during a conflict outside her house, on seeing a soldier lose his hand at her door, gave birth to a daughter with one hand, the other hand being a bleeding stump; he also speaks of the case of the wife of a merchant at Antwerp, who after seeing a soldier's arm shot off at the siege of Ostend gave birth to a daughter with one arm. Plot speaks of a child bearing the figure of a mouse; when pregnant, the mother had been much frightened by one of these animals. Gassendus describes a fetus with the traces of a wound in the same location as one received by the mother. The Lancet speaks of several cases—one of a child with a face resembling a dog whose mother had been bitten; one of a child with one eye blue and the other black, whose mother during confinement had seen a person so marked; of an infant with fins as upper and lower extremities, the mother having seen such a monster; and another, a child born with its feet covered with scalds and burns, whose mother had been badly frightened by fireworks and a descending rocket. There is the history of a woman who while pregnant at seven months with her fifth child was bitten on the right calf by a dog. Ten weeks after, she bore a child with three marks corresponding in size and appearance to those caused by the dog's teeth on her leg. Kerr reports the case of a woman in her seventh month whose daughter fell on a cooking stove, shocking the mother, who suspected fatal burns. The woman was delivered two months later of an infant blistered about the mouth and extremities in a manner similar to the burns of her sister. This infant died on the third day, but another was born fourteen months later with the same blisters. Inflammation set in and nearly all the fingers and toes sloughed of. In a subsequent confinement, long after the mental agitation, a healthy unmarked infant was born.

Hunt describes a case which has since become almost classic of a woman fatally burned, when pregnant eight months, by her clothes catching fire at the kitchen grate. The day after the burns labor began and was terminated by the birth of a well-formed dead female child, apparently blistered and burned in extent and in places corresponding almost exactly to the locations of the mother's injuries. The mother died on the fourth day.

Webb reports the history of a negress who during a convulsion while pregnant fell into a fire, burning the whole front of the abdomen, the front and inside of the thighs to the knees, the external genitals, and the left arm. Artificial delivery was deemed necessary, and a dead child, seemingly burned much like its mother, except less intensely, was delivered. There was also one large blister near the inner canthus of the eye and some large blisters about the neck and throat which the mother did not show. There was no history of syphilis nor of any eruptive fever in the mother, who died on the tenth day with tetanus.

Graham describes a woman of thirty-five, the mother of seven children, who while pregnant was feeding some rabbits, when one of the animals jumped at her with its eyes "glaring" upon her, causing a sudden fright. Her child was born hydrocephalic. Its mouth and face were small and rabbit-shaped. Instead of a nose, it had a fleshy growth 3/4 inch long by 1/4 inch broad, directed upward at an angle of 45 degrees. The space between this and the mouth was occupied by a body resembling an adult eye. Within this were two small, imperfect eyes which moved freely while life lasted (ten minutes). The child's integument was covered with dark, downy, short hair. The woman recovered and afterward bore two normal children.

Parvin mentions an instance of the influence of maternal impression in the causation of a large, vivid, red mark or splotch on the face: "When the mother was in Ireland she was badly frightened by a fire in which some cattle were burned. Again, during the early months of her pregnancy she was frightened by seeing another woman suddenly light the fire with kerosene, and at that time became firmly impressed with the idea that her child would be marked." Parvin also pictures the "turtle-man," an individual with deformed extremities, who might be classed as an ectromelus, perhaps as a phocomelus, or seal-like monster. According to the story, when the mother was a few weeks pregnant her husband, a coarse, rough fisherman, fond of rude jokes, put a large live turtle in the cupboard. In the twilight the wife went to the cupboard and the huge turtle fell out, greatly startling her by its hideous appearance as it fell suddenly to the floor and began to move vigorously.

Copeland mentions a curious case in which a woman was attacked by a rattlesnake when in her sixth month of pregnancy, and gave birth to a child whose arm exhibited the shape and action of a snake, and involuntarily went through snake-like movements. The face and mouth also markedly resembled the head of a snake.

The teeth were situated like a serpent's fangs. The mere mention of a snake filled the child (a man of twenty-nine) with great horror and rage, "particularly in the snake season." Beale gives the history of a case of a child born with its left eye blackened as by a blow, whose mother was struck in a corresponding portion of the face eight hours before confinement. There is on record an account of a young man of twenty-one suffering from congenital deformities attributed to the fact that his mother was frightened by a guinea-pig having been thrust into her face during pregnancy. He also had congenital deformity of the right auricle. At the autopsy, all the skin, tissues, muscles, and bones were found involved. Owen speaks of a woman who was greatly excited ten months previously by a prurient curiosity to see what appearance the genitals of her brother presented after he had submitted to amputation of the penis on account of carcinoma. The whole penis had been removed. The woman stated that from the time she had thus satisfied herself, her mind was unceasingly engaged in reflecting and sympathizing on the forlorn condition of her brother. While in this mental state she gave birth to a son whose penis was entirely absent, but who was otherwise well and likely to live. The other portions of the genitals were perfect and well developed. The appearance of the nephew and the uncle was identical. A most peculiar case is stated by Clerc as occurring in the experience of Kuss of Strasburg. A woman had a negro paramour in America with whom she had had sexual intercourse several times. She was put in a convent on the Continent, where she stayed two years. On leaving the convent she married a white man, and nine months after she gave birth to a dark-skinned child. The supposition was that during her abode in the convent and the nine months subsequently she had the image of her black paramour constantly before her. Loin speaks of a woman who was greatly impressed by the actions of a clown at a circus, and who brought into the world a child that resembled the fantastic features of the clown in a most striking manner.

Mackay describes five cases in which fright produced distinct marks on the fetus. There is a case mentioned in which a pregnant woman was informed that an intimate friend had been thrown from his horse; the immediate cause of death was fracture of the skull, produced by the corner of a dray against which the rider was thrown. The mother was profoundly impressed by the circumstance, which was minutely described to her by an eye-witness. Her child at birth presented a red and sensitive area upon the scalp corresponding in location with the fatal injury in the rider. The child is now an adult woman, and this area upon the scalp remains red and sensitive to pressure, and is almost devoid of hair. Mastin of Mobile, Alabama, reports a curious instance of maternal impression. During the sixth month of the pregnancy of the mother her husband was shot, the ball passing out through the left breast. The woman was naturally much shocked, and remarked to Dr. Mastin: "Doctor, my baby will be ruined, for when I saw the wound I put my hands over my face, and got it covered with blood, and I know my baby will have a bloody face." The child came to term without a bloody face. It had, however, a well-defined spot on the left breast just below the site of exit of the ball from its father's chest. The spot was about the size of a silver half-dollar, and had elevated edges of a bright red color, and was quite visible at the distance of one hundred feet. The authors have had personal communication with Dr. Mastin in regard to this case, which he considers the most positive evidence of a case of maternal impression that he has ever met.

Paternal Impressions.—Strange as are the foregoing cases, those of paternal impression eclipse them. Several are on record, but none are of sufficient authenticity to warrant much discussion on the subject. Those below are given to illustrate the method of report. Stahl, quoted by Steinan, 1843, speaks of the case of a child, the father being a soldier who lost an eye in the war. The child was born with one of its eyes dried up in the orbit, in this respect presenting an appearance like that of the father. Schneider says a man whose wife was expecting confinement dreamt that his oldest son stood beside his bedside with his genitals much mutilated and bleeding. He awoke in a great state of agitation, and a few days later the wife was delivered of a child with exstrophy of the bladder. Hoare recites the curious story of a man who vowed that if his next child was a daughter he would never speak to it. The child proved to be a son, and during the whole of the father's life nothing could induce the son to speak to his father, nor, in fact, to any other male person, but after the father's death he talked fluently to both men and women. Clark reports the birth of a child whose father had a stiff knee-joint, and the child's knee was stiff and bent in exactly the same position as that of its father.

Telegony.—The influence of the paternal seed on the physical and mental constitution of the child is well known. To designate this condition, Telegony is the word that was coined by Weismann in his "Das Keimplasma," and he defines it as "Infection of the Germ," and, at another time, as "Those doubtful instances in which the offspring is said to resemble, not the father, but an early mate of the mother,"—or, in other words, the alleged influence of a previous sire on the progeny produced by a subsequent one from the same mother. In a systematic discussion of telegony before the Royal Medical Society, Edinburgh, on March 1, 1895, Brunton Blaikie, as a means of making the definition of telegony plainer by practical example, prefaced his remarks by citing the classic example which first drew the attention of the modern scientific world to this phenomenon. The facts of this case were communicated in a letter from the Earl of Morton to the President of the Royal Society in 1821, and were as follows: In the year 1816 Lord Morton put a male quagga to a young chestnut mare of 7/8 Arabian blood, which had never before been bred from. The result was a female hybrid which resembled both parents. He now sold the mare to Sir Gore Ousley, who two years after she bore the hybrid put her to a black Arabian horse. During the two following years she had two foals which Lord Morton thus describes: "They have the character of the Arabian breed as decidedly as can be expected when 15/16 of the blood are Arabian, and they are fine specimens of the breed; but both in their color and in the hair of their manes they have a striking resemblance to the quagga. Their color is bay, marked more or less like the quagga in a darker tint. Both are distinguished by the dark line along the ridge of the back, the dark stripes across the forehead, and the dark bars across the back part of the legs." The President of the Royal Society saw the foals and verified Lord Morton's statement.

"Herbert Spencer, in the Contemporary Review for May, 1893, gives several cases communicated to him by his friend Mr. Fookes, whom Spencer says is often appointed judge of animals at agricultural shows. After giving various examples he goes on to say: 'A friend of mine near this had a valuable Dachshund bitch, which most unfortunately had a litter by a stray sheep-dog. The next year the owner sent her on a visit to a pure Dachshund dog, but the produce took quite as much of the first father as the second, and the next year he sent her to another Dachshund, with the same result. Another case: A friend of mine in Devizes had a litter of puppies unsought for, by a setter from a favorite pointer bitch, and after this she never bred any true pointers, no matter what the paternity was.'

"Lord Polwarth, whose very fine breed of Border Leicesters is famed throughout Britain, and whose knowledge on the subject of breeding is great, says that 'In sheep we always consider that if a ewe breeds to a Shrop ram, she is never safe to breed pure Leicesters from, as dun or colored legs are apt to come even when the sire is a pure Leicester. This has been proved in various instances, but is not invariable.' "

Hon. Henry Scott says: "Dog-breeders know this theory well; and if a pure-bred bitch happens to breed to a dog of another breed, she is of little use for breeding pure-bred puppies afterward. Animals which produce large litters and go a short time pregnant show this throwing back to previous sires far more distinctly than others—I fancy dogs and pigs most of all, and probably horses least. The influence of previous sires may be carried into the second generation or further, as I have a cat now which appears to be half Persian (long hair). His dam has very long hair and every appearance of being a half Persian, whereas neither have really any Persian blood, as far as I know, but the grand-dam (a very smooth-haired cat) had several litters by a half-Persian tom-cat, and all her produce since have showed the influence retained. The Persian tom-cat died many years ago, and was the only one in the district, so, although I cannot be absolutely positive, still I think this case is really as stated."

Breeders of Bedlington terriers wish to breed dogs with as powerful jaws as possible. In order to accomplish this they put the Bedlington terrier bitch first to a bull-terrier dog, and get a mongrel litter which they destroy. They now put the bitch to a Bedlington terrier dog and get a litter of puppies which are practically pure, but have much stronger jaws than they would otherwise have had, and also show much of the gameness of the bull-terrier, thus proving that physiologic as well as anatomic characters may be transmitted in this way.

After citing the foregoing examples, Blaikie directs his attention to man, and makes the following interesting remarks:—

"We might expect from the foregoing account of telegony amongst animals that whenever a black woman had a child to a white man, and then married a black man, her subsequent children would not be entirely black. Dr. Robert Balfour of Surinam in 1851 wrote to Harvey that he was continually noticing amongst the colored population of Surinam 'that if a negress had a child or children by a white, and afterward fruitful intercourse with a negro, the latter offspring had generally a lighter color than the parents.' But, as far as I know, this is the only instance of this observation on record. Herbert Spencer has shown that when a pure-bred animal breeds with an animal of a mixed breed, the offspring resembles much more closely the parent of pure blood, and this may explain why the circumstance recorded by Balfour has been so seldom noted. For a negro, who is of very pure blood, will naturally have a stronger influence on the subsequent progeny than an Anglo-Saxon, who comes of a mixed stock. If this be the correct explanation, we should expect that when a white woman married first a black man, and then a white, the children by the white husband would be dark colored. Unfortunately for the proof of telegony, it is very rare that a white woman does marry a black man, and then have a white as second husband; nevertheless, we have a fair number of recorded instances of dark-colored children being born in the above way of white parents.

"Dr. Harvey mentions a case in which 'a young woman, residing in Edinburgh, and born of white (Scottish) parents, but whose mother, some time previous to her marriage, had a natural (mulatto) child by a negro man-servant in Edinburgh, exhibits distinct traces of the negro. Dr. Simpson —afterward Sir James Simpson—whose patient the young woman at one time was, has had no recent opportunities of satisfying himself as to the precise extent to which the negro character prevails in her features; but he recollects being struck with the resemblance, and noticed particularly that the hair had the qualities characteristic of the negro.' Herbert Spencer got a letter from a 'distinguished correspondent' in the United States, who said that children by white parents had been 'repeatedly' observed to show traces of black blood when the women had had previous connection with (i.e., a child by) a negro. Dr. Youmans of New York interviewed several medical professors, who said the above was 'generally accepted as a fact.' Prof. Austin Flint, in 'A Text-book of Human Physiology,' mentioned this fact, and when asked about it said: 'He had never heard the statement questioned.'

"But it is not only in relation to color that we find telegony to have been noticed in the human subject. Dr. Middleton Michel gives a most interesting case in the American Journal of the Medical Sciences for 1868: 'A black woman, mother of several negro children, none of whom were deformed in any particular, had illicit intercourse with a white man, by whom she became pregnant. During gestation she manifested great uneasiness of mind, lest the birth of a mulatto offspring should disclose her conduct. . . . It so happened that her negro husband possessed a sixth digit on each hand, but there was no peculiarity of any kind in the white man, yet when the mulatto child was born it actually presented the deformity of a supernumerary finger.' Taruffi, the celebrated Italian teratologist, in speaking of the subject, says: 'Our knowledge of this strange fact is by no means recent for Fienus, in 1608, said that most of the children born in adultery have a greater resemblance to the legal than to the real father'—an observation that was confirmed by the philosopher Vanini and by the naturalist Ambrosini. From these observations comes the proverb: 'Filium ex adultera excusare matrem a culpa.' Osiander has noted telegony in relation to moral qualities of children by a second marriage. Harvey said that it has long been known that the children by a second husband resemble the first husband in features mind, and disposition. He then gave a case in which this resemblance was very well marked. Orton, Burdach (Traite de Physiologie), and Dr. William Sedgwick have all remarked on this physical resemblance; and Dr. Metcalfe, in a dissertation delivered before this society in 1855, observed that in the cases of widows remarrying the children of the second marriage frequently resemble the first husband.

"An observation probably having some bearing on this subject was made by Count de Stuzeleci (Harvey, loc. cit.). He noticed that when an aboriginal female had had a child by a European, she lost the power of conception by a male of her own race, but could produce children by a white man. He believed this to be the case with many aboriginal races; but it has been disproved, or at all events proved to be by no means a universal law, in every case except that of the aborigines of Australia and New Zealand. Dr. William Sedgwick thought it probable that the unfruitfulness of prostitutes might in some degree be due to the same cause as that of the Australian aborigines who have had children by white men.

"It would seem as though the Israelites had had some knowledge of telegony, for in Deuteronomy we find that when a man died leaving no issue, his wife was commanded to marry her husband's brother, in order that he might 'raise up seed to his brother.' "

We must omit the thorough inquiry into this subject that is offered by Mr. Blaikie. The explanations put forward have always been on one of three main lines:—

(1) The imagination-theory, or, to quote Harvey: "Due to mental causes so operating either on the mind of the female and so acting on her reproductive powers, or on the mind of the male parent, and so influencing the qualities of his semen, as to modify the nutrition and development of the offspring."

(2) Due to a local influence on the reproductive organs of the mother.

(3) Due to a general influence through the fetus on the mother.

Antenatal Pathology.—We have next to deal with the diseases, accidents, and operations that affect the pregnant uterus and its contents; these are rich in anomalies and facts of curious interest, and have been recognized from the earliest times. In the various works usually grouped together under the general designation of "Hippocratic" are to be found the earliest opinions upon the subject of antenatal pathology which the medical literature of Greece has handed down to modern times. That there were medical writers before the time of Hippocrates cannot be doubted, and that the works ascribed to the "Father of Medicine" were immediately followed by those of other physicians, is likewise not to be questioned; but whilst nearly all the writings prior to and after Hippocrates have been long lost to the world, most of those that were written by the Coan physician and his followers have been almost miraculously preserved. As Littre puts it, "Les ecrits hippocratiques demeurent isoles au milieu des debris de l'antique litterature medicale."—(Ballantyne.)

The first to be considered is the transmission of contagious disease to the fetus in utero. The first disease to attract attention was small-pox. Devilliers, Blot, and Depaul all speak of congenital small-pox, the child born dead and showing evidences of the typical small-pox pustulation, with a history of the mother having been infected during pregnancy. Watson reports two cases in which a child in utero had small-pox. In the first case the mother was infected in pregnancy; the other was nursing a patient when seven months pregnant; she did not take the disease, although she had been infected many months before. Mauriceau delivered a woman of a healthy child at full term after she had recovered from a severe attack of this disease during the fifth month of gestation. Mauriceau supposed the child to be immune after the delivery. Vidal reported to the French Academy of Medicine, May, 1871, the case of a woman who gave birth to a living child of about six and one-half months' maturation, which died some hours after birth covered with the pustules of seven or eight days' eruption. The pustules on the fetus were well umbilicated and typical, and could have been nothing but those of small-pox; besides, this disease was raging in the neighborhood at the time. The mother had never been infected before, and never was subsequently. Both parents were robust and neither of them had ever had syphilis. About the time of conception, the early part of December, 1870, the father had suffered from the semiconfluent type, but the mother, who had been vaccinated when a girl, had never been stricken either during or after her husband's sickness. Quirke relates a peculiar instance of a child born at midnight, whose mother was covered with the eruption eight hours after delivery. The child was healthy and showed no signs of the contagion, and was vaccinated at once. Although it remained with its mother all through the sickness, it continued well, with the exception of the ninth day, when a slight fever due to its vaccination appeared. The mother made a good recovery, and the author remarks that had the child been born a short time later, it would most likely have been infected.

Ayer reports an instance of congenital variola in twins. Chantreuil speaks of a woman pregnant with twins who aborted at five and a half months. One of the fetuses showed distinct signs of congenital variola, although the mother and other fetus were free from any symptoms of the disease. In 1853 Charcot reported the birth of a premature fetus presenting numerous variolous pustules together with ulcerations of the derm and mucous membranes and stomach, although the mother had convalesced of the disease some time before. Mitchell describes a case of small-pox occurring three days after birth, the mother not having had the disease since childhood. Shertzer relates an instance of confluent small-pox in the eighth month of pregnancy. The child was born with the disease, and both mother and babe recovered. Among many others offering evidence of variola in utero are Degner, Derham, John Hunter, Blot, Bulkley, Welch, Wright, Digk, Forbes, Marinus, and Bouteiller.

Varicella, Measles, Pneumonia, and even Malaria are reported as having been transmitted to the child in utero. Hubbard attended a woman on March 17, 1878, in her seventh accouchement. The child showed the rash of varicella twenty-four hours after birth, and passed through the regular coarse of chicken-pox of ten days' duration. The mother had no signs of the disease, but the children all about her were infected. Ordinarily the period of incubation is from three to four days, with a premonitory fever of from twenty-four to seventy-two hours' duration, when the rash appears; this case must therefore have been infected in utero. Lomer of Hamburg tells of the case of a woman, twenty-two years, unmarried, pregnant, who had measles in the eighth month, and who gave birth to an infant with measles. The mother was attacked with pneumonia on the fifth day of her puerperium, but recovered; the child died in four weeks of intestinal catarrh. Gautier found measles transmitted from the mother to the fetus in 6 out of 11 cases, there being 2 maternal deaths in the 11 cases.

Netter has observed the case of transmission of pneumonia from a mother to a fetus, and has seen two cases in which the blood from the uterine vessels of patients with pneumonia contained the pneumococcus. Wallick collected a number of cases of pneumonia occurring during pregnancy, showing a fetal mortality of 80 per cent.

Felkin relates two instances of fetal malaria in which the infection was probably transmitted by the male parent. In one case the father near term suffered severely from malaria; the mother had never had a chill. The violent fetal movements induced labor, and the spleen was so large as to retard it. After birth the child had seven malarial paroxysms but recovered, the splenic tumor disappearing.

The modes of infection of the fetus by syphilis, and the infection of the mother, have been well discussed, and need no mention here.

There has been much discussion on the effects on the fetus in utero of medicine administered to the pregnant mother, and the opinions as to the reliability of this medication are so varied that we are in doubt as to a satisfactory conclusion. The effects of drugs administered and eliminated by the mammary glands and transmitted to the child at the breast are well known, and have been witnessed by nearly every physician, and, as in cases of strong metallic purges, etc., need no other than the actual test. However, scientific experiments as to the efficacy of fetal therapeutics have been made from time to time with varying results.

Gusserow of Strasbourg tested for iodin, chloroform, and salicylic acid in the blood and secretions of the fetus after maternal administration just before death.

In 14 cases in which iodin had been administered, he examined the fetal urine of 11 cases; in 5, iodin was present, and in the others, absent. He made some similar experiments on the lower animals. Benicke reports having given salicylic acid just before birth in 25 cases, and in each case finding it in the urine of the child shortly after birth.

At a discussion held in New York some years ago as to the real effect on the fetus of giving narcotics to the mother, Dr. Gaillard Thomas was almost alone in advocating that the effect was quite visible. Fordyce Barker was strongly on the negative side. Henning and Ahlfeld, two German observers, vouch for the opinion of Thomas, and Thornburn states that he has witnessed the effect of nux vomica and strychnin on the fetus shortly after birth. Over fifty years ago, in a memoir on "Placental Phthisis," Sir James Y. Simpson advanced a new idea in the recommendation of potassium chlorate during the latter stages of pregnancy. The efficacy of this suggestion is known, and whether, as Simpson said, it acts by supplying extra oxygen to the blood, or whether the salt itself is conveyed to the fetus, has never been definitely settled.

McClintock, who has been a close observer on this subject, reports some interesting cases. In his first case he tried a mixture of iron perchlorid and potassium chlorate three times a day on a woman who had borne three dead children, with a most successful result. His second case failed, but in a third he was successful by the same medication with a woman who had before borne a dead child. In a fourth case of unsuccessful pregnancy for three consecutive births he was successful. His fifth case was extraordinary: It was that of a woman in her tenth pregnancy, who, with one exception, had always borne a dead child at the seventh or eighth month. The one exception lived a few hours only. Under this treatment he was successful in carrying the woman safely past her time for miscarriage, and had every indication for a normal birth at the time of report. Thornburn believes that the administration of a tonic like strychnin is of benefit to a fetus which, by its feeble heart-beats and movements, is thought to be unhealthy. Porak has recently investigated the passage of substances foreign to the organism through the placenta, and offers an excellent paper on this subject, which is quoted in brief in a contemporary number of Teratologia.

In this important paper, Porak, after giving some historical notes, describes a long series of experiments performed on the guinea-pig in order to investigate the passage of arsenic, copper, lead, mercury, phosphorus, alizarin, atropin, and eserin through the placenta. The placenta shows a real affinity for some toxic substances; in it accumulate copper and mercury, but not lead, and it is therefore through it that the poison reaches the fetus; in addition to its pulmonary, intestinal, and renal functions, it fixes glycogen and acts as an accumulator of poisons, and so resembles in its action the liver; therefore the organs of the fetus possess only a potential activity. The storing up of poisons in the placenta is not so general as the accumulation of them in the liver of the mother. It may be asked if the placenta does not form a barrier to the passage of poisons into the circulation of the fetus; this would seem to be demonstrated by mercury, which was always found in the placenta and never in the fetal organs. In poisoning by lead and copper the accumulation of the poison in the fetal tissues is greater than in the maternal, perhaps from differences in assimilation and disassimilation or from greater diffusion. Whilst it is not an impermeable barrier to the passage of poisons, the placenta offers a varying degree of obstruction: it allows copper and lead to pass easily, arsenic with greater difficulty. The accumulation of toxic substances in the fetus does not follow the same law as in the adult. They diffuse more widely in the fetus. In the adult the liver is the chief accumulatory organ. Arsenic, which in the mother elects to accumulate in the liver, is in the fetus stored up in the skin; copper accumulates in the fetal liver, central nervous system, and sometimes in the skin; lead which is found specially in the maternal liver, but also in the skin, has been observed in the skin, liver, nervous centers, and elsewhere in the fetus. The frequent presence of poisons in the fetal skin demonstrates its physiologic importance. It has probably not a very marked influence on its health. On the contrary, accumulation in the placenta and nerve centers explains the pathogenesis of abortion and the birth of dead fetuses ("mortinatatite") Copper and lead did not cause abortion, but mercury did so in two out of six cases. Arsenic is a powerful abortive agent in the guinea-pig, probably on account of placental hemorrhages. An important deduction is that whilst the placenta is frequently and seriously affected in syphilis, it is also the special seat for the accumulation of mercury. May this not explain its therapeutic action in this disease? The marked accumulation of lead in the central nervous system of the fetus explains the frequency and serious character of saturnine encephalopathic lesions. The presence of arsenic in the fetal skin alone gives an explanation of the therapeutic results of the administration of this substance in skin diseases.

Intrauterine amputations are of interest to the medical man, particularly those cases in which the accident has happened in early pregnancy and the child is born with a very satisfactory and clean stump. Montgomery, in an excellent paper, advances the theory, which is very plausible, that intrauterine amputations are caused by contraction of bands or membranes of organized lymph encircling the limb and producing amputation by the same process of disjunctive atrophy that the surgeons induce by ligature. Weinlechner speaks of a case in which a man devoid of all four extremities was exhibited before the Vienna Medical Society. The amputations were congenital, and on the right side there was a very small stump of the upper arm remaining, admitting the attachment of an artificial apparatus. He was twenty-seven years old, and able to write, to thread a needle, pour water out of a bottle, etc. Cook speaks of a female child born of Indian parents, the fourth birth of a mother twenty-six years old. The child weighed 5 1/2 pounds; the circumference of the head was 14 inches and that of the trunk 13 inches. The upper extremities consisted of perfect shoulder joints, but only 1/4 of each humerus was present. Both sides showed evidences of amputation, the cicatrix on the right side being 1 inch long and on the left 1/4 inch long. The right lower limb was merely a fleshy corpuscle 3/4 inch wide and 1/4 inch long; to the posterior edge was attached a body resembling the little toe of a newly-born infant. On the left side the limb was represented by a fleshy corpuscle 1 inch long and 1/4 inch in circumference, resembling the great toe of an infant. There was no history of shock or injury to the mother. The child presented by the breech, and by the absence of limbs caused much difficulty in diagnosis. The three stages of labor were one and one-half hours, forty-five minutes, and five minutes, respectively. The accompanying illustration shows the appearance of the limbs at the time of report.

Figure 10 represents a negro boy, the victim of intrauterine amputation, who learned to utilize his toes for many purposes. The illustration shows his mode of holding his pen.

There is an instance reported in which a child at full term was born with an amputated arm, and at the age of seventeen the stump was scarcely if at all smaller than the other. Blake speaks of a case of congenital amputation of both the upper extremities. Gillilam a mentions a case that shows the deleterious influence of even the weight of a fetal limb resting on a cord or band. His case was that of a fetus, the product of a miscarriage of traumatic origin; the soft tissues were almost cut through and the bone denuded by the limb resting on one of the two umbilical cords, not encircling it, but in a sling. The cord was deeply imbedded in the tissues.

The coilings of the cord are not limited to compression about the extremities alone, but may even decapitate the head by being firmly wrapped several times about the neck. According to Ballantyne, there is in the treatise De Octimestri Partu, by Hippocrates, a reference to coiling of the umbilical cord round the neck of the fetus. This coiling was, indeed, regarded as one of the dangers of the eighth month, and even the mode of its production is described. It is said that if the cord he extended along one side of the uterus, and the fetus lie more to the other side, then when the culbute is performed the funis must necessarily form a loop round the neck or chest of the infant. If it remain in this position, it is further stated, the mother will suffer later and the fetus will either perish or be born with difficulty. If the Hippocratic writers knew that this coiling is sometimes quite innocuous, they did not in any place state the fact.

The accompanying illustrations show the different ways in which the funis may be coiled, the coils sometimes being as many as 8.

Bizzen mentions an instance in which from strangulation the head of a fetus was in a state of putrefaction, the funis being twice tightly bound around the neck. Cleveland, Cuthbert, and Germain report analogous instances. Matthyssens observed the twisting of the funis about the arm and neck of a fetus the body of which was markedly wasted. There was complete absence of amniotic fluid during labor. Blumenthal presented to the New York Pathological Society an ovum within which the fetus was under going intrauterine decapitation. Buchanan describes a case illustrative of the etiology of spontaneous amputation of limbs in utero Nebinger reports a case of abortion, showing commencing amputation of the left thigh from being encircled by the funis. The death of the fetus was probably due to compression of the cord. Owen mentions an instance in which the left arm and hand of a fetus were found in a state of putrescence from strangulation, the funis being tightly bound around at the upper part. Simpson published an article on spontaneous amputation of the forearm and rudimentary regeneration of the hand in the fetus. Among other contributors to this subject are Avery, Boncour, Brown, Ware, Wrangell, Young, Nettekoven, Martin, Macan, Leopold, Hecker, Gunther, and Friedinger.

Wygodzky finds that the greatest number of coils of the umbilical cord ever found to encircle a fetus are 7 (Baudelocque), 8 (Crede), and 9 (Muller and Gray). His own case was observed this year in Wilna. The patient was a primipara aged twenty. The last period was seen on May 10, 1894. On February 19th the fetal movements suddenly ceased. On the 20th pains set in about two weeks before term. At noon turbid liquor amnii escaped. At 2 P.M., on examination, Wygodzky defined a dead fetus in left occipito-anterior presentation, very high in the inlet. The os was nearly completely dilated, the pains strong. By 4 P.M. the head was hardly engaged in the pelvic cavity. At 7 P.M. it neared the outlet at the height of each pain, but retracted immediately afterward. After 10 P.M. the pains grew weak. At midnight Wygodzky delivered the dead child by expression. Not till then was the cause of delay clear. The funis was very tense and coiled 7 times round the neck and once round the left shoulder; there was also a distinct knot. It measured over 65 inches in length. The fetus was a male, slightly macerated. It weighed over 5 pounds, and was easily delivered entire after division and unwinding of the funis. No marks remained on the neck. The placenta followed ten minutes later and, so far as naked-eye experience indicated, seemed healthy.

Intrauterine fractures are occasionally seen, but are generally the results of traumatism or of some extraordinary muscular efforts on the part of the mother. A blow on the abdomen or a fall may cause them. The most interesting cases are those in which the fractures are multiple and the causes unknown. Spontaneous fetal fractures have been discussed thoroughly, and the reader is referred to any responsible text-book for the theories of causation. Atkinson, De Luna, and Keller report intrauterine fractures of the clavicle. Filippi contributes an extensive paper on the medicolegal aspect of a case of intrauterine fracture of the os cranium. Braun of Vienna reports a case of intrauterine fracture of the humerus and femur. Rodrigue describes a case of fracture and dislocation of the humerus of a fetus in utero. Gaultier reports an instance of fracture of both femora intrauterine. Stanley, Vanderveer, and Young cite instances of intrauterine fracture of the thigh; in the case of Stanley the fracture occurred during the last week of gestation, and there was rapid union of the fragments during lactation. Danyau, Proudfoot, and Smith mention intrauterine fracture of the tibia; in Proudfoot's case there was congenital talipes talus.

Dolbeau describes an instance in which multiple fractures were found in a fetus, some of which were evidently postpartum, while others were assuredly antepartum. Hirschfeld describes a fetus showing congenital multiple fractures. Gross speaks of a wonderful case of Chaupier in which no less than 113 fractures were discovered in a child at birth. It survived twenty-four hours, and at the postmortem examination it was found that some were already solid, some uniting, whilst others were recent. It often happens that the intrauterine fracture is well united at birth. There seems to be a peculiar predisposition of the bones to fracture in the cases in which the fractures are multiple and the cause is not apparent.

The results to the fetus of injuries to the pregnant mother are most diversified. In some instances the marvelous escape of any serious consequences of one or both is almost incredible, while in others the slightest injury is fatal. Guillemont cites the instance of a woman who was killed by a stroke of lightning, but whose fetus was saved; while Fabricius Hildanus describes a case in which there was perforation of the head, fracture of the skull, and a wound of the groin, due to sudden starting and agony of terror of the mother. Here there was not the slightest history of any external violence.

It is a well-known fact that injuries to the pregnant mother show visible effects on the person of the fetus. The older writers kept a careful record of the anomalous and extraordinary injuries of this character and of their effects. Brendelius tells us of hemorrhage from the mouth and nose of the fetus occasioned by the fall of the mother; Buchner mentions a case of fracture of the cranium from fright of the mother; Reuther describes a contusion of the os sacrum and abdomen in the mother from a fall, with fracture of the arm and leg of the fetus from the same cause; Sachse speaks of a fractured tibia in a fetus, caused by a fall of the mother; Slevogt relates an instance of rupture of the abdomen of a fetus by a fall of the mother; the Ephemerides contains accounts of injuries to the fetus of this nature, and among others mentions a stake as having been thrust into a fetus in utero; Verduc offers several examples, one a dislocation of the fetal foot from a maternal fall; Plocquet gives an instance of fractured femur; Walther describes a case of dislocation of the vertebrae from a fall; and there is also a case of a fractured fetal vertebra from a maternal fall. There is recorded a fetal scalp injury, together with clotted blood in the hair, after a fall of the mother: Autenrieth describes a wound of the pregnant uterus, which had no fatal issue, and there is also another similar case on record.

The modern records are much more interesting and wonderful on this subject than the older ones. Richardson speaks of a woman falling down a few weeks before her delivery. Her pelvis was roomy and the birth was easy; but the infant was found to have extensive wounds on the back, reaching from the 3d dorsal vertebra across the scapula, along the back of the humerus, to within a short distance of the elbow. Part of these wounds were cicatrized and part still granulating, which shows that the process of reparation is as active in utero as elsewhere.

Injuries about the genitalia would naturally be expected to exercise some active influence on the uterine contents; but there are many instances reported in which the escape of injury is marvelous. Gibb speaks of a woman, about eight months pregnant, who fell across a chair, lacerating her genitals and causing an escape of liquor amnii. There was regeneration of this fluid and delivery beyond term. The labor was tedious and took place two and a half months after the accident. The mother and the female child did well. Purcell reports death in a pregnant woman from contused wound of the vulva. Morland relates an instance of a woman in the fifth month of her second pregnancy, who fell on the roof of a woodshed by slipping from one of the steps by which she ascended to the roof, in the act of hanging out some clothes to dry. She suffered a wound on the internal surface of the left nympha 1 1/2 inch long and 1/2 inch deep. She had lost about three quarts of blood, and had applied ashes to the vagina to stop the bleeding. She made a recovery by the twelfth day, and the fetal sounds were plainly audible. Cullingworth speaks of a woman who, during a quarrel with her husband, was pushed away and fell between two chairs, knocking one of them over, and causing a trivial wound one inch long in the vagina, close to the entrance. She screamed, there was a gush of blood, and she soon died. The uterus contained a fetus three or four months old, with the membranes intact, the maternal death being due to the varicosity of the pregnant pudenda, the slight injury being sufficient to produce fatal hemorrhage. Carhart describes the case of a pregnant woman, who, while in the stooping position, milking a cow, was impaled through the vagina by another cow. The child was born seven days later, with its skull crushed by the cow's horn. The horn had entered the vagina, carrying the clothing with it.

There are some marvelous cases of recovery and noninterference with pregnancy after injuries from horns of cattle. Corey speaks of a woman of thirty-five, three months pregnant, weighing 135 pounds, who was horned by a cow through the abdominal parietes near the hypogastric region; she was lifted into the air, carried, and tossed on the ground by the infuriated animal. There was a wound consisting of a ragged rent from above the os pubis, extending obliquely to the left and upward, through which protruded the great omentum, the descending and transverse colon, most of the small intestines, as well as the pyloric extremity of the stomach. The great omentum was mangled and comminuted, and bore two lacerations of two inches each. The intestines and stomach were not injured, but there was considerable extravasation of blood into the abdominal cavity. The intestines were cleansed and an unsuccessful attempt was made to replace them. The intestines remained outside of the body for two hours, and the great omentum was carefully spread out over the chest to prevent interference with the efforts to return the intestines. The patient remained conscious and calm throughout; finally deep anesthesia was produced by ether and chloroform, three and a half hours after the accident, and in twenty minutes the intestines were all replaced in the abdominal cavity. The edges were pared, sutured, and the wound dressed. The woman was placed in bed, on the right side, and morphin was administered. The sutures were removed on the ninth day, and the wound had healed except at the point of penetration. The woman was discharged twenty days after, and, incredible to relate, was delivered of a well-developed, full-term child just two hundred and two days from the time of the accident. Both the mother and child did well.

Luce speaks of a pregnant woman who was horned in the lower part of the abdomen by a cow, and had a subsequent protrusion of the intestines through the wound. After some minor complications, the wound healed fourteen weeks after the accident, and the woman was confined in natural labor of a healthy, vigorous child. In this case no blood was found on the cow's horn, and the clothing was not torn, so that the wound must have been made by the side of the horn striking the greatly distended abdomen.

Richard, quoted also by Tiffany, speaks of a woman, twenty-two, who fell in a dark cellar with some empty bottles in her hand, suffering a wound in the abdomen 2 inches above the navel on the left side 8 cm. long. Through this wound a mass of intestines, the size of a man's head, protruded. Both the mother and the child made a good convalescence. Harris cites the instance of a woman of thirty, a multipara, six months pregnant, who was gored by a cow; her intestines and omentum protruded through the rip and the uterus was bruised. There was rapid recovery and delivery at term. Wetmore of Illinois saw a woman who in the summer of 1860, when about six months pregnant, was gored by a cow, and the large intestine and the omentum protruded through the wound. Three hours after the injury she was found swathed in rags wet with a compound solution of whiskey and camphor, with a decoction of tobacco. The intestines were cold to the touch and dirty, but were washed and replaced. The abdomen was sewed up with a darning needle and black linen thread; the woman recovered and bore a healthy child at the full maturity of her gestation. Crowdace speaks of a female pauper, six months pregnant, who was attacked by a buffalo, and suffered a wound about 1 1/2 inch long and 1/2 inch wide just above the umbilicus. Through this small opening 19 inches of intestine protruded. The woman recovered, and the fetal heart-beats could be readily auscultated.

Major accidents in pregnant women are often followed by the happiest results. There seems to be no limit to what the pregnant uterus can successfully endure. Tiffany, who has collected some statistics on this subject, as well as on operations successfully performed during pregnancy, which will be considered later, quotes the account of a woman of twenty-seven, eight months pregnant, who was almost buried under a clay wall. She received terrible wounds about the head, 32 sutures being used in this location alone. Subsequently she was confined, easily bore a perfectly normal female child, and both did well. Sibois describes the case of a woman weighing 190 pounds, who fell on her head from the top of a wall from 10 to 12 feet high. For several hours she exhibited symptoms of fracture of the base of the skull, and the case was so diagnosed; fourteen hours after the accident she was perfectly conscious and suffered terrible pain about the head, neck, and shoulders. Two days later an ovum of about twenty days was expelled, and seven months after she was delivered of a healthy boy weighing 10 1/2 pounds. She had therefore lost after the accident one-half of a double conception.

Verrier has collected the results of traumatism during pregnancy, and summarizes 61 cases. Prowzowsky cites the instance of a patient in the eighth month of her first pregnancy who was wounded by many pieces of lead pipe fired from a gun but a few feet distant. Neither the patient nor the child suffered materially from the accident, and gestation proceeded; the child died on the fourth day after birth without apparent cause. Milner records an instance of remarkable tolerance of injury in a pregnant woman. During her six months of pregnancy the patient was accidentally shot through the abdominal cavity and lower part of the thorax. The missile penetrated the central tendon of the diaphragm and lodged in the lung. The injury was limited by localized pneumonia and peritonitis, and the wound was drained through the lung by free expectoration. Recovery ensued, the patient giving birth to a healthy child sixteen weeks later. Belin mentions a stab-wound in a pregnant woman from which a considerable portion of the epiploon protruded. Sloughing ensued, but the patient made a good recovery, gestation not being interrupted. Fancon describes the case of a woman who had an injury to the knee requiring drainage. She was attacked by erysipelas, which spread over the whole body with the exception of the head and neck; yet her pregnancy was uninterrupted and recovery ensued. Fancon also speaks of a girl of nineteen, frightened by her lover, who threatened to stab her, who jumped from a second-story window. For three days after the fall she had a slight bloody flow from the vulva. Although she was six months pregnant there was no interruption of the normal course of gestation.

Bancroft speaks of a woman who, being mistaken for a burglar, was shot by her husband with a 44-caliber bullet. The missile entered the second and third ribs an inch from the sternum, passed through the right lung, and escaped at the inferior angle of the scapula, about three inches below the spine; after leaving her body it went through a pine door. She suffered much hemorrhage and shock, but made a fair recovery at the end of four weeks, though pregnant with her first child at the seventh month. At full term she was delivered by foot-presentation of a healthy boy. The mother at the time of report was healthy and free from cough, and was nursing her babe, which was strong and bright.

All the cases do not have as happy an issue as most of the foregoing ones, though in some the results are not so bad as might be expected. A German female, thirty-six, while in the sixth month of pregnancy, fell and struck her abdomen on a tub. She was delivered of a normal living child, with the exception that the helix of the left ear was pushed anteriorly, and had, in its middle, a deep incision, which also traversed the antihelix and the tragus, and continued over the cheek toward the nose, where it terminated. The external auditory meatus was obliterated. Gurlt speaks of a woman, seven months pregnant, who fell from the top of a ladder, subsequently losing some blood and water from the vagina. She had also persistent pains in the belly, but there was no deterioration of general health. At her confinement, which was normal, a strong boy was born, wanting the arm below the middle, at which point a white bone protruded. The wound healed and the separated arm came away after birth. Wainwright relates the instance of a woman of forty, who when six months pregnant was run over by railway cars. After a double amputation of the legs she miscarried and made a good recovery. Neugebauer reported the history of a case of a woman who, while near her term of pregnancy, committed suicide by jumping from a window. She ruptured her uterus, and a dead child with a fracture of the parietal bone was found in the abdominal cavity. Staples speaks of a Swede of twenty-eight, of Minnesota, who was accidentally shot by a young man riding by her side in a wagon. The ball entered the abdomen two inches above the crest of the right ilium, a little to the rear of the anterior superior spinous process, and took a downward and forward course. A little shock was felt but no serious symptoms followed. In forty hours there was delivery of a dead child with a bullet in its abdomen. Labor was normal and the internal recovery complete. Von Chelius, quoting the younger Naegele, gives a remarkable instance of a young peasant of thirty-five, the mother of four children, pregnant with the fifth child, who was struck on the belly violently by a blow from a wagon pole. She was thrown down, and felt a tearing pain which caused her to faint. It was found that the womb had been ruptured and the child killed, for in several days it was delivered in a putrid mass, partly through the natural passage and partly through an abscess opening in the abdominal wall. The woman made a good recovery. A curious accident of pregnancy is that of a woman of thirty-eight, advanced eight months in her ninth pregnancy, who after eating a hearty meal was seized by a violent pain in the region of the stomach and soon afterward with convulsions, supposed to have been puerperal. She died in a few hours, and at the autopsy it was found that labor had not begun, but that the pregnancy had caused a laceration of the spleen, from which had escaped four or five pints of blood. Edge speaks of a case of chorea in pregnancy in a woman of twenty-seven, not interrupting pregnancy or retarding safe delivery. This had continued for four pregnancies, but in the fourth abortion took place.

Buzzard had a case of nervous tremor in a woman, following a fall at her fourth month of pregnancy, who at term gave birth to a male child that was idiotic. Beatty relates a curious accident to a fetus in utero. The woman was in her first confinement and was delivered of a small but healthy and strong boy. There was a small puncture in the abdominal parietes, through which the whole of the intestines protruded and were constricted. The opening was so small that he had to enlarge it with a bistoury to replace the bowel, which was dark and congested; he sutured the wound with silver wire, but the child subsequently died.

Tiffany of Baltimore has collected excellent statistics of operations during pregnancy; and Mann of Buffalo has done the same work, limiting himself to operations on the pelvic organs, where interference is supposed to have been particularly contraindicated in pregnancy. Mann, after giving his individual cases, makes the following summary and conclusions:— (1) Pregnancy is not a general bar to operations, as has been supposed.

(2) Union of the denuded surfaces is the rule, and the cicatricial tissue, formed during the earlier months of pregnancy, is strong enough to resist the shock of labor at term.

(3) Operations on the vulva are of little danger to mother or child.

(4) Operations on the vagina are liable to cause severe hemorrhage, but otherwise are not dangerous.

(5) Venereal vegetations or warts are best treated by removal.

(6) Applications of silver nitrate or astringents may be safely made to the vagina. For such application, phenol or iodin should not be used, pure or in strong solution.

(7) Operations on the bladder or urethra are not dangerous or liable to be followed by abortion.

(8) Operations for vesicovaginal fistulae should not be done, as they are dangerous, and are liable to be followed by much hemorrhage and abortion.

(9) Plastic operations may be done in the earlier months of pregnancy with fair prospects of a safe and successful issue.

(10) Small polypi may be treated by torsion or astringents. If cut, there is likely to be a subsequent abortion.

(11) Large polypi removed toward the close of pregnancy will cause hemorrhage.

(12) Carcinoma of the cervix should be removed at once.

A few of the examples on record of operations during pregnancy of special interest, will be given below. Polaillon speaks of a double ovariotomy on a woman pregnant at three months, with the subsequent birth of a living child at term. Gordon reports five successful ovariotomies during pregnancy, in Lebedeff's clinic. Of these cases, 1 aborted on the fifth day, 2 on the fifteenth, and the other 2 continued uninterrupted. He collected 204 cases with a mortality of only 3 per cent; 22 per cent aborted, and 69.4 per cent were delivered at full term.

Kreutzman reports two cases in which ovarian tumors were successfully removed from pregnant subjects without the interruption of gestation. One of these women, a secundipara, had gone two weeks over time, and had a large ovarian cyst, the pedicle of which had become twisted, the fluid in the cyst being sanguineous. May describes an ovariotomy performed during pregnancy at Tottenham Hospital. The woman, aged twenty-two, was pale, diminutive in size, and showed an enormous abdomen, which measured 50 inches in circumference at the umbilicus and 27 inches from the ensiform cartilage to the pubes. At the operation, 36 pints of brown fluid were drawn off. Delivery took place twelve hours after the operation, the mother recovering, but the child was lost. Galabin had a case of ovariotomy performed on a woman in the sixth month of pregnancy without interruption of pregnancy; Potter had a case of double ovariotomy with safe delivery at term; and Storry had a similar case. Jacobson cites a case of vaginal lithotomy in a patient six and a half months pregnant, with normal delivery at full term. Tiffany quotes Keelan's description of a woman of thirty-five, in the eighth month of pregnancy, from whom he removed a stone weighing 12 1/2 ounces and measuring 2 by 2 1/2 inches, with subsequent recovery and continuation of pregnancy. Rydygier mentions a case of obstruction of the intestine during the sixth month of gestation, showing symptoms of strangulation for seven days, in which he performed abdominal section. Recovery of the woman without abortion ensued. The Revue de Chirurgien 1887, contains an account of a woman who suffered internal strangulation, on whom celiotomy was performed; she recovered in twenty-five days, and did not miscarry, which shows that severe injury to the intestine with operative interference does not necessarily interrupt pregnancy. Gilmore, without inducing abortion, extirpated the kidney of a negress, aged thirty-three, for severe and constant pain. Tiffany removed the kidney of a woman of twenty-seven, five months pregnant, without interruption of this or subsequent pregnancies. The child was living. He says that Fancon cites instances of operation without abortion.

Lovort describes an enucleation of the eye in the second month of pregnancy. Pilcher cites the instance of a woman of fifty-eight, eight months in her fourth pregnancy, whose breast and axilla he removed without interruption of pregnancy. Robson, Polaillon, and Coen report similar instances.

Rein speaks of the removal of an enormous echinococcus cyst of the omentum without interruption of pregnancy. Robson reports a multi-locular cyst of the ovary with extensive adhesions of the uterus, removed at the tenth week of pregnancy and ovariotomy performed without any interruption of the ordinary course of labor. Russell cites the instance of a woman who was successfully tapped at the sixth month of pregnancy.

McLean speaks of a successful amputation during pregnancy; Napper, one of the arm; Nicod, one of the arm; Russell, an amputation through the shoulder joint for an injury during pregnancy, with delivery and recovery; and Vesey speaks of amputation for compound fracture of the arm, labor following ten hours afterward with recovery. Keen reports the successful performance of a hip-joint amputation for malignant disease of the femur during pregnancy. The patient, who was five months advanced in gestation, recovered without aborting.

Robson reports a case of strangulated hernia in the third month of pregnancy with stercoraceous vomiting. He performed herniotomy in the femoral region, and there was a safe delivery at full term. In the second month of pregnancy he also rotated an ovarian tumor causing acute symptoms and afterward performed ovariotomy without interfering with pregnancy. Mann quotes Munde in speaking of an instance of removal of elephantiasis of the vulva without interrupting pregnancy, and says that there are many cases of the removal of venereal warts without any interference with gestation. Campbell of Georgia operated inadvertently at the second and third month in two cases of vesicovaginal fistula in pregnant women. The first case showed no interruption of pregnancy, but in the second case the woman nearly died and the fistula remained unhealed. Engelmann operated on a large rectovaginal fistula in the sixth month of pregnancy without any interruption of pregnancy, which is far from the general result. Cazin and Rey both produced abortion by forcible dilatation of the anus for fissure, but Gayet used both the fingers and a speculum in a case at five months and the woman went to term. By cystotomy Reamy removed a double hair-pin from a woman pregnant six and a half months, without interruption, and according to Mann again, McClintock extracted stones from the bladder by the urethra in the fourth month of pregnancy, and Phillips did the same in the seventh month. Hendenberg and Packard report the removal of a tumor weighing 8 3/4 pounds from a pregnant uterus without interrupting gestation.

The following extract from the University Medical Magazine of Philadelphia illustrates the after-effects of abdominal hysteropasy on subsequent pregnancies:—

"Fraipont (Annales de la Societe Medico-Chirurgicale de Liege, 1894) reports four cases where pregnancy and labor were practically normal, though the uterus of each patient had been fixed to the abdominal walls. In two of the cases the hysteropexy had been performed over five years before the pregnancy occurred, and, although the bands of adhesion between the fundus and the parietes must have become very tough after so long a period, no special difficulty was encountered.

In two of the cases the forceps was used, but not on account of uterine inertia; the fetal head was voluminous, and in one of the two cases internal rotation was delayed. The placenta was always expelled easily, and no serious postpartum hemorrhage occurred. Fraipont observed the progress of pregnancy in several of these cases. The uterus does not increase specially in its posterior part, but quite uniformly, so that, as might be expected, the fundus gradually detaches itself from the abdominal wall. Even if the adhesions were not broken down they would of necessity be so stretched as to be useless for their original purpose after delivery. Bands of adhesion could not share in the process of involution. As, however, the uterus undergoes perfect involution, it is restored to its original condition before the onset of the disease which rendered hysteropexy necessary."

The coexistence of an extensive tumor of the uterus with pregnancy does not necessarily mean that the product of conception will be blighted. Brochin speaks of a case in which pregnancy was complicated with fibroma of the uterus, the accouchement being natural at term. Byrne mentions a case of pregnancy complicated with a large uterine fibroid. Delivery was effected at full term, and although there was considerable hemorrhage the mother recovered. Ingleby describes a case of fibrous tumor of the uterus terminating fatally, but not until three weeks after delivery. Lusk mentions a case of pregnancy with fibrocystic tumor of the uterus occluding the cervix. At the appearance of symptoms of eclampsia version was performed and delivery effected, followed by postpartum hemorrhage. The mother died from peritonitis and collapse, but the stillborn child was resuscitated. Roberts reports a case of pregnancy associated with a large fibrocellular polypus of the uterus. A living child was delivered at the seventh month, ecrasement was performed, and the mother recovered.

Von Quast speaks of a fibromyoma removed five days after labor. Gervis reports the removal of a large polypus of the uterus on the fifth day after confinement. Davis describes the spontaneous expulsion of a large polypus two days after the delivery of a fine, healthy, male child. Deason mentions a case of anomalous tumor of the uterus during pregnancy which was expelled after the birth of the child; and Daly also speaks of a tumor expelled from the uterus after delivery. Cathell speaks of a case of pregnancy complicated with both uterine fibroids and measles. Other cases of a similar nature to the foregoing are too numerous to mention. Figure 13, taken from Spiegelberg, shows a large fibroid blocking the pelvis of a pregnant woman.

There are several peculiar accidents and anomalies not previously mentioned which deserve a place here, viz., those of the membranes surrounding the fetus. Brown speaks of protrusion of the membranes from the vulva several weeks before confinement. Davies relates an instance in which there was a copious watery discharge during pregnancy not followed by labor. There is a case mentioned in which an accident and an inopportune dose of ergot at the fifth month of pregnancy were followed by rupture of the amniotic sac, and subsequently a constant flow of watery fluid continued for the remaining three months of pregnancy. The fetus died at the time, and was born in an advanced state of putrefaction, by version, three months after the accident. The mother died five months after of carcinoma of the uterus. Montgomery reports the instance of a woman who menstruated last on May 22, 1850, and quickened on September 26th, and continued well until the 11th of November. At this time, as she was retiring, she became conscious that there was a watery discharge from the vagina, which proved to be liquor amnii. Her health was good. The discharge continued, her size increased, and the motions of the child continued active. On the 18th of January a full-sized eight months' child was born. It had an incessant, wailing, low cry, always of evil augury in new-born infants. The child died shortly after. The daily discharge was about 5 ounces, and had lasted sixty-eight days, making 21 pints in all. The same accident of rupture of the membranes long before labor happened to the patient's mother.

Bardt speaks of labor twenty-three days after the flow of the waters; and Cobleigh one of seventeen days; Bradley relates the history of a case of rupture of the membranes six weeks before delivery. Rains cites an instance in which gestation continued three months after rupture of the membranes, the labor-pains lasting thirty-six hours. Griffiths speaks of rupture of the amniotic sac at about the sixth month of pregnancy with no untoward interruption of the completion of gestation and with delivery of a living child. There is another observation of an accouchement terminating successfully twenty-three days after the loss of the amniotic fluid. Campbell mentions delivery of a living child twelve days after rupture of the membranes. Chesney relates the history of a double collection of waters. Wood reports a case in which there was expulsion of a bag of waters before the rupture of the membranes. Bailly, Chestnut, Bjering, Cowger, Duncan, and others also record premature rupture of the membranes without interruption of pregnancy.

Harris gives an instance of the membranes being expelled from the uterus a few days before delivery at the full term. Chatard, Jr., mentions extrusion of the fetal membranes at the seventh month of pregnancy while the patient was taking a long afternoon walk, their subsequent retraction, and normal labor at term. Thurston tells of a case in which Nature had apparently effected the separation of the placenta without alarming hemorrhage, the ease being one of placenta praevia, terminating favorably by natural processes. Playfair speaks of the detachment of the uterine decidua without the interruption of pregnancy.

Guerrant gives a unique example of normal birth at full term in which the placenta was found in the vagina, but not a vestige of the membranes was noticed. The patient had experienced nothing unusual until within three months of expected confinement, since which time there had been a daily loss of water from the uterus. She recovered and was doing her work. There was no possibility that this was a case of retained secundines.

Anomalies of the Umbilical Cord.—Absence of the membranes has its counterpart in the deficiency of the umbilical cord, so frequently noticed in old reports. The Ephemerides, Osiander, Stark's Archives, Thiebault, van der Wiel, Chatton, and Schurig all speak of it, and it has been noticed since. Danthez speaks of the development of a fetus in spite of the absence of an umbilical cord. Stute reports an observation of total absence of the umbilical cord, with placental insertion near the cervix of the uterus.

There is mentioned a bifid funis. The Ephemerides and van der Wiel speak of a duplex funis. Nolde reports a cord 38 inches long; and Werner cites the instance of a funis 51 inches long. There are modern instances in which the funis has been bifid or duplex, and there is also a case reported in which there were two cords in a twin pregnancy, each of them measuring five feet in length. The Lancet gives the account of a most peculiar pregnancy consisting of a placenta alone, the fetus wanting. What this "placenta" was will always be a matter of conjecture.

Occasionally death of the fetus is caused by the formation of knots in the cord, shutting off the fetal circulation; Gery, Grieve, Mastin, Passot, Piogey, Woets, and others report instances of this nature. Newman reports a curious case of twins, in which the cord of one child was encircled by a knot on the cord of the other. Among others, Latimer and Motte report instances of the accidental tying of the bowel with the funis, causing an artificial anus.

The diverse causes of abortion are too numerous to attempt giving them all, but some are so curious and anomalous that they deserve mention. Epidemics of abortion are spoken of by Fickius, Fischer, and the Ephemerides. Exposure to cold is spoken of as a cause, and the same is alluded to by the Ephemerides; while another case is given as due to exposure white nude. There are several cases among the older writers in which odors are said to have produced abortion, but as analogues are not to be found in modern literature, unless the odor is very poisonous or pungent, we can give them but little credence. The Ephemerides gives the odor of urine as provocative of abortion; Sulzberger, Meyer, and Albertus all mention odors; and Vesti gives as a plausible cause the odor of carbonic vapor. The Ephemerides mentions singultus as a cause of abortion. Mauriceau, Pelargus, and

Valentini mention coughing. Hippocrates mentions the case of a woman who induced abortion by calling excessively loud to some one. Fabrieius Hildanus speaks of abortion following a kick in the region of the coccyx. Gullmannus speaks of an abortion which he attributes to the woman's constant neglect to answer the calls of nature, the rectum being at all times in a state of irritation from her negligence. Hawley mentions abortion at the fourth or fifth month due to the absorption of spirits of turpentine. Solingen speaks of abortion produced by sneezing. Osiander cites an instance in which a woman suddenly arose, and in doing so jolted herself so severely that she produced abortion. Hippocrates speaks of extreme hunger as a cause of abortion. Treuner speaks of great anger and wrath in a woman disturbing her to the extent of producing abortion.

The causes that are observed every day, such tight lacing, excessive venery, fright, and emotions, are too well known to be discussed here. There has been reported a recent case of abortion following a viper-bite, and analogues may be found in the writings of Severinus and Oedman, who mention viper-bites as the cause; but there are so many associate conditions accompanying a snake-bite, such as fright, treatment, etc., any one of which could be a cause in itself, that this is by no means a reliable explanation. Information from India an this subject would be quite valuable.

The Ephemerides speak of bloodless abortion, and there have been modern instances in which the hemorrhage has been hardly noticeable.

Abortion in a twin pregnancy does not necessarily mean the abortion or death of both the products of conception. Chapman speaks of the case of the expulsion of a blighted fetus at the seventh month, the living child remaining to the full term, and being safely delivered, the placenta following. Crisp says of a case of labor that the head of the child was obstructed by a round body, the nature of which he was for some time unable to determine. He managed to push the obstructing body up and delivered a living, full-term child; this was soon followed by a blighted fetus, which was 11 inches long, weighed 12 ounces, with a placenta attached weighing 6 1/2 ounces. It is quite common for a blighted fetus to be retained and expelled at term with a living child, its twin.

Bacon speaks of twin pregnancy, with the death of one fetus at the fourth month and the other delivered at term. Beall reports the conception of twins, with one fetus expelled and the other retained; Beauchamp cites a similar instance. Bothwell describes a twin labor at term, in which one child was living and the other dead at the fifth month and macerated. Belt reports an analogous case. Jameson gives the history of an extraordinary case of twins in which one (dead) child was retained in the womb for forty-nine weeks, the other having been born alive at the expiration of nine months. Hamilton describes a case of twins in which one fetus died from the effects of an injury between the fourth and fifth months and the second arrived at full period. Moore cites an instance in which one of the fetuses perished about the third month, but was not expelled until the seventh, and the other was carried to full term. Wilson speaks of a secondary or blighted fetus of the third month with fatty degeneration of the membranes retained and expelled with its living twin at the eighth month of uterogestation.

There was a case at Riga in 1839 of a robust girl who conceived in February, and in consequence her menses ceased. In June she aborted, but, to her dismay, soon afterward the symptoms of advanced pregnancy appeared, and in November a full-grown child, doubtless the result of the same impregnation as the fetus, was expelled at the fourth month. In 1860 Schuh reported an instance before the Vienna Faculty of Medicine in which a fetus was discharged at the third month of pregnancy and the other twin retained until full term. The abortion was attended with much metrorrhagia, and ten weeks afterward the movements of the other child could be plainly felt and pregnancy continued its course uninterrupted. Bates mentions a twin pregnancy in which an abortion took place at the second month and was followed by a natural birth at full term. Hawkins gives a case of miscarriage, followed by a natural birth at full term; and Newnham cites a similar instance in which there was a miscarriage at the seventh month and a birth at full term.

Worms in the Uterus.—Haines speaks of a most curious case—that of a woman who had had a miscarriage three days previous; she suffered intense pain and a fetid discharge. A number of maggots were seen in the vagina, and the next day a mass about the size of an orange came away from the uterus, riddled with holes, and which contained a number of dead maggots, killed by the carbolic acid injection given soon after the miscarriage. The fact seems inexplicable, but after their expulsion the symptoms immediately ameliorated. This case recalls a somewhat similar one given by the older writers, in which a fetus was eaten by a worm. Analogous are those cases spoken of by Bidel of lumbricoides found in the uterus; by Hole, in which maggots were found in the vagina and uterus; and Simpson, in which the abortion was caused by worms in the womb—if the associate symptoms were trustworthy.

We can find fabulous parallels to all of these in some of the older writings. Pare mentions Lycosthenes' account of a woman in Cracovia in 1494 who bore a dead child which had attached to its back a live serpent, which had gnawed it to death. He gives an illustration showing the serpent in situ. He also quotes the case of a woman who conceived by a mariner, and who, after nine months, was delivered by a midwife of a shapeless mass, followed by an animal with a long neck, blazing eyes, and clawed feet. Ballantyne says that in the writings of Hippocrates there is in the work on "Diseases", which is not usually regarded as genuine, a some what curious statement with regard to worms in the fetus. It is affirmed that flat worms develop in the unborn infant, and the reason given is that the feces are expelled so soon after birth that there would not be sufficient time during extrauterine life for the formation of creatures of such a size. The same remark applies to round worms. The proof of these statements is to be found in the fact that many infants expel both these varieties of parasites with the first stool. It is difficult to know what to make of these opinions; for, with the exception of certain cases in some of the seventeenth and eighteenth century writers, there are no records in medicine of the occurrence of vermes in the infant at birth. It is possible that other things, such as dried pieces of mucus, may have been erroneously regarded as worms.

CHAPTER III

OBSTETRIC ANOMALIES.

General Considerations.—In discussing obstetric anomalies we shall first consider those strange instances in which stages of parturition are unconscious and for some curious reason the pains of labor absent. Some women are anatomically constituted in a manner favorable to child-birth, and pass through the experience in a comparatively easy manner; but to the great majority the throes of labor are anticipated with extreme dread, particularly by the victims of the present fashion of tight lacing.

It seems strange that a physiologic process like parturition should be attended by so much pain and difficulty. Savages in their primitive and natural state seem to have difficulty in many cases, and even animals are not free from it. We read of the ancient wild Irish women breaking the pubic bones of their female children shortly after birth, and by some means preventing union subsequently, in order that these might have less trouble in child-birth—as it were, a modified and early form of symphysiotomy. In consequence of this custom the females of this race, to quote an old English authority, had a "waddling, lamish gesture in their going." These old writers said that for the same reason the women in some parts of Italy broke the coccyxes of their female children. This report is very likely not veracious, because this bone spontaneously repairs itself so quickly and easily. Rodet and Engelmunn, in their most extensive and interesting papers on the modes of accouchement among the primitive peoples, substantiate the fear, pain, and difficulty with which labor is attended, even in the lowest grades of society.

In view of the usual occurrence of pain and difficulty with labor, it seems natural that exceptions to the general rule should in all ages have attracted the attention of medical men, and that literature should be replete with such instances. Pechlin and Muas record instances of painless births. The Ephemerides records a birth as having occurred during asphyxia, and also one during an epileptic attack. Storok also speaks of birth during unconsciousness in an epileptic attack; and Haen and others describe cases occurring during the coma attending apoplectic attacks. King reports the histories of two married women, fond mothers and anticipating the event, who gave birth to children, apparently unconsciously. In the first case, the appearance of the woman verified the assertion; in the second, a transient suspension of the menstrual influence accounted for it. After some months epilepsy developed in this case. Crawford speaks of a Mrs. D., who gave birth to twins in her first confinement at full term, and who two years after aborted at three months. In December, 1868, a year after the abortion, she was delivered of a healthy, living fetus of about five or six months' growth in the following manner: While at stool, she discovered something of a shining, bluish appearance protruding through the external labia, but she also found that when she lay down the tumor disappeared. This tumor proved to be the child, which had been expelled from the uterus four days before, with the waters and membranes intact, but which had not been recognized; it had passed through the os without pain or symptoms, and had remained alive in the vagina over four days, from whence it was delivered, presenting by the foot.

The state of intoxication seems by record of several cases to render birth painless and unconscious, as well as serving as a means of anesthesia in the preanesthetic days.

The feasibility of practising hypnotism in child-birth has been discussed, and Fanton reports 12 cases of parturition under the hypnotic influence. He says that none of the subjects suffered any pain or were aware of the birth, and offers the suggestion that to facilitate the state of hypnosis it should be commenced before strong uterine contractions have occurred.

Instances of parturition or delivery during sleep, lethargies, trances, and similar conditions are by no means uncommon. Heister speaks of birth during a convulsive somnolence, and Osiander of a case during sleep. Montgomery relates the case of a lady, the mother of several children, who on one occasion was unconsciously delivered in sleep. Case relates the instance of a French woman residing in the town of Hopedale, who, though near confinement, attributed her symptoms to over-fatigue on the previous day. When summoned, the doctor found that she had severe lumbar pains, and that the os was dilated to the size of a half-dollar. At ten o'clock he suggested that everyone retire, and directed that if anything of import occurred he should be called. About 4 A.M. the husband of the girl, in great fright, summoned the physician, saying: "Monsieur le Medecin, il y a quelque chose entre les jambes de ma femme," and, to Dr. Case's surprise, he found the head of a child wholly expelled during a profound sleep of the mother. In twenty minutes the secundines followed. The patient, who was only twenty years old, said that she had dreamt that something was the matter with her, and awoke with a fright, at which instant, most probably, the head was expelled. She was afterward confined with the usual labor-pains.

Palfrey speaks of a woman, pregnant at term, who fell into a sleep about eleven o'clock, and dreamed that she was in great pain and in labor, and that sometime after a fine child was crawling over the bed. After sleeping for about four hours she awoke and noticed a discharge from the vagina. Her husband started for a light, but before he obtained it a child was born by a head-presentation. In a few minutes the labor-pains returned and the feet of a second child presented, and the child was expelled in three pains, followed in ten minutes by the placenta. Here is an authentic case in which labor progressed to the second stage during sleep.

Weill describes the case of a woman of twenty-three who gave birth to a robust boy on the 16th of June, 1877, and suckled him eleven months. This birth lasted one hour. She became pregnant again and was delivered under the following circumstances: She had been walking on the evening of September 5th and returned home about eleven o'clock to sleep. About 3 A.M. she awoke, feeling the necessity of passing urine. She arose and seated herself for the purpose. She at once uttered a cry and called her husband, telling him that a child was born and entreating him to send for a physician. Weill saw the woman in about ten minutes and she was in the same position, so he ordered her to be carried to bed. On examining the urinal he found a female child weighing 10 pounds. He tied the cord and cared for the child. The woman exhibited little hemorrhage and made a complete recovery. She had apparently slept soundly through the uterine contractions until the final strong pain, which awoke her, and which she imagined was a call for urination.

Samelson says that in 1844 he was sent for in Zabelsdorf, some 30 miles from Berlin, to attend Hannah Rhode in a case of labor. She had passed easily through eight parturitions. At about ten o'clock in the morning, after a partially unconscious night, there was a sudden gush of blood and water from the vagina; she screamed and lapsed into an unconscious condition. At 10.35 the face presented, soon followed by the body, after which came a great flow of blood, welling out in several waves. The child was a male middle-sized, and was some little time in making himself heard. Only by degrees did the woman's consciousness return. She felt weary and inclined to sleep, but soon after she awoke and was much surprised to know what had happened. She had seven or eight pains in all. Schultze speaks of a woman who, arriving at the period for delivery, went into an extraordinary state of somnolence, and in this condition on the third day bore a living male child.

Berthier in 1859 observed a case of melancholia with delirium which continued through pregnancy. The woman was apparently unconscious of her condition and was delivered without pain. Cripps mentions a case in which there was absence of pain in parturition. Depaul mentions a woman who fell in a public street and was delivered of a living child during a syncope which lasted four hours. Epley reports painless labor in a patient with paraplegia. Fahnestock speaks of the case of a woman who was delivered of a son while in a state of artificial somnambulism, without pain to herself or injury to the child. Among others mentioning painless or unconscious labor are Behrens (during profound sleep), Eger, Tempel, Panis, Agnoia, Blanckmeister, Whitehill, Gillette, Mattei, Murray, Lemoine, and Moglichkeit.

Rapid Parturition Without Usual Symptoms.—Births unattended by symptoms that are the usual precursors of labor often lead to speedy deliveries in awkward places. According to Willoughby, in Darby, February 9, 1667, a poor fool, Mary Baker, while wandering in an open, windy, and cold place, was delivered by the sole assistance of Nature, Eve's midwife, and freed of her afterbirth. The poor idiot had leaned against a wall, and dropped the child on the cold boards, where it lay for more than a quarter of an hour with its funis separated from the placenta. She was only discovered by the cries of the infant. In "Carpenter's Physiology" is described a remarkable case of instinct in an idiotic girl in Paris, who had been seduced by some miscreant; the girl had gnawed the funis in two, in the same manner as is practised by the lower animals. From her mental imbecility it can hardly be imagined that she had any idea of the object of this separation, and it must have been instinct that impelled her to do it. Sermon says the wife of Thomas James was delivered of a lusty child while in a wood by herself. She put the child in an apron with some oak leaves, marched stoutly to her husband's uncle's house a half mile distant, and after two hours' rest went on her journey one mile farther to her own house; despite all her exertions she returned the next day to thank her uncle for the two hours' accommodation. There is related the history of a case of a woman who was delivered of a child on a mountain during a hurricane, who took off her gown and wrapped the child up in it, together with the afterbirth, and walked two miles to her cottage, the funis being unruptured.

Harvey relates a case, which he learned from the President of Munster, Ireland, of a woman with child who followed her husband, a soldier in the army, in daily march. They were forced to a halt by reason of a river, and the woman, feeling the pains of labor approaching, retired to a thicket, and there alone brought forth twins. She carried them to the river, washed them herself, did them up in a cloth, tied them to her back, and that very day marched, barefooted, 12 miles with the soldiers, and was none the worse for her experience. The next day the Deputy of Ireland and the President of Munster, affected by the story, to repeat the words of Harvey, "did both vouchsafe to be godfathers of the infants."

Willoughby relates the account of a woman who, having a cramp while in bed with her sister, went to an outhouse, as if to stool, and was there delivered of a child. She quickly returned to bed, her going and her return not being noticed by her sleeping sister. She buried the child, "and afterward confessed her wickedness, and was executed in the Stafford Gaol, March 31, 1670." A similar instance is related by the same author of a servant in Darby in 1647. Nobody suspected her, and when delivered she was lying in the same room with her mistress. She arose without awakening anyone, and took the recently delivered child to a remote place, and hid it at the bottom of a feather tub, covering it with feathers; she returned without any suspicion on the part of her mistress. It so happened that it was the habit of the Darby soldiers to peep in at night where they saw a light, to ascertain if everything was all right, and they thus discovered her secret doings, which led to her trial at the next sessions at Darby.

Wagner relates the history of a case of great medicolegal interest. An unmarried servant, who was pregnant, persisted in denying it, and took every pains to conceal it. She slept in a room with two other maids, and, on examination, she stated that on the night in question she got up toward morning, thinking to relieve her bowels. For this purpose she secured a wooden tub in the room, and as she was sitting down the child passed rapidly into the empty vessel. It was only then that she became aware of the nature of her pains. She did not examine the child closely, but was certain it neither moved nor cried. The funis was no doubt torn, and she made an attempt to tie it. Regarding the event as a miscarriage, she took up the tub with its contents and carried it to a sand pit about 30 paces distant, and threw the child in a hole in the sand that she found already made. She covered it up with sand and packed it firmly so that the dogs could not get it. She returned to her bedroom, first calling up the man-servant at the stable. She awakened her fellow-servants, and feeling tired sat down on a stool. Seeing the blood on the floor, they asked her if she had made way with the child. She said: "Do you take me for an old sow?" But, having their suspicions aroused, they traced the blood spots to the sand pit. Fetching a spade, they dug up the child, which was about one foot below the surface. On the access of air, following the removal of the sand and turf, the child began to cry, and was immediately taken up and carried to its mother, who washed it and laid it on her bed and soon gave it the breast. The child was healthy with the exception of a club-foot, and must have been under ground at least fifteen minutes and no air could have reached it. It seems likely that the child was born asphyxiated and was buried in this state, and only began to assume independent vitality when for the second time exposed to the air. This curious case was verified to English correspondents by Dr. Wagner, and is of unquestionable authority; it became the subject of a thorough criminal investigation in Germany.

During the funeral procession of Marshal MacMahon in Paris an enormous crowd was assembled to see the cortege pass, and in this crowd was a woman almost at the time of delivery; the jostling which she received in her endeavors to obtain a place of vantage was sufficient to excite contraction, and, in an upright position, she gave birth to a fetus, which fell at her feet. The crowd pushed back and made way for the ambulance officials, and mother and child were carried off, the mother apparently experiencing little embarrassment. Quoted by Taylor, Anderson speaks of a woman accused of child murder, who walked a distance of 28 miles on a single day with her two-days-old child on her back.

There is also a case of a female servant named Jane May, who was frequently charged by her mistress with pregnancy but persistently denied it. On October 26th she was sent to market with some poultry. Returning home, she asked the boy who drove her to stop and allow her to get out. She went into a recess in a hedge. In five minutes she was seen to leave the hedge and follow the cart, walking home, a distance of a mile and a half. The following day she went to work as usual, and would not have been found out had not a boy, hearing feeble cries from the recess of the hedge, summoned a passer-by, but too late to save the child. At her trial she said she did not see her babe breathe nor cry, and she thought by the sudden birth that it must have been a still-born child.

Shortt says that one day, while crossing the esplanade at Villaire, between seven and eight o'clock in the morning, he perceived three Hindoo women with large baskets of cakes of "bratties" on their heads, coming from a village about four miles distant. Suddenly one of the women stood still for a minute, stooped, and to his surprise dropped a fully developed male child to the ground. One of her companions ran into the town, about 100 yards distant, for a knife to divide the cord. A few of the female passers-by formed a screen about the mother with their clothes, and the cord was divided. The after-birth came away, and the woman was removed to the town. It was afterward discovered that she was the mother of two children, was twenty-eight years old, had not the slightest sign of approaching labor, and was not aware of parturition until she actually felt the child between her thighs.

Smith of Madras, in 1862, says he was hastily summoned to see an English lady who had borne a child without the slightest warning. He found the child, which had been born ten minutes, lying close to the mother's body, with the funis uncut. The native female maid, at the lady's orders, had left the child untouched, lifting the bed-clothes to give it air. The lady said that she arose at 5.30 feeling well, and during the forenoon had walked down a long flight of steps across a walk to a small summer-house within the enclosure of her grounds. Feeling a little tired, she had lain down on her bed, and soon experienced a slight discomfort, and was under the impression that something solid and warm was lying in contact with her person. She directed the servant to look below the bed-clothes, and then a female child was discovered. Her other labors had extended over six hours, and were preceded by all the signs distinctive of childbirth, which fact attaches additional interest to the case. The ultimate fate of the child is not mentioned. Smith quotes Wilson, who said he was called to see a woman who was delivered without pain while walking about the house. He found the child on the floor with its umbilical cord torn across.

Langston mentions the case of a woman, twenty-three, who, between 4 and 5 A.M., felt griping pains in the abdomen. Knowing her condition she suspected labor, and determined to go to a friend's house where she could be confined in safety. She had a distance of about 600 yards to go, and when she was about half way she was delivered in an upright position of a child, which fell on the pavement and ruptured its funis in the fall. Shortly after, the placenta was expelled, and she proceeded on her journey, carrying the child in her arms. At 5.50 the physician saw the woman in bed, looking well and free from pain, but complaining of being cold. The child, which was her first, was healthy, well nourished, and normal, with the exception of a slight ecchymosis of the parietal bone on the left side. The funis was lacerated transversely four inches from the umbilicus. Both mother and child progressed favorably. Doubtless the intense cold had so contracted the blood-vessels as to prevent fatal hemorrhage to mother and child. This case has a legal bearing in the supposition that the child had been killed in the fall.

There is reported the case of a woman in Wales, who, while walking with her husband, was suddenly seized with pains, and would have been delivered by the wayside but for the timely help of Madame Patti, the celebrated diva, who was driving by, and who took the woman in her carriage to her palatial residence close by.

It was to be christened in a few days with an appropriate name in remembrance of the occasion. Coleman met an instance in a married woman, who without the slightest warning was delivered of a child while standing near a window in her bedroom. The child fell to the floor and ruptured the cord about one inch from the umbilicus, but with speedy attention the happiest results were attained. Twitchell has an example in the case of a young woman of seventeen, who was suddenly delivered of a child while ironing some clothes. The cord in this case was also ruptured, but the child sustained no injury. Taylor quotes the description of a child who died from an injury to the head caused by dropping from the mother at an unexpected time, while she was in the erect position; he also speaks of a parallel case on record.

Unusual Places of Birth.—Besides those mentioned, the other awkward positions in which a child may be born are so numerous and diversified that mention of only a few can be made here. Colton tells of a painless labor in an Irish girl of twenty-three, who felt a desire to urinate, and while seated on the chamber dropped a child. She never felt a labor-pain, and twelve days afterward rode 20 miles over a rough road to go to her baby's funeral. Leonhard describes the case of a mother of thirty-seven, who had borne six children alive, who was pregnant for the tenth time, and who had miscalculated her pregnancy. During pregnancy she had an attack of small-pox and suffered all through pregnancy with constipation. She had taken a laxative, and when returning to bed from stool was surprised to find herself attached to the stool by a band. The child in the vessel began to cry and was separated from the woman, who returned to bed and suddenly died one-half hour later. The mother was entirely unconscious of the delivery. Westphal mentions a delivery in a water-closet.

Brown speaks of a woman of twenty-six who had a call of nature while in bed, and while sitting up she gave birth to a fine, full-grown child, which, falling on the floor, ruptured the funis. She took her child, lay down with it for some time, and feeling easier, hailed a cab, drove to a hospital with the child in her arms, and wanted to walk upstairs. She was put to bed and delivered of the placenta, there being but little hemorrhage from the cord; both she and her child made speedy recoveries. Thebault reports an instance of delivery in the erect position, with rupture of the funis at the placenta. There was recently a rumor, probably a newspaper fabrication, that a woman while at stool in a railway car gave birth to a child which was found alive on the track afterward.

There is a curious instance on record in which a child was born in a hip-bath and narrowly escaped drowning. The mother was a European woman aged forty, who had borne two children, the last nine years before. She was supposed to have dropsy of the abdomen, and among other treatments was the use of a speculum and caustic applications for inflammation of the womb. The escape of watery fluid for two days was considered evidence of the rupture of an ovarian cyst. At the end of two days, severe pains set in, and a warm hip-bath and an opiate were ordered. While in the bath she bore a fully-matured, living, male child, to the great surprise of herself and her friends. The child might have been drowned had not assistance been close at hand.

Birth by the Rectum.—In some cases in which there is some obstacle to the delivery of a child by the natural passages, the efforts of nature to expel the product of conception lead to an anomalous exit. There are some details of births by the rectum mentioned in the last century by Reta and others. Payne cites the instance of a woman of thirty-three, in labor thirty-six hours, in whom there was a congenital absence of the vaginal orifice. The finger, gliding along the perineum, arrived at a distended anus, just inside of which was felt a fetal head. He anesthetized the patient and delivered the child with forceps, and without perineal rupture. There was little hemorrhage, and the placenta was removed with slight difficulty. Five months later, Payne found an unaltered condition of the perineum and vicinity; there was absence of the vaginal orifice, and, on introducing the finger along the anterior wall of the rectum, a fistula was found, communicating with the vagina; above this point the arrangement and the situation of the parts were normal. The woman had given birth to three still-born children, and always menstruated easily. Coitus always seemed satisfactory, and no suspicion existed in the patient's mind, and had never been suggested to her, of her abnormality.

Harrison saw a fetus delivered by the anus after rupture of the uterus; the membranes came away by the same route. In this case the neck of the uterus was cartilaginous and firmly adherent to the adjacent parts. In seven days after the accouchement the woman had completely regained her health. Vallisneri reports the instance of a woman who possessed two uteruses, one communicating with the vagina, the other with the rectum. She had permitted rectal copulation and had become impregnated in this manner. Louis, the celebrated French surgeon, created a furore by a pamphlet entitled "De partium externarum generationi inservientium in mulieribus naturali vitiosa et morbosa dispositione, etc.," for which he was punished by the Sorbonne, but absolved by the Pope. He described a young lady who had no vaginal opening, but who regularly menstruated by the rectum. She allowed her lover to have connection with her in the only possible way, by the rectum, which, however, sufficed for impregnation, and at term she bore by the rectum a well-formed child. Hunter speaks of a case of pregnancy in a woman with a double vagina, who was delivered at the seventh month by the rectum. Mekeln and Andrews give instances of parturition through the anus.

Morisani describes a case of extrauterine pregnancy with tubal rupture and discharge into the culdesac, in which there was delivery by the rectum. After an attack of severe abdominal pain, followed by hemorrhage, the woman experienced an urgent desire to empty the rectum. The fetal movements ceased, and a recurrence of these symptoms led the patient to go to stool, at which she passed blood and a seromucoid fluid. She attempted manually to remove the offending substances from the rectum, and in consequence grasped the leg of a fetus. She was removed to a hospital, where a fetus nine inches long was removed from the rectum. The rectal opening gradually cicatrized, the sac became obliterated, and the woman left the hospital well.

Birth Through Perineal Perforation.—Occasionally there is perineal perforation during labor, with birth of the child through the opening. Brown mentions a case of rupture of the perineum with birth of a child between the vaginal opening and the anus. Cassidy reports a case of child-birth through the perineum. A successful operation was performed fifteen days after the accident. Dupuytren speaks of the passage of an infant through a central opening of the perineum. Capuron, Gravis, and Lebrun all report accouchement through a perineal perforation, without alteration in the sphincter ani or the fourchet. In his "Diseases of Women" Simpson speaks of a fistula left by the passage of an infant through the perineum. Wilson, Toloshinoff, Stolz, Argles, Demarquay, Harley, Hernu, Martyn, Lamb, Morere, Pollock, and others record the birth of children through perineal perforations.

Birth Through the Abdominal Wall.—Hollerius gives a very peculiar instance in which the abdominal walls gave way from the pressure exerted by the fetus, and the uterus ruptured, allowing the child to be extracted by the hand from the umbilicus; the mother made a speedy recovery. In such cases delivery is usually by means of operative interference (which will be spoken of later), but rarely, as here, spontaneously. Farquharson and Ill both mention rupture of the abdominal parietes during labor.

There have been cases reported in which the recto-vaginal septum has been ruptured, as well as the perineum and the sphincter ani, giving all the appearance of a birth by the anus.

There is an account of a female who had a tumor projecting between the vagina and rectum, which was incised through the intestine, and proved to be a dead child. Saviard reported what he considered a rather unique case, in which the uterus was ruptured by external violence, the fetus being thrown forward into the abdomen and afterward extracted from an umbilical abscess.

Birth of the Fetus Enclosed in the Membranes.—Harvey says that an infant can rest in its membranes several hours after birth without loss of life. Schurig eventrated a pregnant bitch and her puppies lived in their membranes half an hour. Wrisberg cites three observations of infants born closed in their membranes; one lived seven minutes; the other two nine minutes; all breathed when the membranes were cut and air admitted. Willoughby recorded the history of a case which attracted much comment at the time. It was the birth of twins enclosed in their secundines. The sac was opened and, together with the afterbirth, was laid over some hot coals; there was, however, a happy issue, the children recovering and living. Since Willoughby's time several cases of similar interest have been noticed, one in a woman of forty, who had been married sixteen years, and who had had several pregnancies in her early married life and a recent abortion. Her last pregnancy lasted about twenty-eight or twenty-nine weeks, and terminated, after a short labor, by the expulsion of the ovum entire. The membranes had not been ruptured, and still enclosed the fetus and the liquor amnii. On breaking them, the fetus was seen floating on the waters, alive, and, though very diminutive, was perfectly formed. It continued to live, and a day afterward took the breast and began to cry feebly. At six weeks it weighed 2 pounds 2 ounces, and at ten months, 12 pounds, but was still very weak and ill-nourished. Evans has an instance of a fetus expelled enveloped in its membranes entire and unruptured. The membranes were opaque and preternaturally thickened, and were opened with a pair of scissors; strenuous efforts were made to save the child, but to no purpose. The mother, after a short convalescence, made a good recovery. Forman reports an instance of unruptured membranes at birth, the delivery following a single pain, in a woman of twenty-two, pregnant for a second time. Woodson speaks of a case of twins, one of which was born enveloped in its secundines.

Van Bibber was called in great haste to see a patient in labor. He reached the house in about fifteen minutes, and was told by the midwife, a woman of experience, that she had summoned him because of the expulsion from the womb of something the like of which she had never seen before. She thought it must have been some variety of false conception, and had wrapped it up in some flannel. It proved to be a fetus enclosed in its sac, with the placenta, all having been expelled together and intact. He told the nurse to rupture the membranes, and the child, which had been in the unruptured sac for over twenty minutes, began to cry. The infant lived for over a month, but eventually died of bronchitis.

Cowger reports labor at the end of the seventh month without rupture of the fetal sac. Macknus and Rootes speak of expulsion of the entire ovum at the full period of gestation. Roe mentions a case of parturition with unruptured membrane.

Slusser describes the delivery of a full-grown fetus without rupture of the membrane.

"Dry Births."—The reverse of the foregoing are those cases in which, by reason of the deficiency of the waters, the birth is dry. Numerous causes can be stated for such occurrences, and the reader is referred elsewhere for them, the subject being an old one. The Ephemerides speaks of it, and Rudolph discusses its occurrence exhaustively and tells of the difficulties of such a labor. Burrall mentions a case of labor without apparent liquor amnii, delivery being effected by the forceps. Strong records an unusual obstetric case in which there was prolongation of the pregnancy, with a large child, and entire absence of liquor amnii. The case was also complicated with interstitial and subserous fibroids and a contracted pelvis, combined with a posterior position of the occiput and nonrotation of the head. Lente mentions a case of labor without liquor amnii; and Townsend records delivery without any sanguineous discharge. Cosentino mentions a case of the absence of liquor amnii associated with a fetal monstrosity.

Delivery After Death of the Mother.—Curious indeed are those anomalous cases in which the delivery is effected spontaneously after the death of the mother, or when, by manipulation, the child is saved after the maternal decease. Wegelin gives the account of a birth in which version was performed after death and the child successfully delivered. Bartholinus, Wolff, Schenck, Horstius, Hagendorn, Fabricius Hildanus, Valerius, Rolfinck, Cornarius, Boener, and other older writers cite cases of this kind. Pinard gives a most wonderful case. The patient was a woman of thirty-eight who had experienced five previous normal labors. On October 27th she fancied she had labor pains and went to the Lariboisiere Maternite, where, after a careful examination, three fetal poles were elicited, and she was told, to her surprise, of the probability of triplets. At 6 P.M., November 13th, the pains of labor commenced. Three hours later she was having great dyspnea with each pain. This soon assumed a fatal aspect and the midwife attempted to resuscitate the patient by artificial respiration, but failed in her efforts, and then she turned her attention to the fetuses, and, one by one, she extracted them in the short space of five minutes; the last one was born twelve minutes after the mother's death. They all lived (the first two being females), and they weighed from 4 1/4 to 6 1/2 pounds.

Considerable attention has been directed to the advisability of accelerated and forced labor in the dying, in order that the child may be saved. Belluzzi has presented several papers on this subject. Csurgay of Budapest mentions saving the child by forced labor in the death agonies of the mother. Devilliers considers this question from both the obstetric and medicolegal points of view. Hyneaux mentions forcible accouchement practised on both the dead and the dying. Rogowicz advocates artificial delivery by the natural channel in place of Cesarian section in cases of pending or recent death, and Thevenot discussed this question at length at the International Medico-Legal Congress in 1878. Duer presented the question of postmortem delivery in this country.

Kelly reports the history of a woman of forty who died in her eighth pregnancy, and who was delivered of a female child by version and artificial means. Artificial respiration was successfully practised on the child, although fifteen minutes had elapsed from the death of the mother to its extraction. Driver relates the history of a woman of thirty-five, who died in the eighth month of gestation, and who was delivered postmortem by the vagina, manual means only being used. The operator was about to perform Cesarean section when he heard the noise of the membranes rupturing. Thornton reports the extraction of a living child by version after the death of the mother. Aveling has compiled extensive statistics on all varieties of postmortem deliveries, collecting 44 cases of spontaneous expulsion of the fetus after death of the mother.

Aveling states that in 1820 the Council of Cologne sanctioned the placing of a gag in the mouth of a dead pregnant woman, thereby hoping to prevent suffocation of the infant, and there are numerous such laws on record, although most of them pertain to the performance of Cesarean section immediately after death.

Reiss records the death of a woman who was hastily buried while her husband was away, and on his return he ordered exhumation of her body, and on opening the coffin a child's cry was heard. The infant had evidently been born postmortem. It lived long afterward under the name of "Fils de la terre." Willoughby mentions the curious instance in which rumbling was heard from the coffin of a woman during her hasty burial. One of her neighbors returned to the grave, applied her ear to the ground, and was sure she heard a sighing noise. A soldier with her affirmed her tale, and together they went to a clergyman and a justice, begging that the grave be opened. When the coffin was opened it was found that a child had been born, which had descended to her knees. In Derbyshire, to this day, may be seen on the parish register: "April ye 20, 1650, was buried Emme, the wife of Thomas Toplace, who was found delivered of a child after she had lain two hours in the grave."

Johannes Matthaeus relates the case of a buried woman, and that some time afterward a noise was heard in the tomb. The coffin was immediately opened, and a living female child rolled to the feet of the corpse. Hagendorn mentions the birth of a living child some hours after the death of the mother. Dethardingius mentions a healthy child born one-half hour after the mother's death. In the Gentleman's Magazine there is a record of an instance, in 1759, in which a midwife, after the death of a woman whom she had failed to deliver, imagined that she saw a movement under the shroud and found a child between its mother's legs. It died soon after. Valerius Maximus says that while the body of the mother of Gorgia Epirotas was being carried to the grave, a loud noise was heard to come from the coffin and on examination a live child was found between the thighs,— whence arose the proverb: "Gorgiam prius ad funus elatum, quam natum fuisse."

Other cases of postmortem delivery are less successful, the delivery being delayed too late for the child to be viable. The first of Aveling's cases was that of a pregnant woman who was hanged by a Spanish Inquisitor in 1551 While still hanging, four hours later, two children were said to have dropped from her womb. The second case was of a woman of Madrid, who after death was shut in a sepulcher. Some months after, when the tomb was opened, a dead infant was found by the side of the corpse. Rolfinkius tells of a woman who died during parturition, and her body being placed in a cellar, five days later a dead boy and girl were found on the bier. Bartholinus is accredited with the following: Three midwives failing to deliver a woman, she died, and forty-eight hours after death her abdomen swelled to such an extent as to burst her grave-clothes, and a male child, dead, was seen issuing from the vagina. Bonet tells of a woman, who died in Brussels in 1633, who, undelivered, expired in convulsions on Thursday. On Friday abdominal movements in the corpse were seen, and on Sunday a dead child was found hanging between the thighs. According to Aveling, Herman of Berne reports the instance of a young lady whose body was far advanced in putrefaction, from which was expelled an unbroken ovum containing twins. Even the placenta showed signs of decomposition. Naumann relates the birth of a child on the second day after the death of the mother. Richter of Weissenfels, in 1861, reported the case of a woman who died in convulsions, and sixty hours after death an eight months' fetus came away. Stapedius writes to a friend of a fetus being found dead between the thighs of a woman who expired suddenly of an acute disease. Schenk mentions that of a woman, dying at 5 P.M., a child having two front teeth was born at 3 A.M. Veslingius tells of a woman dying of epilepsy on June 6, 1630, from whose body, two days later, issued a child. Wolfius relates the case of a woman dying in labor in 1677. Abdominal movements being seen six hours after death, Cesarean section was suggested, but its performance was delayed, and eighteen hours after a child was spontaneously born. Hoyer of Mulhausen tells of a child with its mouth open and tongue protruding, which was born while the mother was on the way to the grave. Bedford of Sydney, according to Aveling, relates the story of a case in which malpractice was suspected on a woman of thirty-seven, who died while pregnant with her seventh child. The body was exhumed, and a transverse rupture of the womb six inches long above the cervix was found, and the body of a dead male child lay between the thighs. In 1862, Lanigan tells of a woman who was laid out for funeral obsequies, and on removal of the covers for burial a child was found in bed with her. Swayne is credited with the description of the death of a woman whom a midwife failed to deliver. Desiring an inquest, the coroner had the body exhumed, when, on opening the coffin, a well-developed male infant was found parallel to and lying on the lower limbs, the cord and placenta being entirely unattached from the mother.

Some time after her decease Harvey found between the thighs of a dead woman a dead infant which had been expelled postmortem. Mayer relates the history of a case of a woman of forty-five who felt the movement of her child for the fourth time in the middle of November. In the following March she had hemoptysis, and serious symptoms of inflammation in the right lung following, led to her apparent death on the 31st of the month. For two days previous to her death she had failed to perceive the fetal movements. She was kept on her back in a room, covered up and undisturbed, for thirty-six hours, the members of the family occasionally visiting her to sprinkle holy water on her face. There was no remembrance of cadaveric distortion of the features or any odor. When the undertakers were drawing the shroud on they noticed a half-round, bright-red, smooth-looking body between the genitals which they mistook for a prolapsed uterus. Early on April 2d, a few hours before interment, the men thought to examine the swelling they had seen the day before. A second look showed it to be a dead female child, now lying between the thighs and connected with the mother by the umbilical cord. The interment was stopped, and Mayer was called to examine the body, but with negative results, though the signs of death were not plainly visible for a woman dead fifty-eight hours. By its development the body of the fetus confirmed the mother's account of a pregnancy of twenty-one weeks. Mayer satisfies himself at least that the mother was in a trance at the time of delivery and died soon afterward.

Moritz gives the instance of a woman dying in pregnancy, undelivered, who happened to be disinterred several days after burial. The body was in an advanced state of decomposition, and a fetus was found in the coffin. It was supposed that the pressure of gas in the mother's body had forced the fetus from the uterus. Ostmann speaks of a woman married five months, who was suddenly seized with rigors, headache, and vomiting. For a week she continued to do her daily work, and in addition was ill-treated by her husband. She died suddenly without having any abdominal pain or any symptoms indicative of abortion. The body was examined twenty-four hours after death and was seen to be dark, discolored, and the abdomen distended. There was no sanguineous discharge from the genitals, but at the time of raising the body to place it in the coffin, a fetus, with the umbilical cord, escaped from the vagina. There seemed to have been a rapid putrefaction in this ease, generating enough pressure of gas to expel the fetus as well as the uterus from the body. This at least is the view taken by Hoffman and others in the solution of these strange cases.

Antepartum Crying of the Child.—There are on record fabulous cases of children crying in the uterus during pregnancy, and all sorts of unbelievable stories have been constructed from these reported occurrences. Quite possible, however, and worthy of belief are the cases in which the child has been heard to cry during the progress of parturition—that is, during delivery. Jonston speaks of infants crying in the womb, and attempts a scientific explanation of the fact. He also quotes the following lines in reference to this subject:—

> "Mirandum foetus nlaterna clausus in alvo
> Dicitur insuetos ore dedisse sonos.
> Causa subest; doluit se angusta sede telleri
> Et cupiit magnae cernere moliis opus.
> Aut quia quaerendi studio vis fessa parentum
> Aucupii aptas innuit esse manus."

The Ephemerides gives examples of the child hiccoughing in the uterus. Cases of crying before delivery, some in the vagina, some just before the complete expulsion of the head from the os uteri, are very numerous in the older writers; and it is quite possible that on auscultation of the pregnant abdomen fetal sounds may have been exaggerated into cries. Bartholinus, Borellus, Boyle, Buchner, Paullini, Mezger, Riolanus, Lentillus, Marcellus Donatus, and Wolff all speak of children crying before delivery; and Mazinus relates the instance of a puppy whose feeble cries could be heard before expulsion from the bitch. Osiander fully discusses the subject of infants crying during parturition.

McLean describes a case in which he positively states that a child cried lustily in utero during application of the forceps. He compared the sound as though from a voice in the cellar. This child was in the uterus, not in the vagina, and continued the crying during the whole of the five minutes occupied by delivery.

Cesarean Section.—Although the legendary history of Cesarean section is quite copious, it is very seldom that we find authentic records in the writings of the older medical observers. The works of Hippocrates, Aretxeus, Galen, Celsus, and Aetius contain nothing relative to records of successful Cesarean sections. However, Pliny says that Scipio Africanus was the first and Manlius the second of the Romans who owed their lives to the operation of Cesarean section; in his seventh book he says that Julius Caesar was born in this way, the fact giving origin to his name. Others deny this and say that his name came from the thick head of hair which he possessed. It is a frequent subject in old Roman sculpture, and there are many delineations of the birth of Bacchus by Cesarean section from the corpse of Semele. Greek mythology tells us of the birth of Bacchus in the following manner: After Zeus burnt the house of Semele, daughter of Cadmus, he sent Hermes in great haste with directions to take from the burnt body of the mother the fruit of seven months. This child, as we know, was Bacchus. Aesculapius, according to the legend of the Romans, had been excised from the belly of his dead mother, Corinis, who was already on the funeral pile, by his benefactor, Apollo; and from this legend all products of Cesarean sections were regarded as sacred to Apollo, and were thought to have been endowed with sagacity and bravery.

Old records tell us that one of the kings of Navarre was delivered in this way, and we also have records of the birth of the celebrated Doge, Andreas Doria, by this method. Jane Seymour was supposed to have been delivered of Edward VI by Cesarean section, the father, after the consultation of the physicians was announced to him, replying: "Save the child by all means, for I shall be able to get mothers enough." Robert II of Scotland was supposed to have been delivered in this way after the death of his mother, Margery Bruce, who was killed by being thrown from a horse. Shakespere's immortal citation of Macduff, "who was from his mother's womb untimely ripped," must have been such a case, possibly crudely done, perchance by cattle-horn. Pope Gregory XIV was said to have been taken from his mother's belly after her death. The Philosophical Transactions, in the last century contain accounts of Cesarean section performed by an ignorant butcher and also by a midwife; and there are many records of the celebrated case performed by Jacob Nufer, a cattle gelder, at the beginning of the sixteenth century.

By the advent of antisepsis and the improvements of Porro and others, Cesarean section has come to be a quite frequent event, and a record of the successful cases would hardly be considered a matter of extraordinary interest, and would be out of the province of this work, but a citation of anomalous cases will be given. Baldwin reports a case of Cesarean section on a typical rachitic dwarf of twenty-four, who weighed 100 pounds and was only 47 1/2 inches tall. It was the ninth American case, according to the calculation of Harris, only the third successful one, and the first successful one in Ohio. The woman had a uniformly contracted pelvis whose anteroposterior diameter was about 1 1/4 inches. The hygienic surroundings for the operation were not of the best, as the woman lived in a cellar. Tait's method of performing the operation was determined upon and successfully performed. Convalescence was prompt, and in three weeks the case was dismissed. The child was a female of 7 1/2 pounds which inherited the deformities of its mother. It thrived for nine and a half months, when it died of angina Ludovici. Figure 15 represents the mother and child.

Harris gives an account of an operation upon a rachitic dwarf who was impregnated by a large man, a baby weighing 14 pounds and measuring 20 inches being delivered by the knife. St. Braun gives the account of a Porro-Cesarean operation in the case of a rachitic dwarf 3 feet 10 inches tall, in which both the mother and child recovered. Munde speaks of twins being delivered by Cesarean section. Franklin gives the instance of a woman delivered at full term of a living child by this means, in whom was also found a dead fetus. It lay behind the stump of the amputated cervix, in the culdesac of Douglas. The patient died of hemorrhage.

Croston reports a case of Cesarean section on a primipara of twenty-four at full term, with the delivery of a double female monster weighing 12 1/2 pounds. This monster consisted of two females of about the same size, united from the sternal notch to the navel, having one cord and one placenta. It was stillborn. The diagnosis was made before operation by vaginal examination. In a communication to Croston, Harris remarked that this was the first successful Cesarean section for double monstrous conception in America, and added that in 1881 Collins and Leidy performed the same operation without success.

Instances of repeated Cesarean section were quite numerous, and the pride of the operators noteworthy, before the uterus was removed at the first operation, as is now generally done. Bacque reports two sections in the same woman, and Bertrandi speaks of a case in which the operation was successfully executed many times in the same woman. Rosenberg reports three cases repeated successfully by Leopold of Dresden. Skutsch reports a case in which it was twice performed on a woman with a rachitic pelvis, and who the second time was pregnant with twins; the children and mother recovered. Zweifel cites an instance in which two Cesarean sections were performed on a patient, both of the children delivered being in vigorous health. Stolz relates a similar case. Beck gives an account of a Cesarean operation twice on the same woman; in the first the child perished, but in the second it survived. Merinar cites an instance of a woman thrice opened. Parravini gives a similar instance. Charlton gives an account of the performance carried out successfully four times in the same woman; Chisholm mentions a case in which it was twice performed. Michaelis of Kiel gives an instance in which he performed the same operation on a woman four times, with successful issues to both mother and children, despite the presence of peritonitis the last time. He had operated in 1826, 1830, 1832, and 1836. Coe and Gueniot both mention cases in which Cesarean section had been twice performed with successful terminations as regards both mothers and children. Rosenberg tabulates a number of similar cases from medical literature.

Cases of Cesarean section by the patient herself are most curious, but may be readily believed if there is any truth in the reports of the operation being done in savage tribes. Felkin gives an account of a successful case performed in his presence, with preservation of the lives of both mother and child, by a native African in Kahura, Uganda Country. The young girl was operated on in the crudest manner, the hemorrhage being checked by a hot iron. The sutures were made by means of seven thin, hot iron spikes, resembling acupressure-needles, closing the peritoneum and skin. The wound healed in eleven days, and the mother made a complete recovery. Thomas Cowley describes the case of a negro woman who, being unable to bear the pains of labor any longer, took a sharp knife and made a deep incision in her belly—deep enough to wound the buttocks of her child, and extracted the child, placenta and all. A negro horse-doctor was called, who sewed the wound up in a manner similar to the way dead bodies are closed at the present time.

Barker gives the instance of a woman who, on being abused by her husband after a previous tedious labor, resolved to free herself of the child, and slyly made an incision five inches long on the left side of the abdomen with a weaver's knife. When Barker arrived the patient was literally drenched with blood and to all appearance dead. He extracted a dead child from the abdomen and bandaged the mother, who lived only forty hours. In his discourses on Tropical Diseases Moseley speaks of a young negress in Jamaica who opened her uterus and extracted therefrom a child which lived six days; the woman recovered. Barker relates another case in Rensselaer County, N.Y., in which the incision was made with the razor, the woman likewise recovering. There is an interesting account of a poor woman at Prischtina, near the Servian frontier, who, suffering greatly from the pains of labor, resolved to open her abdomen and uterus. She summoned a neighbor to sew up the incision after she had extracted the child, and at the time of report, several months later, both the mother and child were doing well.

Madigan cites the case of a woman of thirty-four, in her seventh confinement, who, while temporarily insane, laid open her abdomen with a razor, incised the uterus, and brought out a male child. The abdominal wound was five inches long, and extended from one inch above the umbilicus straight downward. There was little or no bleeding and the uterus was firmly contracted. She did not see a physician for three hours. The child was found dead and, with the placenta, was lying by her side. The neighbors were so frightened by the awful sight that they ran away, or possibly the child might have been saved by ligature of the funis. Not until the arrival of the clergyman was anything done, and death ultimately ensued.

A most wonderful case of endurance of pain and heroism was one occurring in Italy, which attracted much European comment at the time. A young woman, illegitimately pregnant, at full term, on March 28th, at dawn, opened her own abdomen on the left side with a common knife such as is generally used in kitchens. The wound measured five inches, and was directed obliquely outward and downward. She opened the uterus in the same direction, and endeavored to extract the fetus. To expedite the extraction, she drew out an arm and amputated it, and finding the extraction still difficult, she cut off the head and completely emptied the womb, including the placenta. She bound a tight bandage around her body and hid the fetus in a straw mattress. She then dressed herself and attended to her domestic duties. She afterward mounted a cart and went into the city of Viterbo, where she showed her sister a cloth bathed in blood as menstrual proof that she was not pregnant. On returning home, having walked five hours, she was seized with an attack of vomiting and fainted. The parents called Drs. Serpieri and Baliva, who relate the case. Thirteen hours had elapsed from the infliction of the wound, through which the bulk of the intestines had been protruding for the past six hours. The abdomen was irrigated, the toilet made, and after the eighteenth day the process of healing was well progressed, and the woman made a recovery after her plucky efforts to hide her shame.

Cases like the foregoing excite no more interest than those on record in which an abdominal section has been accidental, as, for instance, by cattle-horns, and the fetus born through the wound. Zuboldie speaks of a case in which a fetus was born from the wound made by a bull's horn in the mother's abdomen. Deneux describes a case in which the wound made by the horn was not sufficiently large to permit the child's escape, but it was subsequently brought through the opening. Pigne speaks of a woman of thirty-eight, who in the eighth month of her sixth pregnancy was gored by a bull, the horn effecting a transverse wound 27 inches long, running from one anterior spine to the other. The woman was found cold and insensible and with an imperceptible pulse. The small intestines were lying between the thighs and covered with coagulated blood. In the process of cleansing, a male child was expelled spontaneously through a rent in the uterus. The woman was treated with the usual precautions and was conscious at midday. In a month she was up. She lived twenty years without any inconvenience except that due to a slight hernia on the left side. The child died at the end of a fortnight.

In a very exhaustive article Harris of Philadelphia has collected nearly all the remaining cases on record, and brief extracts from some of them will be given below. In Zaandam, Holland, 1647, a farmer's wife was tossed by a furious bull. Her abdomen was ripped open, and the child and membranes escaped. The child suffered no injuries except a bruised upper lip and lived nine months. The mother died within forty hours of her injuries. Figure 19 taken from an engraving dated 1647, represents an accouchement by a mad bull, possibly the same case. In Dillenberg, Germany, in 1779, a multipara was gored by an ox at her sixth month of pregnancy; the horn entered the right epigastric region, three inches from the linea alba, and perforated the uterus. The right arm of the fetus protruded; the wound was enlarged and the fetus and placenta delivered. Thatcher speaks of a woman who was gored by a cow in King's Park, and both mother and child were safely delivered and survived.

In the Parish of Zecoytia, Spain, in 1785, Marie Gratien was gored by an ox in the superior portion of her epigastrium, making a wound eight inches long which wounded the uterus in the same direction. Dr. Antonio di Zubeldia and Don Martin Monaco were called to take charge of the case. While they were preparing to effect delivery by the vagina, the woman, in an attack of singultus, ruptured the line of laceration and expelled the fetus, dead. On the twenty-first day the patient was doing well. The wound closed at the end of the sixteenth week. The woman subsequently enjoyed excellent health and, although she had a small ventral hernia, bore and nursed two children.

Marsh cites the instance of a woman of forty-two, the mother of eight children, who when eight months pregnant was horned by a cow. Her clothes were not torn, but she felt that the child had slipped out, and she caught it in her dress. She was seen by some neighbors twelve yards from the place of accident, and was assisted to her house. The bowels protruded and the child was separated from the funis. A physician saw the woman three-quarters of an hour afterward and found her pulseless and thoroughly exhausted. There was considerable but not excessive loss of blood, and several feet of intestine protruded through the wound. The womb was partially inverted through the wound, and the placenta was still attached to the inverted portion. The wound in the uterus was Y-shaped. The mother died in one and a half hours from the reception of her injuries, but the child was uninjured.

Scott mentions the instance of a woman thirty-four years old who was gored by an infuriated ox while in the ninth month of her eighth pregnancy. The horn entered at the anterior superior spinous process of the ilium, involving the parietes and the uterus. The child was extruded through the wound about half an hour after the occurrence of the accident. The cord was cut and the child survived and thrived, though the mother soon died. Stalpart tells the almost incredible story of a soldier's wife who went to obtain water from a stream and was cut in two by a cannonball while stooping over. A passing soldier observed something to move in the water, which, on investigation, he found to be a living child in its membranes. It was christened by order of one Cordua and lived for some time after.

Postmortem Cesarean Section.—The possibility of delivering a child by Cesarean section after the death of the mother has been known for a long time to the students of medicine. In the olden times there were laws making compulsory the opening of the dead bodies of pregnant women shortly after death. Numa Pompilius established the first law, which was called "les regia," and in later times there were many such ordinances. A full description of these laws is on record. Life was believed possible after a gestation of six months or over, and, as stated, some famous men were supposed to have been born in this manner. Francois de Civile, who on great occasions signed himself "trois fois enterre et trois fois par le grace de Dieu ressucite," saw the light of the world by a happy Cesarean operation on his exhumed mother. Fabricius Hildanus and Boarton report similar instances. Bourton cites among others the case of an infant who was found living twelve hours after the death of his mother. Dufour and Mauriceau are two older French medical writers who discuss this subject. Flajani speaks of a case in which a child was delivered at the death of its mother, and some of the older Italian writers discuss the advisability of the operation in the moribund state before death actually ensues. Heister writes of the delivery of the child after the death of the mother by opening the abdomen and uterus

Harris relates several interesting examples. In Peru in 1794 a Sambi woman was killed by lightning, and the next day the abdomen was opened by official command and a living child was extracted. The Princess von Swartzenberg, who was burned to death at a ball in Paris in 1810, was said to have had a living child removed from her body the next day. Like all similar instances, this was proved to be false, as her body was burned beyond the possibility of recognition, and, besides, she was only four months pregnant. Harris mentions another case of a young woman who threw herself from the Pont Neuf into the Seine. Her body was recovered, and a surgeon who was present seized a knife from a butcher standing by and extracted a living child in the presence of the curious spectators. Campbell discusses this subject most thoroughly, though he advances no new opinions upon it.

Duer tabulates the successful results of a number of cases of Cesarean section after death as follows:—

Children extracted between 1 and 5 minutes after death of the mother, 21

"	"	10 and 15	"	"	"	"	"	"	13
"	"	15 and 30	"	"	"	"	"	"	2
"	"	1 hour	"	"	"	"	"	"	2
"	"	2 hours	"	"	"	"	"	"	2

Garezky of St. Petersburg collected reports of 379 cases of Cesarean section after death with the following results: 308 were extracted dead; 37 showed signs of life; 34 were born alive. Of the 34, only 5 lived for any length of time. He concludes that if extracted within five or six minutes after death, they may be born alive; if from six to ten minutes, they may still be born alive, though asphyxiated; if from ten to twenty-six minutes, they will be highly asphyxiated. In a great number of these cases the infant was asphyxiated or dead in one minute. Of course, if the death is sudden, as by apoplexy, accident, or suicide, the child's chances are better. These statistics seem conscientious and reliable, and we are safe in taking them as indicative of the usual result, which discountenances the old reports of death as taking place some time before extraction.

Peuch is credited with statistics showing that in 453 operations 101 children gave signs of life, but only 45 survived.

During the Commune of Paris, Tarnier, one night at the Maternite, was called to an inmate who, while lying in bed near the end of pregnancy, had been killed by a ball which fractured the base of the skull and entered the brain. He removed the child by Cesarean section and it lived for several days. In another case a pregnant woman fell from a window for a distance of more than 30 feet, instant death resulting; thirty minutes at least after the death of the mother an infant was removed, which, after some difficulty, was resuscitated and lived for thirteen years. Tarnier states that delivery may take place three-quarters of an hour or even an hour after the death of the mother, and he also quotes an extraordinary case by Hubert of a successful Cesarean operation two hours after the mother's death; the woman, who was eight months pregnant, was instantly killed while crossing a railroad track.

Hoffman records the case of a successful Cesarean section done ten minutes after death. The patient was a woman of thirty-six, in her eighth month of pregnancy, who was suddenly seized with eclampsia, which terminated fatally in ten hours. Ten minutes after her last respiration the Cesarean section was performed and a living male child delivered. This infant was nourished with the aid of a spoon, but it died in twenty-five hours in consequence of its premature birth and enfeebled vitality.

Green speaks of a woman, nine months pregnant, who was run over by a heavily laden stage-coach in the streets of Southwark. She died in about twenty minutes, and in about twenty minutes more a living child was extracted from her by Cesarean section. There was a similar case in the Hopital St. Louis, in Paris, in 1829; but in this case the child was born alive five minutes after death. Squire tells of a case in which the mother died of dilatation of the aorta, and in from twenty to thirty minutes the child was saved. In comment on this case Aveling is quoted as saying that he believed it possible to save a child one hour after the death of the mother. No less an authority than Playfair speaks of a case in which a child was born half an hour after the death of the mother. Beckman relates the history of a woman who died suddenly in convulsions. The incision was made about five minutes after death, and a male child about four pounds in weight was extracted. The child exhibited feeble heart-contractions and was despaired of. Happily, after numerous and persistent means of resuscitation, applied for about two and a half hours, regular respirations were established and the child eventually recovered. Walter reports a successful instance of removal of the child after the death of the mother from apoplexy.

Cleveland gives an account of a woman of forty-seven which is of special interest. The mother had become impregnated five months after the cessation of menstruation, and a uterine sound had been used in ignorance of the impregnation at this late period. The mother died, and one hour later a living child was extracted by Cesarean section. There are two other recent cases recorded of extraction after an hour had expired from the death. One is cited by Veronden in which the extraction was two hours after death, a living child resulting, and the other by Blatner in which one hour had elapsed after death, when the child was taken out alive.

Cases of rupture of the uterus during pregnancy from the pressure of the contents and delivery of the fetus by some unnatural passage are found in profusion through medical literature, and seem to have been of special interest to the older observers. Benivenius saw a case in which the uterus ruptured and the intestines protruded from the vulva. An instance similar to the one recorded by Benivenius is also found in the last century in Germany. Bouillon and Desbois, two French physicians of the last century, both record examples of the uterus rupturing in the last stages of pregnancy and the mother recovering. Schreiber gives an instance of rupture of the uterus occasioned by the presence of a 13-pound fetus, and there is recorded the account of a rupture caused by a 20-pound fetus that made its way into the abdomen. We find old accounts of cases of rupture of the uterus with birth by the umbilicus and the recovery of the woman. Vespre describes a case in which the uterus was ruptured by the feet of the fetus.

Farquharson has an account of a singular case in midwifery in which abdomen ruptured from the pressure of the fetus; and quite recently Geoghegan illustrates the possibilities of uterine pressure in pregnancy by a postmortem examination after a fatal parturition, in which the stomach was found pushed through the diaphragm and lying under the left clavicle. Heywood Smith narrates the particulars of a case of premature labor at seven months in which rupture of the uterus occurred and, notwithstanding the fact that the case was complicated by placenta praevia, the patient recovered.

Rupture of the uterus and recovery does not necessarily prevent subsequent successful pregnancy and delivery by the natural channels. Whinery relates an instance of a ruptured uterus in a healthy Irish woman of thirty-seven from whom a dead child was extracted by abdominal section and who was safely delivered of a healthy female child about one year afterward. Analogous to this case is that of Lawrence, who details the instance of a woman who had been delivered five times of dead children; she had a very narrow pelvis and labor was always induced at the eighth month to assure delivery. In her sixth pregnancy she had miscalculated her time, and, in consequence, her uterus ruptured in an unexpected parturition, but she recovered and had several subsequent pregnancies.

Occasionally there is a spontaneous rupture of the vagina during the process of parturition, the uterus remaining intact. Wiltshire reports such a case in a woman who had a most prominent sacrum; the laceration was transverse and quite extensive, but the woman made a good recovery. Schauta pictures an exostosis on the promontory of the sacrum. Blenkinsop cites an instance in which the labor was neither protracted nor abnormally severe, yet the rupture of the vagina took place with the escape of the child into the abdomen of the mother, and was from thence extracted by Cesarean section. A peculiarity of this case was the easy expulsion from the uterus, no instrumental or other manual interference being attempted and the uterus remaining perfectly intact.

In some cases there is extensive sloughing of the genitals after parturition with recovery far beyond expectation. Gooch mentions a case in which the whole vagina sloughed, yet to his surprise the patient recovered. Aetius and Benivenius speak of recovery in such cases after loss of the whole uterus. Cazenave of Bordeaux relates a most marvelous case in which a primipara suffered in labor from an impacted head. She was twenty-five, of very diminutive stature, and was in labor a long time. After labor, sloughing of the parts commenced and progressed to such an extent that in one month there were no traces of the labia, nymphae, vagina, perineum, or anus. There was simply a large opening extending from the meatus urinarius to the coccyx. The rectovaginal septum, the lower portion of the rectum, and the neck of the bladder were obliterated. The woman survived, although she always experienced great difficulty in urination and in entirely emptying the rectum. A similar instance is reported in a woman of thirty who was thirty-six hours in labor. The fundus of the uterus descended into the vagina and the whole uterine apparatus was removed. The lower part of the rectum depended between the labia; in the presence of the physician the nurse drew this out and it separated at the sphincter ani. On examining the parts a single opening was seen, as in the preceding case, from the pubes to the coccyx. Some time afterward the end of the intestine descended several inches and hung loosely on the concave surface of the rectum. A sponge was introduced to support the rectum and prevent access of air. The destruction of the parts was so complete and the opening so large as to bring into view the whole inner surface of the pelvis, in spite of which, after prolonged suppuration, the wound cicatrized from behind forward and health returned, except as regards the inconvenience of feces and urine. Milk-secretion appeared late and lasted two months without influencing the other functions.

There are cases in which, through the ignorance of the midwife or the physician, prolapsed pelvic organs are mistaken for afterbirth and extracted. There have been instances in which the whole uterus and its appendages, not being recognized, have been dragged out. Walters cites the instance of a woman of twenty-two, who was in her third confinement. The midwife in attendance, finding the afterbirth did not come away, pulled at the funis, which broke at its attachment. She then introduced her hand and tore away what proved to be the whole of the uterus, with the right ovary and fallopian tube, a portion of the round ligament, and the left tube and ovarian ligament attached to it. A large quantity of omentum protruded from the vulva and upper part of the vagina, and an enormous rent was left. Walters saw the woman twenty-one hours afterward, and ligated and severed the protruding omentum. On the twenty-eighth day, after a marvelous recovery, she was able to drive to the Royal Berkshire Hospital, a distance of five miles. At the time of report, two years and six months after the mutilation, she was in perfect health. Walters looked into the statistics of such cases and found 36 accidental removals of the uterus in the puerperium with 14 recoveries. All but three of these were without a doubt attended by previous inversion of the uterus.

A medical man was tried for manslaughter in 1878 because he made a similar mistake. He had delivered a woman by means of the forceps, and, after delivery, brought away what he thought a tumor. This "tumor" consisted of the uterus, with the placenta attached to the fundus, the funis, a portion of the lateral ligament, containing one ovary and about three inches of vagina. The uterus was not inverted. A horrible case, with similar results, happened in France, and was reported by Tardieu. A brutal peasant, whose wife was pregnant, dragged out a fetus of seven months, together with the uterus and the whole intestinal canal, from within 50 cm. of the pylorus to within 8 cm. of the ileocecal valve. The woman was seen three-quarters of an hour after the intestines had been found in the yard (where the brute had thrown them), still alive and reproaching her murderer. Hoffman cites an instance in which a midwife, in her anxiety to extract the afterbirth, made traction on the cord, brought out the uterus, ovaries, and tubes, and tore the vulva and perineum as far as the anus.

Woodson tells the story of a negress who was four months pregnant, and who, on being seized with severe uterine pains in a bath, succeeded in seizing the fetus and dragging it out, but inverting the uterus in the operation. There is a case recorded of a girl of eighteen, near her labor, who, being driven from her house by her father, took refuge in a neighboring house, and soon felt the pains of child-birth. The accoucheur was summoned, pronounced them false pains, and went away. On his return he found the girl dying, with her uterus completely inverted and hanging between her legs. This unfortunate maiden had been delivered while standing upright, with her elbows on the back of a chair. The child suddenly escaped, bringing with it the uterus, but as the funis ruptured the child fell to the floor. Wagner pictures partial prolapse of the womb in labor.

It would too much extend this chapter to include the many accidents incident to labor, and only a few of especial interest will be given. Cases like rupture of an aneurysm during labor, extensive hemorrhage, the entrance of air into the uterine veins and sinuses, and common lacerations will be omitted, together with complicated births like those of double monsters, etc., but there are several other cases that deserve mention. Eldridge gives an instance of separation of the symphysis pubis during labor,—a natural symphysiotomy. A separation of 3/4 inch could be discerned at the symphysis, and in addition the sacroiliac synchondrosis was also quite movable. The woman had not been able to walk in the latter part of her pregnancy. The child weighed 10 1/2 pounds and had a large head in a remarkably advanced stage of ossification, with the fontanelles nearly closed. Delivery was effected, though during the passage of the head the pubes separated to such an extent that Eldridge placed two fingers between them. The mother recovered, and had perfect union and normal locomotion.

Sanders reports a case of the separation of the pubic bones in labor. Studley mentions a case of fracture of the pelvis during instrumental delivery. Humphreys cites a most curious instance. The patient, it appears, had a large exostosis on the body of the pubes which, during parturition, was forced through the walls of the uterus and bladder, resulting in death. Kilian reports four cases of death from perforation of the uterus in this manner. Schauta pictures such an exostosis.

Chandler relates an instance in which there was laceration of the liver during parturition; and Hubbard records a case of rupture of the spleen after labor.

Symphysiotomy is an operation consisting of division of the pubic symphysis in order to facilitate delivery in narrow pelves. This operation has undergone a most remarkable revival during the past two years. It originated in a suggestion by Pineau in his work on surgery in 1598, and in 1665 was first performed by La Courvee upon a dead body in order to save the child, and afterward by Plenk, in 1766, for the same purpose. In 1777 Sigault first proposed the operation on the living, and Ferrara was the one to carry out, practically, the proposition,— although Sigault is generally considered to be the first symphysiotormist, and the procedure is very generally known as the "Sigaultean operation." From Ferrara's time to 1858, when the operation had practically died out, it had been performed 85 times, with a recorded mortality of 33 per cent. In 1866 the Italians, under the leadership of Morisani of Naples, revived the operation, and in twenty years had performed it 70 times with a mortality of 24 per cent. Owing to rigid antiseptic technic, the last 38 of these operations (1886 to 1891) showed a mortality of only 50 per cent, while the infant-mortality was only 10 2/3 per cent. The modern history of this operation is quite interesting, and is very completely reviewed by Hirst and Dorland.

In November, 1893, Hirst reported 212 operations since 1887, with a maternal mortality of 12.73 per cent and a fetal mortality of 28 per cent. In his later statistics Morisani gives 55 cases with 2 maternal deaths and 1 infantile death, while Zweifel reports 14 cases from the Leipzig clinic with no maternal death and 2 fetal deaths, 1 from asphyxia and 1 from pneumonia, two days after birth. All the modern statistics are correspondingly encouraging.

Irwin reports a case in which the firm attachment of the fetal head to the uterine parietes rendered delivery without artificial aid impossible, and it was necessary to perform craniotomy. The right temporal region of the child adhered to the internal surface of the neck of the uterus, being connected by membranes. The woman was forty-four years old, and the child was her fourth.

Delay in the Birth of the Second Twin.—In twin pregnancies there is sometimes a delay of many days in the birth of a second child, even to such an extent as to give suspicion of superfetation. Pignot speaks of one twin two months before the other. De Bosch speaks of a delay of seventeen days; and there were 2 cases on record in France in the last century, one of which was delayed ten days, and the other showed an interval of seven weeks between the delivery of the twins. There is an old case on record in which there was an interval of six weeks between deliveries; Jansen gives an account of three births in ten months; Pinart mentions a case with an interval of ten days; Thilenius, one of thirteen days; and Ephemerides, one of one week. Wildberg describes a case in which one twin was born two months after the other, and there was no secretion of milk until after the second birth. A full description of Wildberg's case is given in another journal in brief, as follows: A woman, eighteen months married, was in labor in the eighth month of pregnancy. She gave birth to a child, which, though not fully matured, lived. There was no milk-secretion in her breasts, and she could distinctly feel the movements of another child; her abdomen increased in size. After two months she had another labor, and a fully developed and strong child was born, much heavier than the first. On the third day after, the breasts became enlarged, and she experienced considerable fever. It was noticeable in this case that a placenta was discharged a quarter of an hour after the first birth. Irvine relates an instance of thirty-two days' delay; and Pfau one of seven days'.

Carson cites the instance of a noblewoman of forty, the mother of four children, who was taken ill about two weeks before confinement was expected, and was easily delivered of a male child, which seemed well formed, with perfect nails, but weakly. After the birth the mother never became healthy or natural in appearance. She was supposed to be dying of dropsy, but after forty-four days the mystery was cleared by the birth of a fine, well-grown, and healthy daughter. Both mother and child did well.

Addison describes the case of a woman who was delivered of a healthy male child, and everything was well until the evening of the fourth day, when intense labor-pains set in, and well-formed twins about the size of a pigeon's egg were born. In this strange case, possibly an example of superfetation, the patient made a good recovery and the first child lived. A similar case is reported by Lumby in which a woman was delivered on January 18th, by a midwife, of a full-grown and healthy female child. On the third day she came down-stairs and resumed her ordinary duties, which she continued until February 4th (seventeen days after). At this time she was delivered of twins, a boy and a girl, healthy and well-developed. The placenta was of the consistency of jelly and had to be scooped away with the hand. The mother and children did well. This woman was the mother of ten children besides the product of this conception, and at the latter occurrence had entire absence of pains and a very easy parturition.

Pincott had a case with an interval of seven weeks between the births; Vale 1 of two months; Bush 1 of seventeen days; and Burke 1 with an interval of two months. Douglas cites an instance of twins being born four days apart. Bessems of Antwerp, in 1866, mentions a woman with a bicornate uterus who bore two twins at fifty-four days' interval.

CHAPTER IV

PROLIFICITY.

General Historic Observations.—Prolificity is a much discussed subject, for besides its medical and general interest it is of importance in social as well as in political economy. Superfluous population was a question that came to consciousness early; Aristotle spoke of legislation to prevent the increase of population and the physical and mental deterioration of the race,—he believed in a population fixed as regards numbers,—and later Lycurgus transformed these precepts into a terrible law. Strabonius reports that the inhabitants of Cathea brought their infants at the age of two months before a magistrate for inspection. The strong and promising were preserved and the weak destroyed. The founders of the Roman Empire followed a similar usage. With great indignation Seneca, Ovid, and Juvenal reproved this barbarity of the Romans. With the domination of Christianity this custom gradually diminished, and Constantine stopped it altogether, ordering succor to the people too poor to rear their own children. The old Celts were so jealous of their vigor that they placed their babes on a shield in the river, and regarded those that the waves respected as legitimate and worthy to become members of their clans. In many of the Oriental countries, where the population is often very excessive and poverty great, the girl babies of the lower classes were destroyed. At one time the crocodiles, held sacred in the Nile, were given the surplus infants. By destroying the females the breeding necessarily diminished, and the number of the weaker and dependent classes became less. In other countries persons having children beyond their ability to support were privileged to sell them to citizens, who contracted to raise them on condition that they became their slaves.

General Law, and the Influence of War.—In the increase of the world's population, although circumstances may for the time alter it, a general average of prolificity has, in the long run, been maintained. In the history of every nation artificial circumstances, such as fashion, war, poverty, etc., at some period have temporarily lowered the average of prolificity; but a further search finds another period, under opposite circumstances, which will more than compensate for it. The effect of a long-continued war or wars on generation and prolificity has never been given proper consideration. In such times marriages become much less frequent; the husbands are separated from their wives for long periods; many women are left widows; the females become in excess of the males; the excitement of the times overtops the desire for sexual intercourse, or, if there is the same desire, the unprolific prostitute furnishes the satisfaction; and such facts as these, coupled with many similar ones, soon produce an astonishing effect upon the comparative birth-rate and death-rate of the country. The resources of a country, so far as concerns population, become less as the period of peace-disturbance is prolonged. Mayo-Smith quotes von Mayr in the following example of the influence of the war of 1870-71 on the birth-rate in Bavaria,—the figures for births are thrown back nine months, so as to show the time of conception: Before the war under normal conception the number of births was about 16,000 per month. During the war it sank to about 2000 per month. Immediately on the cessation of hostilities it arose to its former number, while the actual return of the troops brought an increase of 2000 per month. The maximum was reached in March, 1872, when it was 18,450. The war of 1866 seems to have passed over Germany without any great influence, the birth-rate in 1865 being 39.2; in 1866, 39.4; in 1867, 38.3; in 1868, 38.4. On the other hand, while the birth-rate in 1870 was 40.1, in 1871 it was only 35.9; in 1872 it recovered to 41.1, and remained above 41 down to 1878. Von Mayr believes the war had a depressing influence upon the rate apart from the mere absence of the men, as shown in the fact that immediately upon the cessation of hostilities it recovered in Bavaria, although it was several months before the return of the troops.

Mayo-Smith, in remarking on the influence of war on the marriage-rate, says that in 1866 the Prussian rate fell from 18.2 to 15.6, while the Austrian rate fell from 15.5 to 13.0. In the war of 1870-71 the Prussian rate fell from 17.9 in 1869 to 14.9 in 1870 and 15.9 in 1871; but in the two years after peace was made it rose to 20.6 and 20.2, the highest rates ever recorded. In France the rate fell from 16.5 to 12.1 and 14.4, and then rose to 19.5 and 17.7, the highest rates ever recorded in France.

Influence of Rural and Urban Life.—Rural districts are always very prolific, and when we hear the wails of writers on "Social Economy," bemoaning the small birth-rates of their large cities, we need have no fear for urban extinction, as emigration from the country by many ambitious sons and daughters, to avail themselves of the superior advantages that the city offers, will not only keep up but to a certain point increase the population, until the reaction of overcrowding, following the self-regulating law of compensation, starts a return emigration.

The effect of climate and race on prolificity, though much spoken of, is not so great a factor as supposed. The inhabitants of Great Britain are surpassed by none in the point of prolificity; yet their location is quite northern. The Swedes have always been noted for their fecundity. Olaf Rudbeck says that from 8 to 12 was the usual family number, and some ran as high as 25 or 30. According to Lord Kames, in Iceland before the plague (about 1710) families of from 15 to 20 were quite common. The old settlers in cold North America were always blessed with large families, and Quebec is still noted for its prolificity. There is little difference in this respect among nations, woman being limited about the same everywhere, and the general average of the range of the productive function remaining nearly identical in all nations. Of course, exception must be made as to the extremes of north or south.

Ancient and Modern Prolificity.—Nor is there much difference between ancient and modern times. We read in the writings of Aristotle, Pliny, and Albucasis of the wonderful fertility of the women of Egypt, Arabia, and other warm countries, from 3 to 6 children often being born at once and living to maturity; but from the wonder and surprise shown in the narration of these facts, they were doubtless exceptions, of which parallels may be found in the present day. The ancient Greek and Roman families were no larger than those of to-day, and were smaller in the zenith of Roman affluence, and continued small until the period of decadence.

Legal Encouragement of Prolificity.—In Quebec Province, Canada, according to a Montreal authority, 100 acres of land are allotted to the father who has a dozen children by legitimate marriage. The same journal states that, stimulated by the premium offered, families of 20 or more are not rare, the results of patriotic efforts. In 1895, 1742 "chefs de famille" made their claim according to the conditions of the law, and one, Paul Bellanger, of the River du Loup, claimed 300 acres as his premium, based on the fact that he was the father of 36 children. Another claimant, Monsieur Thioret de Sainte Genevieve, had been presented by his wife, a woman not yet thirty years old, with 17 children. She had triplets twice in the space of five years and twins thrice in the mean time. It is a matter of conjecture what the effect would be of such a premium in countries with a lowering birth-rate, and a French medical journal, quoting the foregoing, regretfully wishes for some countrymen at home like their brothers in Quebec.

Old Explanations of Prolificity.—The old explanation of the causation of the remarkable exceptions to the rules of prolificity was similar to that advanced by Empedocles, who says that the greater the quantity of semen, the greater the number of children at birth. Pare, later, uses a similar reason to explain the causation of monstrosities, grouping them into two classes, those due to deficiency of semen, such as the acephalous type, and those due to excess, such as the double monsters. Hippocrates, in his work on the "Nature of the Infant," tells us that twins are the result of a single coitus, and we are also informed that each infant has a chorion; so that both kinds of plural gestation (monochorionic and dichorionic) were known to the ancients. In this treatise it is further stated that the twins may be male or female, or both males or both females; the male is formed when the semen is thick and strong.

The greatest number of children at a single birth that it is possible for a woman to have has never been definitely determined. Aristotle gives it as his opinion that one woman can bring forth no more than 5 children at a single birth, and discredits reports of multiplicity above this number; while Pliny, who is not held to be so trustworthy, positively states that there were authentic records of as many as 12 at a birth. Throughout the ages in which superstitious distortion of facts and unquestioning credulity was unchecked, all sorts of incredible accounts of prolificity are found. Martin Cromerus, a Polish historian, quoted by Pare, who has done some good work in statistical research on this subject, says a that Margaret, of a noble and ancient family near Cracovia, the wife of Count Virboslaus, brought forth 36 living children on January 20, 1296.

The celebrated case of Countess Margaret, daughter of Florent IV, Earl of Holland, and spouse of Count Hermann of Henneberg, was supposed to have occurred just before this, on Good Friday, 1278. She was at this time forty-two years of age, and at one birth brought forth 365 infants, 182 males, 182 females, and 1 hermaphrodite. They were all baptized in two large brazen dishes by the Bishop of Treras, the males being called John, the females Elizabeth. During the last century the basins were still on exhibition in the village church of Losdun, and most of the visitors to Hague went out to see them, as they were reckoned one of the curiosities of Holland. The affliction was ascribed to the curse of a poor woman who, holding twins in her arms, approached the Countess for aid. She was not only denied alms, but was insulted by being told that her twins were by different fathers, whereupon the poor woman prayed God to send the Countess as many children as there were days in the year. There is room for much speculation as to what this case really was. There is a possibility that it was simply a case of hydatidiform or multiple molar pregnancy, elaborated by an exhaustive imagination and superstitious awe. As late as 1799 there was a woman of a town of

Andalusia who was reported to have been delivered of 16 male infants, 7 of which were alive two months later.

Mayo-Smith remarks that the proportion of multiple births is not more than 1 per cent of the total number of parturitions. The latest statistics, by Westergaard, give the following averages to number of cases of 100 births in which there were 2 or more at a birth:—

Sweden,	1.45
Germany,	1.24
Bavaria,	1.38
Denmark,	1.34
Holland,	1.30
Prussia,	1.26
Scotland,	1.22
Norway,	1.32
Saxony,	1.20
Italy,	1.21
Austria,	1.17
Switzerland,	1.16
France,	0.99
Belgium,	0.97
Spain,	0.85

In Prussia, from 1826 to 1880, there were 85 cases of quadruplets and 3 cases of 5 at a birth.

The most extensive statistics in regard to multiple births are those of Veit, who reviews 13,000,000 births in Prussia. According to his deductions, twins occur once in 88 births; triplets, once in 7910; and quadruplets, once in 371,126. Recent statistics supplied by the Boards of Health of New York and Philadelphia place the frequency of twin births in these cities at 1 in every 120 births, while in Bohemia twins occur once in about 60 births, a proportion just twice as great. Of 150,000 twin pregnancies studied by Veit, in one-third both children were boys; in slightly less than one-third both were girls; in the remaining third both sexes were represented.

Authentic records of 5 and 6 at a birth are extremely rare and infinitesimal in proportion. The reputed births in excess of 6 must be looked on with suspicion, and, in fact, in the great majority of reports are apocryphal.

The examples of multiple births of a single pregnancy will be taken up under their respective numbers, several examples of each being given, together with the authorities. Many twin and triplet brothers have figured prominently in history, and, in fact, they seem especially favored. The instance of the Horatii and the Curatii, and their famous battle, on which hung the fate of Rome and Alba, is familiar to every one, their strength and wisdom being legendary with the Romans.

Twins and triplets, being quite common, will not be considered here, although there are 2 cases of interest of the latter that deserve citation. Sperling reports 2 instances of triplets; in the first there was 1 placenta and chorion, 2 amnions, and the sex was the same; in the second case, in which the sexes were different, there were 3 placentas, 3 chorions, and 3 amnions. What significance this may have is only a matter of conjecture. Petty describes a case of triplets in which one child was born alive, the other 2 having lost their vitality three months before. Mirabeau has recently found that triple births are most common (1 to 6500) in multiparous women between thirty and thirty-four years of age. Heredity seems to be a factor, and duplex uteruses predispose to multiple births. Ross reports an instance of double uterus with triple pregnancy.

Quadruplets are supposed to occur once in about every 400,000 births. There are 72 instances recorded in the Index Catalogue of the Surgeon General's Library, U. S. A., up to the time of compilation, not including the subsequent cases in the Index Medicus. At the Hotel-Dieu, in Paris, in 108,000 births, covering a period of sixty years, mostly in the last century, there was only one case of quadruplets. The following extract of an account of the birth of quadruplets is given by Dr. De Leon of Ingersoll, Texas:—

"I was called to see Mrs. E. T. Page, January 10, 1890, about 4 o'clock A.M.; found her in labor and at full time, although she assured me that her 'time' was six weeks ahead. At 8 o'clock A.M. I delivered her of a girl baby; I found there were triplets, and so informed her. At 11 A.M. I delivered her of the second girl, after having rectified presentation, which was singular, face, hands, and feet all presented; I placed in proper position and practised 'version.' This child was 'still-born,' and after considerable effort by artificial respiration it breathed and came around 'all right.' The third girl was born at 11.40 A.M. This was the smallest one of the four. In attempting to take away the placenta, to my astonishment I found the feet of another child. At 1 P.M. this one was born; the head of this child got firmly impacted at the lower strait, and it was with a great deal of difficulty and much patient effort that it was finally disengaged; it was blocked by a mass of placenta and cords. The first child had its own placenta; the second and third had their placenta; the fourth had also a placenta. They weighed at birth in the aggregate 19 1/2 pounds without clothing; the first weighed 6 pounds; the second 5 pounds; the third 4 1/2 pounds; the fourth 4 pounds. Mrs. Page is a blonde, about thirty-six years old, and has given birth to 14 children, twins three times before this, one pair by her first husband. She has been married to Page three years, and has had 8 children in that time. I have waited on her each time. Page is an Englishman, small, with dark hair, age about twenty-six, and weighs about 115 pounds. They are in St. Joseph, Mo., now, having contracted with Mr. Uffner of New York to travel and exhibit themselves in Denver, St. Joseph, Omaha, and Nebraska City, then on to Boston, Mass., where they will spend the summer."

There is a report from Canada of the birth of 4 living children at one time. The mother, a woman of thirty-eight, of small stature, weighing 100 pounds, had 4 living children of the ages of twelve, ten, eight, and seven years, respectively. She had aborted at the second month, and at full term was delivered of 2 males, weighing, respectively, 4 pounds 9 1/4 ounces and 4 pounds 3 ounces; and of 2 females, weighing 4 pounds 3 ounces and 3 pounds 13 3/4 ounces, respectively. There was but one placenta, and no more exhaustion or hemorrhage than at a single birth. The father weighed 169 pounds, was forty-one years old, and was 5 feet 5 inches tall, healthy and robust. The Journal of St. Petersburg, a newspaper of the highest standard, stated that at the end of July, 1871, a Jewish woman residing in Courland gave birth to 4 girls, and again, in May, 1872, bore 2 boys and a girl; the mother and the 7 children, born within a period of ten months, were doing well at the time of the report. In the village of Iwokina, on May 26, 1854, the wife of a peasant bore 4 children at a birth, all surviving. Bousquet speaks of a primiparous mother, aged twenty-four, giving birth to 4 living infants, 3 by the breech and 1 by the vertex, apparently all in one bag of membranes. They were nourished by the help of 3 wet-nurses. Bedford speaks of 4 children at a birth, averaging 5 pounds each, and all nursing the mother.

Quintuplets are quite rare, and the Index Catalogue of the Surgeon General's Library, U. S. A., gives only 19 cases, reports of a few of which will be given here, together with others not given in the Catalogue, and from less scientific though reliable sources. In the year 1731 there was one case of quintuplets in Upper Saxony and another near Prague, Bohemia. In both of these cases the children were all christened and had all lived to maturity. Garthshore speaks of a healthy woman, Margaret Waddington, giving birth to 5 girls, 2 of which lived; the 2 that lived weighed at birth 8 pounds 12 ounces and 9 pounds, respectively. He discusses the idea that woman was meant to bear more than one child at a birth, using as his argument the existence of the double nipple and mamma, to which might be added the not infrequent occurrence of polymazia.

In March, 1736, in a dairy cellar in the Strand, London, a poor woman gave birth to 3 boys and 9 girls. In the same journal was reported the birth at Wells, Somersetshire, in 1739, of 4 boys and a girl, all of whom were christened and were healthy. Pare in 1549 gives several instances of 5 children at a birth, and Pliny reports that in the peninsula of Greece there was a woman who gave birth to quintuplets on four different occasions. Petritus, a Greek physician, speaks of the birth of quintuplets at the seventh month. Two males and one female were born dead, being attached to the same placenta; the others were united to a common placenta and lived three days. Chambon mentions an instance of 5 at a birth. Not far from Berne, Switzerland, the wife of John Gelinger, a preacher in the Lordship of Berne, brought forth twins, and within a year after she brought forth quintuplets, 3 sons and 2 daughters. There is a similar instance reported in 1827 of a woman of twenty-seven who, having been delivered of twins two years before, was brought to bed with 5 children, 3 boys and 2 girls. Their length was from 15 1/2 to 16 1/2 inches. Although regularly formed, they did not seem to have reached maturity. The mother was much exhausted, but recovered. The children appeared old-looking, had tremulous voices, and slept continually; during sleep their temperatures seemed very low.

Kennedy showed before the Dublin Pathological Society 5 fetuses with the involucra, the product of an abortion at the third month. At Naples in 1839 Giuseppa Califani gave birth to 5 children; and about the same time Paddock reported the birth in Franklin County, Pa., of quintuplets. The Lancet relates an account of the birth of quintuplets, 2 boys and 3 girls, by the wife of a peasant on March 1, 1854. Moffitt records the birth at Monticello, Ill., of quintuplets. The woman was thirty-five years of age; examination showed a breech presentation; the second child was born by a foot-presentation, as was the third, but the last was by a head-presentation. The combined weight was something over 19 pounds, and of the 5, 3 were still-born, and the other 2 died soon after birth. The Elgin Courant (Scotland), 1858, speaks of a woman named Elspet Gordon, at Rothes, giving birth to 3 males and 2 females. Although they were six months' births, the boys all lived until the following morning. The girls were still-born. One of the boys had two front teeth when born. Dr. Dawson of Rothes is the obstetrician mentioned in this case.

The following recent instance is given with full details to illustrate the difficulties attending the births of quintuplets. Stoker has reported the case of a healthy woman, thirty-five years old, 5 feet 1 inch high, and of slight build, whom he delivered of 5 fetuses in the seventh month of pregnancy, none of the children surviving. The patient's mother had on two occasions given birth to twins. The woman herself had been married for six years and had borne 4 children at full term, having no difficulty in labor. When she came under observation she computed that she had been pregnant for six months, and had had her attention attracted to the unusually large size of her abdomen. She complained of fixed pain in the left side of the abdomen on which side she thought she was larger. Pains set in with regularity and the labor lasted eight and three-quarter hours. After the rupture of the membranes the first child presented by the shoulder. Version was readily performed; the child was dead (recently). Examination after the birth of the first child disclosed the existence of more than one remaining fetus. The membranes protruded and became tense with each contraction. The presentation was a transverse one. In this case also there was little difficulty in effecting internal version. The child lived a couple of hours. The third fetus was also enclosed in a separate sac, which had to be ruptured. The child presented by the breech and was delivered naturally, and lived for an hour. In the fourth case the membranes had likewise to be ruptured, and alarming hemorrhage ensued. Version was at once practised, but the chin became locked with that of the remaining fetus. There was some difficulty and considerable delay in freeing the children, though the extent of locking was not at any time formidable. The child was dead (recently). The fifth fetus presented by the head and was delivered naturally. It lived for half an hour. The placenta was delivered about five minutes after the birth of the last child, and consisted of two portions united by a narrow isthmus. One, the smaller, had two cords attached centrally and close together; the other, and larger, had two cords attached in a similar way and one where it was joined to the isthmus. The organ appeared to be perfectly healthy. The cord of the fourth child was so short that it had to be ligated in the vagina. The children were all females and of about the same size, making a total weight of 8 pounds. The mother rallied quickly and got on well.

Trustworthy records of sextuplets are, of course, extremely scarce. There are few catalogued at Washington, and but two authentic cases are on record in the United States. On December 30, 1831, a woman in Dropin was delivered of 6 daughters, all living, and only a little smaller than usual in size. The mother was not quite twenty years old, but was of strong constitution. The 6 lived long enough to be baptized, but died the evening of their births. There was a case a of sextuplets in Italy in 1844. In Maine, June 27, 1847, a woman was delivered of 6 children, 2 surviving and, together with the mother, doing well. In 1885 there was reported the birth of sextuplets in Lorca, Spain, of which only one survived. At Dallas, Texas, in 1888, Mrs. George Hirsh of Navarro County gave birth to 6 children, the mother and the children all doing well. There were 4 boys and 2 girls, and they were all perfect, well formed, but rather small.

Valsalli gives an instance which is quoted by the Medical News without giving the authority. Valsalli's account, which differs slightly from the account in the Medical News, is briefly as follows: While straining at stool on the one hundred and fifteenth day of pregnancy the membranes ruptured and a foot prolapsed, no pain having been felt before the accident. A fetus was delivered by the midwife. Valsalli was summoned and found the woman with an enormously distended abdomen, within which were felt numerous fetal parts; but no fetal heart-sounds or movements were noticed. The cervix was only slightly dilated, and, as no pains were felt, it was agreed to wait. On the next day the membranes were ruptured and 4 more fetuses were delivered. Traction on the umbilical cord started hemorrhage, to check which the physician placed his hand in the uterine cavity. In this most arduous position he remained four hours until assistance from Lugano came. Then, in the presence of the three visiting physicians, a sixth amniotic sac was delivered with its fetus. The woman had a normal convalescence, and in the following year gave birth to healthy, living twins. The News says the children all moved vigorously at birth; there were 4 males and 2 females, and for the 6 there was only one placenta The mother, according to the same authority, was thirty-six years of age, and was in her second pregnancy.

Multiple Births over Six.—When we pass sextuplets the records of multiple births are of the greatest rarity and in modern records there are almost none. There are several cases mentioned by the older writers whose statements are generally worthy of credence, which, however incredible, are of sufficient interest at least to find a place in this chapter. Albucasis affirms that he knew of the birth of seven children at one time; and d'Alechampius reports that Bonaventura, the slave of one Savelli, a gentleman of Siena, gave birth to 7 children, 4 of whom were baptized. At the Parish of San Ildefonso, Valladolid, Julianna, wife of Benito Quesada, gave birth to 3 children in one day, and during the following night to 4 more. Sigebert, in his Chronicles, says that the mother of the King of Lombardy had borne 7 children at a birth. Borellus says that in 1650 the lady of the then present Lord Darre gave birth to eight perfect children at one parturition and that it was the unusual event of the country.

Mrs. Timothy Bradlee of Trumbull County, Ohio, in 1872 is reported to have given birth to 8 children at one time. They were healthy and living, but quite small. The mother was married six years previously and then weighed 273 pounds. She had given birth to 2 pairs of twins, and, with these 3 boys and 5 girls, she had borne 12 children in six years. She herself was a triplet and her father and her mother were of twin births and one of her grandmothers was the mother of 5 pairs of twins. This case was most celebrated and was much quoted, several British journals extracting it.

Watering of Maregnac speaks of the simultaneous birth of 8 children at one time. When several months pregnant the woman was seized with colicky pains and thought them a call of nature. She went into a vineyard to answer it, and there, to her great astonishment, gave birth to 8 fetuses. Watering found them enclosed in a sac, and thought they probably had died from mutual pressure during growth. The mother made a good recovery.

In 1755 Seignette of Dijon reports the simultaneous birth of nine children. Franciscus Picus Mirandulae, quoted by Pare, says that one Dorothea, an Italian, bore 20 children at 2 confinements, the first time bearing 9 and the second time eleven. He gives a picture of this marvel of prolificity, in which her belly is represented as hanging down to her knees, and supported by a girdle from the neck. In the Annals, History, and Guide to Leeds and York, according to Walford, there is mention of Ann Birch, who in 1781 was delivered of 10 children. One daughter, the sole survivor of the 10, married a market gardener named Platt, who was well known in Leeds. Jonston quotes Baytraff as saying that he knew of a case in which 9 children were born simultaneously; and also says that the Countess of Altdorf gave birth to twelve at one birth. Albucasis mentions a case of fifteen well-formed children at a birth. According to Le Brun, Gilles de Trazegines, who accompanied Saint Louis to Palestine, and who was made Constable of France, was one of thirteen infants at a simultaneous accouchement. The Marquise, his mother, was impregnated by her husband before his departure, and during his absence had 13 living children. She was suspected by the native people and thought to be an adulteress, and some of the children were supposed to be the result of superfetation. They condemned them all to be drowned, but the Marquis appeared upon the scene about this time and, moved by compassion, acknowledged all 13. They grew up and thrived, and took the name of Trazegines, meaning, in the old language, 13 drowned, although many commentaries say that "gines" was supposed to mean in the twelfth century "nes," or, in full, the interpretation would be "13 born."

Cases in which there is a repetition of multiple births are quite numerous, and sometimes so often repeated as to produce a family the size of which is almost incredible. Aristotle is credited with saying that he knew the history of a woman who had quintuplets four times. Pliny's case of quintuplets four times repeated has been mentioned; and Pare, who may be believed when he quotes from his own experience, says that the wife of the last Lord de Maldemeure, who lived in the Parish of Seaux, was a marvel of prolificity. Within a year after her marriage she gave birth to twins; in the next year to triplets; in the third year to quadruplets; in the fourth year to quintuplets, and in the fifth year bore sextuplets; in this last labor she died. The then present Lord de Maldemeure, he says, was one of the final sextuplets. This case attracted great notice at the time, as the family was quite noble and very well known. Seaux, their home, was near Chambellay. Picus Mirandulae gathered from the ancient Egyptian inscriptions that the women of Egypt brought forth sometimes 8 children at a birth, and that one woman bore 30 children in 4 confinements. He also cites, from the history of a certain Bishop of Necomus, that a woman named Antonia, in the Territory of Mutina, Italy, now called Modena, had brought forth 40 sons before she was forty years of age, and that she had had 3 and 4 at a birth. At the auction of the San Donato collection of pictures a portrait of Dianora Frescobaldi, by one of the Bronzinos in the sixteenth century, sold for about $3000. At the bottom of this portrait was an inscription stating that she was the mother of 52 children. This remarkable woman never had less than 3 at a birth, and tradition gives her as many as 6.

Merriman quotes a case of a woman, a shopkeeper named Blunet, who had 21 children in 7 successive births. They were all born alive, and 12 still survived and were healthy. As though to settle the question as to whom should be given the credit in this case, the father or the mother, the father experimented upon a female servant, who, notwithstanding her youth and delicateness, gave birth to 3 male children that lived three weeks. According to despatches from Lafayette, Indiana, investigation following the murder, on December 22, 1895, of Hester Curtis, an aged woman of that city, developed the rather remarkable fact that she had been the mother of 25 children, including 7 pairs of twins.

According to a French authority the wife of a medical man at Fuentemajor, in Spain, forty-three years of age, was delivered of triplets 13 times. Puech read a paper before the French Academy in which he reports 1262 twin births in Nimes from 1790 to 1875, and states that of the whole number in 48 cases the twins were duplicated, and in 2 cases thrice repeated, and in one case 4 times repeated.

Warren gives an instance of a lady, Mrs. M——, thirty-two years of age, married at fourteen, who, after the death of her first child, bore twins, one living a month and the other six weeks. Later she again bore twins, both of whom died. She then miscarried with triplets, and afterward gave birth to 12 living children, as follows: July 24, 1858, 1 child; June 30, 1859, 2 children; March 24, 1860, 2 children; March 1, 1861, 3 children; February 13, 1862, 4 children; making a total of 21 children in eighteen years, with remarkable prolificity in the later pregnancies. She was never confined to her bed more than three days, and the children were all healthy.

A woman in Schlossberg, Germany, gave birth to twins; after a year, to triplets, and again, in another year, to 3 fairly strong boys. In the State Papers, Domestic Series, Charles I, according to Walford, appears an extract from a letter from George Garrard to Viscount Conway, which is as follows: "Sir John Melton, who entertained you at York, hath buried his wife, Curran's daughter. Within twelve months she brought him 4 sons and a daughter, 2 sons last summer, and at this birth 2 more and a daughter, all alive." Swan mentions a woman who gave birth to 6 children in seventeen months in 2 triple pregnancies. The first terminated prematurely, 2 children dying at once, the other in five weeks. The second was uneventful, the 3 children living at the time of the report. Rockwell gives the report of a case of a woman of twenty-eight, herself a twin, who gave birth to twins in January, 1879. They died after a few weeks, and in March, 1880, she again bore twins, one living three and the other nine weeks. On March 12, 1881, she gave birth to triplets. The first child, a male, weighed 7 pounds; the second, a female, 6 1/4 pounds; the third, a male, 5 1/2 pounds. The third child lived twenty days, the other two died of cholera infantum at the sixth month, attributable to the bottle-feeding. Banerjee gives the history of a case of a woman of thirty being delivered of her fourth pair of twins. Her mother was dead, but she had 3 sisters living, of one of which she was a twin, and the other 2 were twins. One of her sisters had 2 twin terms, 1 child surviving; like her own children, all were females. A second sister had a twin term, both males, 1 surviving. The other sister aborted female twins after a fall in the eighth month of pregnancy. The name of the patient was Mussamat Somni, and she was the wife of a respectable Indian carpenter.

There are recorded the most wonderful accounts of prolificity, in which, by repeated multiple births, a woman is said to have borne children almost beyond belief. A Naples correspondent to a Paris Journal gives the following: "About 2 or 3 stations beyond Pompeii, in the City of Nocera, lives Maddalena Granata, aged forty-seven, who was married at twenty-eight, and has given birth to 52 living and dead children, 49 being males. Dr. de Sanctis, of Nocera, states that she has had triplets 15 times."

Peasant Kirilow was presented to the Empress of Russia in 1853, at the age of seventy years. He had been twice married, and his first wife had presented him with 57 children, the fruits of 21 pregnancies. She had quadruplets four times, triplets seven times, and twins thrice. By his second wife he had 15 children, twins six times, and triplets once. This man, accordingly, was the father of 72 children, and, to magnify the wonder, all the children were alive at the time of presentation. Herman, in some Russian statistics, relates the instance of Fedor Vassilet, a peasant of the Moscow Jurisdiction, who in 1872, at the age of seventy-five years, was the father of 87 children. He had been twice married; his first wife bore him 69 children in 27 accouchements, having twins sixteen times, triplets seven times, and quadruplets four times, but never a single birth. His second wife bore him 18 children in 8 accouchements. In 1872, 83 of the 87 children were living. The author says this case is beyond all question, as the Imperial Academy of St. Petersburg, as well as the French Academy, have substantial proof of it. The family are still living in Russia, and are the object of governmental favors. The following fact is interesting from the point of exaggeration, if for nothing else: "The New York Medical Journal is accredited with publishing the following extract from the history of a journey to Saragossa, Barcelona, and Valencia, in the year 1585, by Philip II of Spain. The book was written by Henrique Cock, who accompanied Philip as his private secretary. On page 248 the following statements are to be found: At the age of eleven years, Margarita Goncalez, whose father was a Biscayian, and whose mother was French, was married to her first husband, who was forty years old. By him she had 78 boys and 7 girls. He died thirteen years after the marriage, and, after having remained a widow two years, the woman married again. By her second husband, Thomas Gchoa, she had 66 boys and 7 girls. These children were all born in Valencia, between the fifteenth and thirty-fifth year of the mother's age, and at the time when the account was written she was thirty-five years old and pregnant again. Of the children, 47 by the first husband and 52 by the second were baptized; the other births were still or premature. There were 33 confinements in all.

Extreme Prolificity by Single Births.—The number of children a woman may bring forth is therefore not to be accurately stated; there seems to be almost no limit to it, and even when we exclude those cases in which remarkable multiplicity at each birth augments the number, there are still some almost incredible cases on record. The statistics of the St. Pancras Royal Dispensary, 1853, estimated the number of children one woman may bear as from 25 to 69. Eisenmenger relates the history of a case of a woman in the last century bearing 51 children, and there is another case in which a woman bore 44 children, all boys. Atkinson speaks of a lady married at sixteen, dying when she was sixty-four, who had borne 39 children, all at single births, by one husband, whom she survived. The children, 32 daughters and 7 sons, all attained their majority. There was a case of a woman in America who in twenty-six years gave birth to 22 children, all at single births. Thoresby in his "History of Leeds," 1715, mentions three remarkable cases—one the wife of Dr. Phineas Hudson, Chancellor of York, as having died in her thirty-ninth year of her twenty-fourth child; another of Mrs. Joseph Cooper, as dying of her twenty-sixth child, and, lastly, of Mrs. William Greenhill, of a village in Hertford, England, who gave birth to 39 children during her life. Brand, a writer of great repute, in his "History of Newcastle," quoted by Walford, mentions as a well attested fact the wife of a Scotch weaver who bore 62 children by one husband, all of whom lived to be baptized.

A curious epitaph is to be seen at Conway, Carnarvonshire—

"Here lieth the body of Nicholas Hookes, of Conway, gentleman, who was one-and-fortieth child of his father, William Hookes, Esq., by Alice, his wife, and the father of 27 children. He died 20th of March, 1637."

On November 21, 1768, Mrs. Shury, the wife of a cooper, in Vine Street, Westminster, was delivered of 2 boys, making 26 by the same husband. She had previously been confined with twins during the year.

It would be the task of a mathematician to figure the possibilities of paternity in a man of extra long life who had married several prolific women during his prolonged period of virility. A man by the name of Pearsons of Lexton, Nottingham, at the time of the report had been married 4 times. By his first 3 wives he had 39 children and by his last 14, making a total of 53. He was 6 feet tall and lived to his ninety-sixth year. We have already mentioned the two Russian cases in which the paternity was 72 and 87 children respectively, and in "Notes and Queries," June 21, 1856, there is an account of David Wilson of Madison, Ind., who had died a few years previously at the age of one hundred and seven. He had been 5 times married and was the father of 47 children, 35 of whom were living at the time of his death.

On a tomb in Ely, Cambridgeshire, there is an inscription saying that Richard Worster, buried there, died on May 11, 1856, the tomb being in memory of his 22 sons and 5 daughters.

Artaxerxes was supposed to have had 106 children; Conrad, Duke of Moscow, 80; and in the polygamous countries the number seems incredible. Herotinus was said to have had 600; and Jonston also quotes instances of 225 and even of 650 in the Eastern countries.

Recently there have been published accounts of the alleged experiments of Luigi Erba, an Italian gentleman of Perugia, whose results have been announced. About forty years of age and being quite wealthy, this bizarre philanthropist visited various quarters of the world, securing women of different races; having secured a number sufficient for his purposes, he retired with them to Polynesia, where he is accredited with maintaining a unique establishment with his household of females. In 1896, just seven years after the experiment commenced, the reports say he is the father of 370 children.

The following is a report from Raleigh, N.C., on July 28, 1893, to the New York Evening Post:—

"The fecundity of the negro race has been the subject of much comment and discussion. A case has come to light in this State that is one of the most remarkable on record. Moses Williams, a negro farmer, lives in the eastern section of this State. He is sixty-five years old (as nearly as he can make out), but does not appear to be over fifty. He has been married twice, and by the two wives has had born to him 45 children. By the first wife he had 23 children, 20 of whom were girls and 3 were boys. By the second wife he had 22 children—20 girls and 2 boys. He also has about 50 grand-children. The case is well authenticated."

We also quote the following, accredited to the "Annals of Hygiene:"—

"Were it not part of the records of the Berks County courts, we could hardly credit the history of John Heffner, who was accidentally killed some years ago at the age of sixty-nine. He was married first in 1840. In eight years his wife bore him 17 children. The first and second years of their marriage she gave birth to twins. For four successive years afterward she gave birth to triplets. In the seventh year she gave birth to one child and died soon afterward. Heffner engaged a young woman to look after his large brood of babies, and three months later she became the second Mrs. Heffner. She presented her husband with 2 children in the first two years of her wedded life. Five years later she had added 10 more to the family, having twins 5 times. Then for three years she added but 1 a year. At the time of the death of the second wife 12 of the 32 children had died. The 20 that were left did not appear to be any obstacle to a young widow with one child consenting to become the third wife of the jolly little man, for he was known as one of the happiest and most genial of men, although it kept him toiling like a slave to keep a score of mouths in bread. The third Mrs. Heffner became the mother of 9 children in ten years, and the contentment and happiness of the couple were proverbial. One day, in the fall of 1885, the father of the 41 children was crossing a railroad track and was run down by a locomotive and instantly killed. His widow and 24 of the 42 children are still living."

Many Marriages.—In this connection it seems appropriate to mention a few examples of multimarriages on record, to give an idea of the possibilities of the extent of paternity. St. Jerome mentions a widow who married her twenty-second husband, who in his time had taken to himself 20 loving spouses. A gentleman living in Bordeaux in 1772 had been married 16 times. DeLongueville, a Frenchman, lived to be one hundred and ten years old, and had been joined in matrimony to 10 wives, his last wife bearing him a son in his one hundred and first year.

Possible Descendants.—When we indulge ourselves as to the possible number of living descendants one person may have, we soon get extraordinary figures. The Madrid Estafette states that a gentleman, Senor Lucas Nequeiras Saez, who emigrated to America seventy years previously, recently returned to Spain in his own steamer, and brought with him his whole family, consisting of 197 persons. He had been thrice married, and by his first wife had 11 children at 7 births; by his second wife, 19 at 13 births, and by his third wife, 7 at 6 births. The youngest of the 37 was thirteen years old and the eldest seventy. This latter one had a son aged forty-seven and 16 children besides. He had 34 granddaughters, 45 grandsons, 45 great granddaughters, 39 great grandsons, all living. Senor Saez himself was ninety-three years old and in excellent health.

At Litchfield, Conn., there is said to be the following inscription:—

"Here lies the body of Mrs. Mary, wife of Dr. John Bull, Esq. She died November 4, 1778, aetat. ninety, having had 13 children, 101 grandchildren, 274 great grandchildren, and 22 great-great grandchildren, a total of 410; surviving, 336."

In Esher Church there is an inscription, scarcely legible, which records the death of the mother of Mrs. Mary Morton on April 18, 1634, and saying that she was the wonder of her sex and age, for she lived to see nearly 400 issued from her loins.

The following is a communication to "Notes and Queries," March 21, 1891: "Mrs. Mary Honeywood was daughter and one of the coheiresses of Robert Waters, Esq., of Lenham, in Kent. She was born in 1527; married in February, 1543, at sixteen years of age, to her only husband, Robert Honeywood, Esq., of Charing, in Kent. She died in the ninety-third year of her age, in May, 1620. She had 16 children of her own body, 7 sons and 9 daughters, of whom one had no issue, 3 died young—the youngest was slain at Newport battle, June 20, 1600. Her grandchildren, in the second generation, were 114; in the third, 228, and in the fourth, 9; so that she could almost say the same as the distich doth of one of the Dalburg family of Basil: 'Rise up, daughter and go to thy daughter, for thy daughter's daughter hath a daughter.'

"In Markshal Church, in Essex, on Mrs. Honeywood's tomb is the following inscription: 'Here lieth the body of Mary Waters, the daughter and coheir of Robert Waters, of Lenham, in Kent, wife of Robert Honeywood, of Charing, in

Kent, her only husband, who had at her decease, lawfully descended from her, 367 children, 16 of her own body, 114 grandchildren, 228 in the third generation, and 9 in the fourth. She lived a most pious life and died at Markshal, in the ninety-third year of her age and the forty-fourth of her widowhood, May 11, 1620.' (From 'Curiosities for the Ingenious,' 1826.)   S. S. R."

Animal prolificity though not finding a place in this work, presents some wonderful anomalies.

In illustration we may note the following: In the Illustrated London News, May 11, 1895, is a portrait of "Lady Millard," a fine St. Bernard bitch, the property of Mr. Thorp of Northwold, with her litter of 21 puppies, born on February 9, 1896, their sire being a magnificent dog—"Young York." There is quoted an incredible account of a cow, the property of J. N. Sawyer of Ohio, which gave birth to 56 calves, one of which was fully matured and lived, the others being about the size of kittens; these died, together with the mother. There was a cow in France, in 1871, delivered of 5 calves.

CHAPTER V

MAJOR TERATA.

Monstrosities have attracted notice from the earliest time, and many of the ancient philosophers made references to them. In mythology we read of Centaurs, impossible beings who had the body and extremities of a beast; the Cyclops, possessed of one enormous eye; or their parallels in Egyptian myths, the men with pectoral eyes,—the creatures "whose heads do beneath their shoulders grow;" and the Fauns, those sylvan deities whose lower extremities bore resemblance to those of a goat. Monsters possessed of two or more heads or double bodies are found in the legends and fairy tales of every nation. Hippocrates, his precursors, Empedocles and Democritus, and Pliny, Aristotle, and Galen, have all described monsters, although in extravagant and ridiculous language.

Ballantyne remarks that the occasional occurrence of double monsters was a fact known to the Hippocratic school, and is indicated by a passage in De morbis muliebribus, in which it is said that labor is gravely interfered with when the infant is dead or apoplectic or double. There is also a reference to monochorionic twins (which are by modern teratologists regarded as monstrosities) in the treatise De Superfoetatione, in which it is stated that "a woman, pregnant with twins, gives birth to them both at the same time, just as she has conceived them; the two infants are in a single chorion."

Ancient Explanations of Monstrosities.—From the time of Galen to the sixteenth century many incredible reports of monsters are seen in medical literature, but without a semblance of scientific truth. There has been little improvement in the mode of explanation of monstrous births until the present century, while in the Middle Ages the superstitions were more ludicrous and observers more ignorant than before the time of Galen. In his able article on the teratologic records of Chaldea, Ballantyne makes the following trite statements: "Credulity and superstition have never been the peculiar possession of the lower types of civilization only, and the special beliefs that have gathered round the occurrence of teratologic phenomena have been common to the cultured Greek and Roman of the past, the ignorant peasant of modern times, and the savage tribes of all ages. Classical writings, the literature of the Middle Ages, and the popular beliefs of the present day all contain views concerning teratologic subjects which so closely resemble those of the Chaldean magi as to be indistinguishable from them. Indeed, such works as those of Obsequens, Lycosthenes, Licetus, and Ambroise Pare only repeat, but with less accuracy of description and with greater freedom of imagination, the beliefs of ancient Babylon. Even at the present time the most impossible cases of so-called 'maternal impressions' are widely scattered through medical literature; and it is not very long since I received a letter from a distinguished member of the profession asking me whether, in my opinion, I thought it possible for a woman to give birth to a dog. Of course, I do not at all mean to infer that teratology has not made immense advances within recent times, nor do I suggest that on such subjects the knowledge of the magi can be compared with that of the average medical student of the present; but what I wish to emphasize is that, in the literature of ancient Babylonia, there are indications of an acquaintance with structural defects and malformations of the human body which will compare favorably with even the writings of the sixteenth century of the Christian era."

Many reasons were given for the existence of monsters, and in the Middle Ages these were as faulty as the descriptions themselves. They were interpreted as divinations, and were cited as forebodings and examples of wrath, or even as glorifications of the Almighty. The semi-human creatures were invented or imagined, and cited as the results of bestiality and allied forms of sexual perversion prevalent in those times. We find minute descriptions and portraits of these impossible results of wicked practices in many of the older medical books. According to Pare there was born in 1493, as the result of illicit intercourse between a woman and a dog, a creature resembling in its upper extremities its mother, while its lower extremities were the exact counterpart of its canine father. This particular case was believed by Bateman and others to be a precursor to the murders and wickedness that followed in the time of Pope Alexander I. Volateranus, Cardani, and many others cite instances of this kind. Lycosthenes says that in the year 1110, in the bourg of Liege, there was found a creature with the head, visage, hands, and feet of a man, and the rest of the body like that of a pig. Pare quotes this case and gives an illustration. Rhodiginus mentions a shepherd of Cybare by the name of Cratain, who had connection with a female goat and impregnated her, so that she brought forth a beast with a head resembling that of the father, but with the lower extremities of a goat. He says that the likeness to the father was so marked that the head-goat of the herd recognized it, and accordingly slew the goatherd who had sinned so unnaturally.

In the year 1547, at Cracovia, a very strange monster was born, which lived three days. It had a head shaped like that of a man; a nose long and hooked like an elephant's trunk; the hands and feet looking like the web-foot of a goose; and a tail with a hook on it. It was supposed to be a male, and was looked upon as a result of sodomy. Rueff says that the procreation of human beings and beasts is brought about—

(1) By the natural appetite;

(2) By the provocation of nature by delight;

(3) By the attractive virtue of the matrix, which in beasts and women is alike.

Plutarch, in his "Lesser Parallels," says that Aristonymus Ephesius, son of Demonstratus, being tired of women, had carnal knowledge with an ass, which in the process of time brought forth a very beautiful child, who became the maid Onoscelin. He also speaks of the origin of the maiden Hippona, or as he calls her, Hippo, as being from the connection of a man with a mare. Aristotle mentions this in his paradoxes, and we know that the patron of horses was Hippona. In Helvetia was reported the existence of a colt (whose mother had been covered by a bull) that was half horse and half bull. One of the kings of France was supposed to have been presented with a colt with the hinder part of a hart, and which could outrun any horse in the kingdom. Its mother had been covered by a hart.

Writing in 1557, Lycosthenes reports the mythical birth of a serpent by a woman. It is quite possible that some known and classified type of monstrosity was indicated here in vague terms. In 1726 Mary Toft, of Godalming, in Surrey, England, achieved considerable notoriety throughout Surrey, and even over all England, by her extensively circulated statements that she bore rabbits. Even at so late a day as this the credulity of the people was so great that many persons believed in her. The woman was closely watched, and being detected in her maneuvers confessed her fraud. To show the extent of discussion this case called forth, there are no less than nine pamphlets and books in the Surgeon-General's library at Washington devoted exclusively to this case of pretended rabbit-breeding. Hamilton in 1848, and Hard in 1884, both report the births in this country of fetal monstrosities with heads which showed marked resemblance to those of dogs. Doubtless many of the older cases of the supposed results of bestiality, if seen to-day, could be readily classified among some of our known forms of monsters. Modern investigation has shown us the sterile results of the connections between man and beast or between beasts of different species, and we can only wonder at the simple credulity and the imaginative minds of our ancestors. At one period certain phenomena of nature, such as an eclipse or comet, were thought to exercise their influence on monstrous births. Rueff mentions that in Sicily there happened a great eclipse of the sun, and that women immediately began to bring forth deformed and double-headed children.

Before ending these preliminary remarks, there might be mentioned the marine monsters, such as mermaids, sea-serpents, and the like, which from time to time have been reported; even at the present day there are people who devoutly believe that they have seen horrible and impossible demons in the sea. Pare describes and pictures a monster, at Rome, on November 3, 1520, with the upper portion of a child apparently about five or six years old, and the lower part and ears of a fishlike animal. He also pictures a sea-devil in the same chapter, together with other gruesome examples of the power of imagination.

Early Teratology.—Besides such cases as the foregoing, we find the medieval writers report likely instances of terata, as, for instance, Rhodiginus, who speaks of a monster in Italy with two heads and two bodies; Lycosthenes saw a double monster, both components of which slept at the same time; he also says this creature took its food and drink simultaneously in its two mouths. Even Saint Augustine says that he knew of a child born in the Orient who, from the belly up, was in all parts double.

The first evidences of a step toward classification and definite reasoning in regard to the causation of monstrosities were evinced by Ambroise Pare in the sixteenth century, and though his ideas are crude and some of his phenomena impossible, yet many of his facts and arguments are worthy of consideration. Pare attributed the cause of anomalies of excess to an excessive quantity of semen, and anomalies of default to deficiency of the same fluid. He has collected many instances of double terata from reliable sources, but has interspersed his collection with accounts of some hideous and impossible creatures, such as are illustrated in the accompanying figure, which shows a creature that was born shortly after a battle of Louis XII, in 1512; it had the wings, crest, and lower extremity of a bird and a human head and trunk; besides, it was an hermaphrodite, and had an extra eye in the knee. Another illustration represents a monstrous head found in an egg, said to have been sent for examination to King Charles at Metz in 1569. It represented the face and visage of a man, with small living serpents taking the place of beard and hair. So credulous were people at this time that even a man so well informed as Pare believed in the possibility of these last two, or at least represented them as facts. At this time were also reported double hermaphroditic terata, seemingly without latter-day analogues. Rhodiginus speaks of a two-headed monster born in Ferrari, Italy, in 1540, well formed, and with two sets of genitals, one male and the other female. Pare gives a picture of twins, born near Heidelberg in 1486, which had double bodies joined back to back; one of the twins had the aspect of a female and the other of a male, though both had two sets of genitals.

Scientific Teratology.—About the first half of the eighteenth century what might be called the positive period of teratology begins. Following the advent of this era come Mery, Duverney, Winslow, Lemery, and Littre. In their works true and concise descriptions are given and violent attacks are made against the ancient beliefs and prejudices. From the beginning of the second half of the last century to the present time may be termed the scientific epoch of teratology. We can almost with a certainty start this era with the names of Haller, Morgagni, Geoffroy-Saint-Hilaire, and Meckel, who adduced the explanations asked for by Harvey and Wolff. From the appearance of the treatise by Geoffroy-Saint-Hilaire, teratology has made enormous strides, and is to-day well on the road to becoming a science. Hand in hand with embryology it has been the subject of much investigation in this century, and to enumerate the workers of the present day who have helped to bring about scientific progress would be a task of many pages. Even in the artificial production of monsters much has been done, and a glance at the work of Dareste well repays the trouble. Essays on teratogenesis, with reference to batrachians, have been offered by Lombardini; and by Lereboullet and Knoch with reference to fishes. Foll and Warynski have reported their success in obtaining visceral inversion, and even this branch of the subject promises to become scientific.

Terata are seen in the lower animals and always excite interest. Pare gives the history of a sheep with three heads, born in 1577; the central head was larger than the other two, as shown in the accompanying illustration. Many of the Museums of Natural History contain evidences of animal terata. At Hallae is a two-headed mouse; the Conant Museum in Maine contains the skeleton of an adult sheep with two heads; there was an account of a two-headed pigeon published in France in 1734; Leidy found a two-headed snake in a field near Philadelphia; Geoffroy Saint-Hilaire and Conant both found similar creatures, and there is one in the Museum at Harvard; Wyman saw a living double-headed snake in the Jardin des Plantes in Paris in 1853, and many parallel instances are on record.

Classification.—We shall attempt no scientific discussion of the causation or embryologic derivation of the monster, contenting ourselves with simple history and description, adding any associate facts of interest that may be suggested. For further information, the reader is referred to the authors cited or to any of the standard treatises on teratology.

Many classifications of terata have been offered, and each possesses some advantage. The modern reader is referred to the modification of the grouping of Geoffroy-Saint-Hilaire given by Hirst and Piersol, or those of Blanc and Guinard. For convenience, we have adopted the following classification, which will include only those monsters that have LIVED AFTER BIRTH, and who have attracted general notice or attained some fame in their time, as attested by accounts in contemporary literature.

CLASS 1.—Union of several fetuses. CLASS 2.—Union of two distinct fetuses by a connecting band. CLASS 3.—Union of two distinct fetuses by an osseous junction of the cranial bones. CLASS 4.—Union of two distinct fetuses in which one or more parts are eliminated by the junction. CLASS 5.—Fusion of two fetuses by a bony union of the ischii. CLASS 6.—Fusion of two fetuses below the umbilicus into a common lower extremity. CLASS 7.—Bicephalic monsters. CLASS 8.—Parasitic monsters. CLASS 9.—Monsters with a single body and double lower extremities. CLASS 10.—Diphallic terata. CLASS 11.—Fetus in fetu, and dermoid cysts. CLASS 12.—Hermaphrodites.

CLASS I.—Triple Monsters.—Haller and Meckel were of the opinion that no cases of triple monsters worthy of credence are on record, and since their time this has been the popular opinion. Surely none have ever lived. Licetus describes a human monster with two feet and seven heads and as many arms. Bartholinus speaks of a three-headed monster who after birth gave vent to horrible cries and expired. Borellus speaks of a three-headed dog, a veritable Cerberus. Blasius published an essay on triple monsters in 1677. Bordenave is quoted as mentioning a human monster formed of three fetuses, but his description proves clearly that it was only the union of two. Probably the best example of this anomaly that we have was described by Galvagni at Cattania in 1834. This monster had two necks, on one of which was a single head normal in dimensions. On the other neck were two heads, as seen in the accompanying illustration. Geoffroy-Saint-Hilaire mentions several cases, and Martin de Pedro publishes a description of a case in Madrid in 1879. There are also on record some cases of triple monster by inclusion which will be spoken of later. Instances in the lower animals have been seen, the three-headed sheep of Pare, already spoken of, being one.

CLASS II.—Double Monsters.—A curious mode of junction, probably the most interesting, as it admits of longer life in these monstrosities, is that of a simple cartilaginous band extending between two absolutely distinct and different individuals. The band is generally in the sternal region. In 1752 there was described a remarkable monstrosity which consisted of conjoined twins, a perfect and an imperfect child, connected at their ensiform cartilages by a band 4 inches in circumference. The Hindoo sisters, described by Dr. Andrew Berry, lived to be seven years old; they stood face to face, with their chests 6 1/2 inches and their pubes 8 1/2 inches apart. Mitchell describes the full-grown female twins, born at Newport, Ky., called the Newport twins. The woman who gave birth to them became impregnated, it is said, immediately after seeing the famous Siamese twins, and the products of this pregnancy took the conformation of those celebrated exhibitionists.

Perhaps the best known of all double monsters were the Siamese twins. They were exhibited all over the globe and had the additional benefit and advertisement of a much mooted discussion as to the advisability of their severance, in which opinions of the leading medical men of all nations were advanced. The literature on these famous brothers is simply stupendous. The amount of material in the Surgeon General's library at Washington would surprise an investigator. A curious volume in this library is a book containing clippings, advertisements, and divers portraits of the twins. It will be impossible to speak at all fully on this subject, but a short history and running review of their lives will be given: Eng and Chang were born in Siam about May, 1811. Their father was of Chinese extraction and had gone to Siam and there married a woman whose father was also a Chinaman. Hence, for the most part, they were of Chinese blood, which probably accounted for their dark color and Chinese features. Their mother was about thirty-five years old at the time of their birth and had borne 4 female children prior to Chang and Eng. She afterward had twins several times, having eventually 14 children in all. She gave no history of special significance of the pregnancy, although she averred that the head of one and the feet of the other were born at the same time. The twins were both feeble at birth, and Eng continued delicate, while Chang thrived. It was only with difficulty that their lives were saved, as Chowpahyi, the reigning king, had a superstition that such freaks of nature always presaged evil to the country. They were really discovered by Robert Hunter, a British merchant at Bangkok, who in 1824 saw them boating and stripped to the waist. He prevailed on the parents and King Chowpahyi to allow them to go away for exhibition. They were first taken out of the country by a certain Captain Coffin. The first scientific description of them was given by Professor J. C. Warren, who examined them in Boston, at the Harvard University, in 1829. At that time Eng was 5 feet 2 inches and Chang 5 feet 1 1/2 inches in height. They presented all the characteristics of Chinamen and wore long black queues coiled thrice around their heads, as shown by the accompanying illustration. After an eight-weeks' tour over the Eastern States they went to London, arriving at that port November 20, 1829. Their tour in France was forbidden on the same grounds as the objection to the exhibition of Ritta-Christina, namely, the possibility of causing the production of monsters by maternal impressions in pregnant women. After their European tour they returned to the United States and settled down as farmers in North Carolina, adopting the name of Bunker. When forty-four years of age they married two sisters, English women, twenty-six and twenty-eight years of age, respectively. Domestic infelicity soon compelled them to keep the wives at different houses, and they alternated weeks in visiting each wife. Chang had six children and Eng five, all healthy and strong. In 1869 they made another trip to Europe, ostensibly to consult the most celebrated surgeons of Great Britain and France on the advisability of being separated. It was stated that a feeling of antagonistic hatred after a quarrel prompted them to seek "surgical separation," but the real cause was most likely to replenish their depleted exchequer by renewed exhibition and advertisement.

A most pathetic characteristic of these illustrious brothers was the affection and forbearance they showed for each other until shortly before their death. They bore each other's trials and petty maladies with the greatest sympathy, and in this manner rendered their lives far more agreeable than a casual observer would suppose possible. They both became Christians and members or attendants of the Baptist Church.

Figure 31 is a representation of the Siamese twins in old age. On each side of them is a son. The original photograph is in the Mutter Museum, College of Physicians, Philadelphia.

The feasibility of the operation of separating them was discussed by many of the leading men of America, and Thompson, Fergusson, Syme, Sir J. Y. Simpson, Nelaton, and many others in Europe, with various reports and opinions after examination. These opinions can be seen in full in nearly any large medical library. At this time they had diseased and atheromatous arteries, and Chang, who was quite intemperate, had marked spinal curvature, and shortly afterward became hemiplegic. They were both partially blind in their two anterior eyes, possibly from looking outward and obliquely. The point of junction was about the sterno-siphoid angle, a cartilaginous band extending from sternum to sternum. In 1869 Simpson measured this band and made the distance on the superior aspect from sternum to sternum 4 1/2 inches, though it is most likely that during the early period of exhibition it was not over 3 inches. The illustration shows very well the position of the joining band.

The twins died on January 17, 1874, and a committee of surgeons from the College of Physicians of Philadelphia, consisting of Doctors Andrews, Allen, and Pancoast, went to North Carolina to perform an autopsy on the body, and, if possible, to secure it. They made a long and most interesting report on the results of their trip to the College. The arteries, as was anticipated, were found to have undergone calcareous degeneration. There was an hepatic connection through the band, and also some interlacing diaphragmatic fibers therein. There was slight vascular intercommunication of the livers and independence of the two peritoneal cavities and the intestines. The band itself was chiefly a coalescence of the xyphoid cartilages, surrounded by areolar tissue and skin.

The "Orissa sisters," or Radica-Doddica, shown in Europe in 1893, were similar to the Siamese twins in conformation. They were born in Orissa, India, September, 1889, and were the result of the sixth pregnancy, the other five being normal. They were healthy girls, four years of age, and apparently perfect in every respect, except that, from the ensiform cartilage to the umbilicus, they were united by a band 4 inches long and 2 inches wide. The children when facing each other could draw their chests three or four inches apart, and the band was so flexible that they could sit on either side of the body. Up to the date mentioned it was not known whether the connecting band contained viscera. A portrait of these twins was shown at the World's Fair in Chicago.

In the village of Arasoor, district of Bhavany, there was reported a monstrosity in the form of two female children, one 34 inches and the other 33 3/4 inches high, connected by the sternum. They were said to have had small-pox and to have recovered. They seemed to have had individual nervous systems, as when one was pinched the other did not feel it, and while one slept the other was awake. There must have been some vascular connection, as medicine given to one affected both.

Fig. 36 shows a mode of cartilaginous junction by which each component of a double monster may be virtually independent.

Operations on Conjoined Twins.—Swingler speaks of two girls joined at the xiphoid cartilage and the umbilicus, the band of union being 1 1/2 inches thick, and running below the middle of it was the umbilical cord, common to both. They first ligated the cord, which fell off in nine days, and then separated the twins with the bistoury. They each made early recovery and lived.

In the Ephemerides of 1690 Konig gives a description of two Swiss sisters born in 1689 and united belly to belly, who were separated by means of a ligature and the operation afterward completed by an instrument. The constricting band was formed by a coalition of the xiphoid cartilages and the umbilical vessels, surrounded by areolar tissue and covered with skin. Le Beau says that under the Roman reign, A. D. 945, two male children were brought from Armenia to Constantinople for exhibition. They were well formed in every respect and united by their abdomens. After they had been for some time an object of great curiosity, they were removed by governmental order, being considered a presage of evil. They returned, however, at the commencement of the reign of Constantine VII, when one of them took sick and died. The surgeons undertook to preserve the other by separating him from the corpse of his brother, but he died on the third day after the operation.

In 1866 Boehm gives an account of Guzenhausen's case of twins who were united sternum to sternum. An operation for separation was performed without accident, but one of the children, already very feeble, died three days after; the other survived. The last attempt at an operation like this was in 1881, when Biaudet and Buginon attempted to separate conjoined sisters (Marie-Adele) born in Switzerland on June 26th. Unhappily, they were very feeble and life was despaired of when the operation was performed, on October 29th. Adele died six hours afterward, and Marie died of peritonitis on the next day.

CLASS III.—Those monsters joined by a fusion of some of the cranial bones are sometimes called craniopagi. A very ancient observation of this kind is cited by Geoffroy-Saint-Hilaire. These two girls were born in 1495, and lived to be ten years old. They were normal in every respect, except that they were joined at the forehead, causing them to stand face to face and belly to belly. When one walked forward, the other was compelled to walk backward; their noses almost touched, and their eyes were directed laterally. At the death of one an attempt to separate the other from the cadaver was made, but it was unsuccessful, the second soon dying; the operation necessitated opening the cranium and parting the meninges. Bateman said that in 1501 there was living an instance of double female twins, joined at the forehead. This case was said to have been caused in the following manner: Two women, one of whom was pregnant with the twins at the time, were engaged in an earnest conversation, when a third, coming up behind them, knocked their heads together with a sharp blow. Bateman describes the death of one of the twins and its excision from the other, who died subsequently, evidently of septic infection. There is a possibility that this is merely a duplication of the account of the preceding case with a slight anachronism as to the time of death.

At a foundling hospital in St. Petersburg there were born two living girls, in good health, joined by the heads. They were so united that the nose of one, if prolonged, would strike the ear of the other; they had perfectly independent existences, but their vascular systems had evident connection.

Through extra mobility of their necks they could really lie in a straight line, one sleeping on the side and the other on the back. There is a report a of two girls joined at their vertices, who survived their birth. With the exception of this junction they were well formed and independent in existence. There was no communication of the cranial cavities, but simply fusion of the cranial bones covered by superficial fascia and skin. Daubenton has seen a case of union at the occiput, but further details are not quoted.

CLASS IV.—The next class to be considered is that in which the individuals are separate and well formed, except that the point of fusion is a common part, eliminating their individual components in this location. The pygopagous twins belong in this section. According to Bateman, twins were born in 1493 at Rome joined back to back, and survived their birth. The same authority speaks of a female child who was born with "2 bellies, 4 arms, 4 legs, 2 heads, and 2 sets of privates, and was exhibited throughout Italy for gain's sake." The "Biddenden Maids" were born in Biddenden, Kent, in 1100. Their names were Mary and Eliza Chulkhurst, and their parents were fairly well-to-do people. They were supposed to have been united at the hips and the shoulders, and lived until 1134. At the death of one it was proposed to separate them, but the remaining sister refused, saying, "As we came together, we will also go together," and, after about six hours of this Mezentian existence, they died. They bequeathed to the churchwardens of the parish and their successors land to the extent of 20 acres, at the present time bringing a rental of about $155.00 annually, with the instructions that the money was to be spent in the distribution of cakes (bearing the impression of their images, to be given away on each Easter Sunday to all strangers in Biddenden) and also 270 quartern loaves, with cheese in proportion, to all the poor in said parish. Ballantyne has accompanied his description of these sisters by illustrations, one of which shows the cake. Heaton gives a very good description of these maids; and a writer in "Notes and Queries" of March 27, 1875, gives the following information relative to the bequest:—

"On Easter Monday, at Biddenden, near Staplehurst, Kent, there is a distribution, according to ancient custom, of 'Biddenden Maids' cakes,' with bread and cheese, the cost of which is defrayed from the proceeds of some 20 acres of land, now yielding L35 per annum. and known as the 'Bread and Cheese Lands.' About the year 1100 there lived Eliza and Mary Chulkhurst, who were joined together after the manner of the Siamese twins, and who lived for thirty-four years, one dying, and then being followed by her sister within six hours. They left by their will the lands above alluded to and their memory is perpetuated by imprinting on the cakes their effigies 'in their habit as they lived.' The cakes, which are simple flour and water, are four inches long by two inches wide, and are much sought after as curiosities. These, which are given away, are distributed at the discretion of the church-wardens, and are nearly 300 in number. The bread and cheese amounts to 540 quartern loaves and 470 pounds of cheese. The distribution is made on land belonging to the charity, known as the Old Poorhouse. Formerly it used to take place in the Church, immediately after the service in the afternoon, but in consequence of the unseemly disturbance which used to ensue the practice was discontinued. The Church used to be filled with a congregation whose conduct was occasionally so reprehensible that sometimes the church-wardens had to use their wands for other purposes than symbols of office. The impressions of the maids 'on the cakes are of a primitive character, and are made by boxwood dies cut in 1814. They bear the date 1100, when Eliza and Mary Chulkhurst are supposed to have been born, and also their age at death, thirty-four years."

Ballantyne has summed up about all there is to be said on this national monstrosity, and his discussion of the case from its historic as well as teratologic standpoint is so excellent that his conclusions will be quoted—

"It may be urged that the date fixed for the birth of the Biddenden Maids is so remote as to throw grave doubt upon the reality of the occurrence. The year 1100 was, it will be remembered, that in which William Rufus was found dead in the New Forest, 'with the arrow either of a hunter or an assassin in his breast.' According to the Anglo-Saxon Chronicle, several 'prodigies' preceded the death of this profligate and extravagant monarch. Thus it is recorded that 'at Pentecost blood was observed gushing from the earth at a certain town of Berkshire, even as many asserted who declared that they had seen it. And after this, on the morning after Lammas Day, King William was shot.' Now, it is just possible that the birth of the Biddenden Maids may have occurred later, but have been antedated by the popular tradition to the year above mentioned. For such a birth would, in the opinion of the times, be regarded undoubtedly as a most evident prodigy or omen of evil. Still, even admitting that the date 1100 must be allowed to stand, its remoteness from the present time is not a convincing argument against a belief in the real occurrence of the phenomenon; for of the dicephalic Scottish brothers, who lived in 1490, we have credible historic evidence. Further, Lycosthenes, in his "Chronicon Prodigiorum atque Ostentorum", published in 1557, states, upon what authority I know not, that in the year 1112 joined twins resembling the Biddenden phenomenon in all points save in sex were born in England. The passage is as follows: 'In Anglia natus est puer geminus a clune ad superiores partes ita divisus, ut duo haberet capita, duo corpora integra ad renes cum suis brachiis, qui baptizatus triduo supervixit.' It is just possible that in some way or other this case has been confounded with the story of Biddenden; at any rate, the occurrence of such a statement in Lycosthenes' work is of more than passing interest. Had there been no bequest of land in connection with the case of the Kentish Maids, the whole affair would probably soon have been forgotten.

"There is, however, one real difficulty in accepting the story handed down to us as authentic,—the nature of the teratologic phenomenon itself. All the records agree in stating that the Maids were joined together at the shoulders and hips, and the impression on the cakes and the pictures on the 'broadsides' show this peculiar mode of union, and represent the bodies as quite separate in the space between the above-named points. The Maids are shown with four feet and two arms, the right and left respectively, whilst the other arms (left and right) are fused together at the shoulder according to one illustration, and a little above the elbow according to another. Now, although it is not safe to say that such an anomaly is impossible, I do not know of any case of this peculiar mode of union; but it may be that, as Prof. A. R. Simpson has suggested, the Maids had four separate arms, and were in the habit of going about with their contiguous arms round each other's necks, and that this gave rise to the notion that these limbs were united. If this be so, then the teratologic difficulty is removed, for the case becomes perfectly comparable with the well-known but rare type of double terata known as the pygopagous twins, which is placed by Taruffi with that of the ischiopagous twins in the group dicephalus lecanopagus. Similar instances, which are well known to students of teratology, are the Hungarian sisters (Helen and Judith), the North Carolina twins (Millie and Christine), and the Bohemian twins (Rosalie and Josepha Blazek). The interspace between the thoraces may, however, have simply been the addition of the first artist who portrayed the Maids (from imagination?); then it may be surmised that they were ectopagous twins.

"Pygopagous twins are fetuses united together in the region of the nates and having each its own pelvis. In the recorded cases the union has been usually between the sacra and coccyges, and has been either osseous or (more rarely) ligamentous. Sometimes the point of junction was the middle line posteriorly, at other times it was rather a posterolateral union; and it is probable that in the Biddenden Maids it was of the latter kind; and it is likely, from the proposal made to separate the sisters after the death of one, that it was ligamentous in nature.

"If it be granted that the Biddenden Maids were pygopagous twins, a study of the histories of other recorded cases of this monstrosity serves to demonstrate many common characters. Thus, of the 8 cases which Taruffi has collected, in 7 the twins were female; and if to these we add the sisters Rosalie and Josepha Blazek and the Maids, we have 10 cases, of which 9 were girls. Again, several of the pygopagous twins, of whom there are scientific records, survived birth and lived for a number of years, and thus resembled the Biddenden terata. Helen and Judith, for instance, were twenty-three years old at death; and the North Carolina twins, although born in 1851, are still alive. There is, therefore, nothing inherently improbable in the statement that the Biddenden Maids lived for thirty-four years. With regard also to the truth of the record that the one Maid survived her sister for six hours, there is confirmatory evidence from scientifically observed instances, for Joly and Peyrat (Bull. de l'Acad. Med., iii., pp. 51 and 383, 1874) state that in the case seen by them the one infant lived ten hours after the death of the other. It is impossible to make any statement with regard to the internal structure of the Maids or to the characters of their genital organs, for there is absolutely no information forthcoming upon these points. It may simply be said, in conclusion, that the phenomenon of Biddenden is interesting not only on account of the curious bequest which arose out of it, but also because it was an instance of a very rare teratologic type, occurring at a very early period in our national history."

Possibly the most famous example of twins of this type were Helen and Judith, the Hungarian sisters, born in 1701 at Szony, in Hungary. They were the objects of great curiosity, and were shown successively in Holland, Germany, Italy, France, England, and Poland. At the age of nine they were placed in a convent, where they died almost simultaneously in their twenty-second year. During their travels all over Europe they were examined by many prominent physiologists, psychologists, and naturalists; Pope and several minor poets have celebrated their existence in verse; Buffon speaks of them in his "Natural History," and all the works on teratology for a century or more have mentioned them. A description of them can be best given by a quaint translation by Fisher of the Latin lines composed by a Hungarian physician and inscribed on a bronze statuette of them: —

Two sisters wonderful to behold, who have thus grown as one, That naught their bodies can divide, no power beneath the sun. The town of Szoenii gave them birth, hard by far-famed Komorn, Which noble fort may all the arts of Turkish sultans scorn. Lucina, woman's gentle friend, did Helen first receive; And Judith, when three hours had passed, her mother's womb did leave. One urine passage serves for both;—one anus, so they tell; The other parts their numbers keep, and serve their owners well. Their parents poor did send them forth, the world to travel through, That this great wonder of the age should not be hid from view. The inner parts concealed do lie hid from our eyes, alas! But all the body here you view erect in solid brass.

They were joined back to back in the lumbar region, and had all their parts separate except the anus between the right thigh of Helen and the left of Judith and a single vulva. Helen was the larger, better looking, the more active, and the more intelligent. Judith at the age of six became hemiplegic, and afterward was rather delicate and depressed. They menstruated at sixteen and continued with regularity, although one began before the other. They had a mutual affection, and did all in their power to alleviate the circumstances of their sad position. Judith died of cerebral and pulmonary affections, and Helen, who previously enjoyed good health, soon after her sister's first indisposition suddenly sank into a state of collapse, although preserving her mental faculties, and expired almost immediately after her sister. They had measles and small-pox simultaneously, but were affected in different degree by the maladies. The emotions, inclinations, and appetites were not simultaneous. Eccardus, in a very interesting paper, discusses the physical, moral, and religious questions in reference to these wonderful sisters, such as the advisability of separation, the admissibility of matrimony, and, finally, whether on the last day they would rise as joined in life, or separated.

There is an account of two united females, similar in conjunction to the "Hungarian sisters," who were born in Italy in 1700. They were killed at the age of four months by an attempt of a surgeon to separate them.

In 1856 there was reported to have been born in Texas, twins after the manner of Helen and Judith, united back to back, who lived and attained some age. They were said to have been of different natures and dispositions, and inclined to quarrel very often.

Pancoast gives an extensive report of Millie-Christine, who had been extensively exhibited in Europe and the United States. They were born of slave parents in Columbus County, N.C., July 11, 1851; the mother, who had borne 8 children before, was a stout negress of thirty-two, with a large pelvis. The presentation was first by the stomach and afterward by the breech. These twins were united at the sacra by a cartilaginous or possibly osseous union. They were exhibited in Paris in 1873, and provoked as much discussion there as in the United States. Physically, Millie was the weaker, but had the stronger will and the dominating spirit. They menstruated regularly from the age of thirteen. One from long habit yielded instinctively to the other's movements, thus preserving the necessary harmony. They ate separately, had distinct thoughts, and carried on distinct conversations at the same time. They experienced hunger and thirst generally simultaneously, and defecated and urinated nearly at the same times. One, in tranquil sleep, would be wakened by a call of nature of the other. Common sensibility was experienced near the location of union. They were intelligent and agreeable and of pleasant appearance, although slightly under size; they sang duets with pleasant voices and accompanied themselves with a guitar; they walked, ran, and danced with apparent ease and grace. Christine could bend over and lift Millie up by the bond of union.

A recent example of the pygopagus type was Rosa-Josepha Blazek, born in Skerychov, in Bohemia, January 20, 1878. These twins had a broad bony union in the lower part of the lumbar region, the pelvis being obviously completely fused. They had a common urethral and anal aperture, but a double vaginal orifice, with a very apparent septum. The sensation was distinct in each, except where the pelves joined. They were exhibited in Paris in 1891, being then on an exhibition tour around the world. Rosa was the stronger, and when she walked or ran forward she drew her sister with her, who must naturally have reversed her steps. They had independent thoughts and separate minds; one could sleep while the other was awake. Many of their appetites were different, one preferring beer, the other wine; one relished salad, the other detested it, etc. Thirst and hunger were not simultaneous. Baudoin describes their anatomic construction, their mode of life, and their mannerisms and tastes in a quite recent article. Fig. 42 is a reproduction of an early photograph of the twins, and Fig. 43 represents a recent photograph of these "Bohemian twins," as they are now called.

The latest record we have of this type of monstrosity is that given by Tynberg to the County Medical Society of New York, May 27, 1895. The mother was present with the remarkable twins in her arms, crying at the top of their voices. These two children were born at midnight on April 15th. Tynberg remarked that he believed them to be distinct and separate children, and not dependent on a common arterial system; he also expressed his intention of separating them, but did not believe the operation could be performed with safety before another year. Jacobi describes in full Tynberg's instance of pygopagus. He says the confinement was easy; the head of one was born first, soon followed by the feet and the rest of the twins. The placenta was single and the cord consisted of two branches. The twins were united below the third sacral vertebrae in such a manner that they could lie alongside of each other. They were females, and had two vaginae, two urethrae four labia minora, and two labia majora, one anus, but a double rectum divided by a septum. They micturated independently but defecated simultaneously. They virtually lived separate lives, as one might be asleep while the other cried, etc.

CLASS V.—While instances of ischiopagi are quite numerous, few have attained any age, and, necessarily, little notoriety. Pare speaks of twins united at the pelves, who were born in Paris July 20, 1570. They were baptized, and named Louis and Louise. Their parents were well known in the rue des Gravelliers. According to Bateman, and also Rueff, in the year 1552 there were born, not far from Oxford, female twins, who, from the description given, were doubtless of the ischiopagus type. They seldom wept, and one was of a cheerful disposition, while the other was heavy and drowsy, sleeping continually. They only lived a short time, one expiring a day before the other. Licetus speaks of Mrs. John Waterman, a resident of Fishertown, near Salisbury, England, who gave birth to a double female monster on October 26, 1664, which evidently from the description was joined by the ischii. It did not nurse, but took food by both the mouths; all its actions were done in concert; it was possessed of one set of genitourinary organs; it only lived a short while. Many people in the region flocked to see the wonderful child, whom Licetus called "Monstrum Anglicum." It is said that at the same accouchement the birth of this monster was followed by the birth of a well-formed female child, who survived. Geoffroy-Saint-Hilaire quotes a description of twins who were born in France on October 7, 1838, symmetrically formed and united at their ischii. One was christened Marie-Louise, and the other Hortense-Honorine. Their avaricious parents took the children to Paris for exhibition, the exposures of which soon sacrificed their lives. In the year 1841 there was born in the island of Ceylon, of native parents, a monstrous child that was soon brought to Columbo, where it lived only two months. It had two heads and seemed to have duplication in all its parts except the anus and male generative organs. Montgomery speaks of a double child born in County Roscommon, Ireland, on the 24th of July, 1827. It had two heads, two chests with arms complete, two abdominal and pelvic cavities united end to end, and four legs, placed two on either side. It had only one anus, which was situated between the thighs. One of the twins was dark haired and was baptized Mary, while the other was a blonde and was named Catherine. These twins felt and acted independently of each other; they each in succession sucked from the breast or took milk from the spoon, and used their limbs vigorously. One vomited without affecting the other, but the feces were discharged through a common opening.

Goodell speaks of Minna and Minnie Finley, who were born in Ohio and examined by him. They were fused together in a common longitudinal axis, having one pelvis, two heads, four legs, and four arms. One was weak and puny and the other robust and active; it is probable that they had but one rectum and one bladder. Goodell accompanies his description by the mention of several analogous cases. Ellis speaks of female twins, born in Millville, Tenn., and exhibited in New York in 1868, who were joined at the pelves in a longitudinal axis. Between the limbs on either side were to be seen well-developed female genitals, and the sisters had been known to urinate from both sides, beginning and ending at the same time.

Huff details a description of the "Jones twins," born on June 24, 1889, in Tipton County, Indiana, whose spinal columns were in apposition at the lower end. The labor, of less than two hours' duration, was completed before the arrival of the physician. Lying on their mother's back, they could both nurse at the same time. Both sets of genitals and ani were on the same side of the line of union, but occupied normal positions with reference to the legs on either side. Their weight at birth was 12 pounds and their length 22 inches. Their mother was a medium-sized brunette of 19, and had one previous child then living at the age of two; their father was a finely formed man 5 feet 10 inches in height. The twins differed in complexion and color of the eyes and hair. They were publicly exhibited for some time, and died February 19 and 20, 1891, at St. John's Hotel, Buffalo, N.Y. Figure 45 shows their appearance several months after birth.

CLASS VI.—In our sixth class, the first record we have is from the Commentaries of Sigbert, which contains a description of a monstrosity born in the reign of the Emperor Theodosius, who had two heads, two chests with four arms attached, but a single lower extremity. The emotions, affections, and appetites were different. One head might be crying while the other laughed, or one feeding while the other was sleeping. At times they quarreled and occasionally came to blows. This monster is said to have lived two years, one part dying four days before the other, which evinced symptoms of decay like its inseparable neighbor.

Roger of Wendover says that in Lesser Brittany and Normandy, in 1062, there was seen a female monster, consisting of two women joined about the umbilicus and fused into a single lower extremity. They took their food by two mouths but expelled it at a single orifice. At one time, one of the women laughed, feasted, and talked, while the other wept, fasted, and kept a religious silence. The account relates how one of them died, and the survivor bore her dead sister about for three years before she was overcome by the oppression and stench of the cadaver. Batemen describes the birth of a boy in 1529, who had two heads, four ears, four arms, but only two thighs and two legs. Buchanan speaks at length of the famous "Scottish Brothers," who were the cynosure of the eyes of the Court of James III of Scotland. This monster consisted of two men, ordinary in appearance in the superior extremities, whose trunks fused into a single lower extremity. The King took diligent care of their education, and they became proficient in music, languages, and other court accomplishments. Between them they would carry on animated conversations, sometimes merging into curious debates, followed by blows. Above the point of union they had no synchronous sensations, while below, sensation was common to both. This monster lived twenty-eight years, surviving the royal patron, who died June, 1488. One of the brothers died some days before the other, and the survivor, after carrying about his dead brother, succumbed to "infection from putrescence." There was reported to have been born in Switzerland a double headed male monster, who in 1538, at the age of thirty, was possessed of a beard on each face, the two bodies fused at the umbilicus into a single lower extremity. These two twins resembled one another in contour and countenance. They were so joined that at rest they looked upon one another. They had a single wife, with whom they were said to have lived in harmony. In the Gentleman's Magazine about one hundred and fifty years since there was given the portrait and description of a double woman, who was exhibited all over the large cities of Europe. Little can be ascertained anatomically of her construction, with the exception that it was stated that she had two heads, two necks, four arms, two legs, one pelvis, and one set of pelvic organs.

The most celebrated monster of this type was Ritta-Christina, who was born in Sassari, in Sardinia, March 23, 1829. These twins were the result of the ninth confinement of their mother, a woman of thirty-two. Their superior extremities were double, but they joined in a common trunk at a point a little below the mammae. Below this point they had a common trunk and single lower extremities. The right one, christened Ritta, was feeble and of a sad and melancholy countenance; the left, Christina, was vigorous and of a gay and happy aspect. They suckled at different times, and sensations in the upper extremities were distinct. They expelled urine and feces simultaneously, and had the indications in common. Their parents, who were very poor, brought them to Paris for the purpose of public exhibition, which at first was accomplished clandestinely, but finally interdicted by the public authorities, who feared that it would open a door for psychologic discussion and speculation. This failure of the parents to secure public patronage increased their poverty and hastened the death of the children by unavoidable exposure in a cold room. The nervous system of the twins had little in common except in the line of union, the anus, and the sexual organs, and Christina was in good health all through Ritta's sickness; when Ritta died, her sister, who was suckling at the mother's breast, suddenly relaxed hold and expired with a sigh. At the postmortem, which was secured with some difficulty on account of the authorities ordering the bodies to be burned, the pericardium was found single, covering both hearts. The digestive organs were double and separate as far as the lower third of the ilium, and the cecum was on the left side and single, in common with the lower bowel. The livers were fused and the uterus was double. The vertebral columns, which were entirely separate above, were joined below by a rudimentary os innorminatum. There was a junction between the manubrium of each. Sir Astley Cooper saw a monster in Paris in 1792 which, by his description, must have been very similar to Ritta-Christina.

The Tocci brothers were born in 1877 in the province of Turin, Italy. They each had a well-formed head, perfect arms, and a perfect thorax to the sixth rib; they had a common abdomen, a single anus, two legs, two sacra, two vertebral columns, one penis, but three buttocks, the central one containing a rudimentary anus. The right boy was christened Giovanni-Batista, and the left Giacomo. Each individual had power over the corresponding leg on his side, but not over the other one. Walking was therefore impossible. All their sensations and emotions were distinctly individual and independent. At the time of the report, in 1882, they were in good health and showed every indication of attaining adult age. Figure 48 represents these twins as they were exhibited several years ago in Germany.

McCallum saw two female children in Montreal in 1878 named Marie-Rosa Drouin. They formed a right angle with their single trunk, which commenced at the lower part of the thorax of each. They had a single genital fissure and the external organs of generation of a female. A little over three inches from the anus was a rudimentary limb with a movable articulation; it measured five inches in length and tapered to a fine point, being furnished with a distinct nail, and it contracted strongly to irritation. Marie, the left child, was of fair complexion and more strongly developed than Rosa. The sensations of hunger and thirst were not experienced at the same time, and one might be asleep while the other was crying. The pulsations and the respiratory movements were not synchronous. They were the products of the second gestation of a mother aged twenty-six, whose abdomen was of such preternatural size during pregnancy that she was ashamed to appear in public. The order of birth was as follows: one head and body, the lower extremity, and the second body and head.

CLASS VII.—There are many instances of bicephalic monsters on record. Pare mentions and gives an illustration of a female apparently single in conformation, with the exception of having two heads and two necks. The Ephemerides, Haller, Schenck, and Archenholz cite examples, and there is an old account of a double-headed child, each of whose heads were baptized, one called Martha and the other Mary. One was of a gay and the other a sad visage, and both heads received nourishment; they only lived a couple of days. There is another similar record of a Milanese girl who had two heads, but was in all other respects single, with the exception that after death she was found to have had two stomachs. Besse mentions a Bavarian woman of twenty-six with two heads, one of which was comely and the other extremely ugly; Batemen quotes what is apparently the same case— a woman in Bavaria in 1541 with two heads, one of which was deformed, who begged from door to door, and who by reason of the influence of pregnant women was given her expenses to leave the country.

A more common occurrence of this type is that in which there is fusion of the two heads. Moreau speaks of a monster in Spain which was shown from town to town.

Its heads were fused; it had two mouths and two noses; in each face an eye well conformed and placed above the nose; there was a third eye in the middle of the forehead common to both heads; the third eye was of primitive development and had two pupils. Each face was well formed and had its own chin. Buffon mentions a cat, the exact analogue of Moreau's case. Sutton speaks of a photograph sent to Sir James Paget in 1856 by William Budd of Bristol. This portrays a living child with a supernumerary head, which had mouth, nose, eyes, and a brain of its own. The eyelids were abortive, and as there was no orbital cavity the eyes stood out in the form of naked globes on the forehead. When born, the corneas of both heads were transparent, but then became opaque from exposure. The brain of the supernumerary head was quite visible from without, and was covered by a membrane beginning to slough. On the right side of the head was a rudimentary external ear. The nurse said that when the child sucked some milk regurgitated through the supernumerary mouth. The great physiologic interest in this case lies in the fact that every movement and every act of the natural face was simultaneously repeated by the supernumerary face in a perfectly consensual manner, i.e., when the natural mouth sucked, the second mouth sucked; when the natural face cried, yawned, or sneezed, the second face did likewise; and the eyes of the two heads moved in unison. The fate of the child is not known.

Home speaks of a child born in Bengal with a most peculiar fusion of the head. The ordinary head was nearly perfect and of usual volume, but fused with its vertex and reversed was a supernumerary head. Each head had its own separate vessels and brain, and each an individual sensibility, but if one had milk first the other had an abundance of saliva in its mouth. It narrowly escaped being burned to death at birth, as the midwife, greatly frightened by the monstrous appearance, threw it into the fire to destroy it, from whence it was rescued, although badly burned, the vicious conformation of the accessory head being possibly due to the accident. At the age of four it was bitten by a venomous serpent and, as a result, died. Its skull is in the possession of the Royal College of Surgeons in London.

The following well-known story of Edward Mordake, though taken from lay sources, is of sufficient notoriety and interest to be mentioned here:—

"One of the weirdest as well as most melancholy stories of human deformity is that of Edward Mordake, said to have been heir to one of the noblest peerages in England. He never claimed the title, however, and committed suicide in his twenty-third year. He lived in complete seclusion, refusing the visits even of the members of his own family. He was a young man of fine attainments, a profound scholar, and a musician of rare ability. His figure was remarkable for its grace, and his face—that is to say, his natural face—was that of an Antinous. But upon the back of his head was another face, that of a beautiful girl, 'lovely as a dream, hideous as a devil.' The female face was a mere mask, 'occupying only a small portion of the posterior part of the skull, yet exhibiting every sign of intelligence, of a malignant sort, however.' It would be seen to smile and sneer while Mordake was weeping. The eyes would follow the movements of the spectator, and the lips would 'gibber without ceasing.' No voice was audible, but Mordake avers that he was kept from his rest at night by the hateful whispers of his 'devil twin,' as he called it, 'which never sleeps, but talks to me forever of such things as they only speak of in hell. No imagination can conceive the dreadful temptations it sets before me. For some unforgiven wickedness of my forefathers I am knit to this fiend—for a fiend it surely is. I beg and beseech you to crush it out of human semblance, even if I die for it.' Such were the words of the hapless Mordake to Manvers and Treadwell, his physicians. In spite of careful watching he managed to procure poison, whereof he died, leaving a letter requesting that the 'demon face' might be destroyed before his burial, 'lest it continues its dreadful whisperings in my grave.' At his own request he was interred in a waste place, without stone or legend to mark his grave."

A most curious case was that of a Fellah woman who was delivered at Alexandria of a bicephalic monster of apparently eight months' pregnancy. This creature, which was born dead, had one head white and the other black the change of color commencing at the neck of the black head. The bizarre head was of negro conformation and fully developed, and the colored skin was found to be due to the existence of pigment similar to that found in the black race. The husband of the woman had a light brown skin, like an ordinary Fellah man, and it was ascertained that there were some negro laborers in port during the woman's pregnancy; but no definite information as to her relations with them could be established, and whether this was a case of maternal impression or superfetation can only be a matter of conjecture.

Fantastic monsters, such as acephalon, paracephalon, cyclops, pseudencephalon, and the janiceps, prosopthoracopagus, disprosopus, etc., although full of interest, will not be discussed here, as none are ever viable for any length of time, and the declared intention of this chapter is to include only those beings who have lived.

CLASS VIII.—The next class includes the parasitic terata, monsters that consist of one perfect body, complete in every respect, but from the neighborhood of whose umbilicus depends some important portion of a second body. Pare, Benivenius, and Columbus describe adults with acephalous monsters attached to them. Schenck mentions 13 cases, 3 of which were observed by him. Aldrovandus shows 3 illustrations under the name of "monstrum bicorpum monocephalon."

Bustorf speaks of a case in which the nates and lower extremities of one body proceeded out of the abdomen of the other, which was otherwise perfect. Reichel and Anderson mention a living parasitic monster, the inferior trunk of one body proceeding from the pectoral region of the other.

Pare says that there was a man in Paris in 1530, quite forty years of age, who carried about a parasite without a head, which hung pendant from his belly. This individual was exhibited and drew great crowds. Pare appends an illustration, which is, perhaps, one of the most familiar in all teratology. He also gives a portrait of a man who had a parasitic head proceeding from his epigastrium, and who was born in Germany the same year that peace was made with the Swiss by King Francis. This creature lived to manhood and both heads were utilized in alimentation. Bartholinus details a history of an individual named Lazarus-Joannes Baptista Colloredo, born in Genoa in 1617, who exhibited himself all over Europe. From his epigastrium hung an imperfectly developed twin that had one thigh, hands, body, arms, and a well-formed head covered with hair, which in the normal position hung lowest. There were signs of independent existence in the parasite, movements of respiration, etc., but its eyes were closed, and, although saliva constantly dribbled from its open mouth, nothing was ever ingested. The genitals were imperfect and the arms ended in badly formed hands. Bartholinus examined this monster at twenty-two, and has given the best report, although while in Scotland in 1642 he was again examined, and accredited with being married and the father of several children who were fully and admirably developed. Moreau quotes a case of an infant similar in conformation to the foregoing monster, who was born in Switzerland in 1764, and whose supernumerary parts were amputated by means of a ligature. Winslow reported before the Academie Royale des Sciences the history of a girl of twelve who died at the Hotel-Dieu in 1733. She was of ordinary height and of fair conformation, with the exception that hanging from the left flank was the inferior half of another girl of diminutive proportions. The supernumerary body was immovable, and hung so heavily that it was said to be supported by the hands or by a sling. Urine and feces were evacuated at intervals from the parasite, and received into a diaper constantly worn for this purpose. Sensibility in the two was common, an impression applied to the parasite being felt by the girl. Winslow gives an interesting report of the dissection of this monster, and mentions that he had seen an Italian child of eight who had a small head proceeding from under the cartilage of the third left rib. Sensibility was common, pinching the ear of the parasitic head causing the child with the perfect head to cry. Each of the two heads received baptism, one being named John and the other Matthew. A curious question arose in the instance of the girl, as to whether the extreme unction should be administered to the acephalous fetus as well as to the child.

In 1742, during the Ambassadorship of the Marquis de l'Hopital at Naples, he saw in that city an aged man, well conformed, with the exception that, like the little girl of Winslow, he had the inferior extremities of a male child growing from his epigastric region. Haller and Meckel have also observed cases like this. Bordat described before the Royal Institute of France, August, 1826, a Chinaman, twenty-one years of age, who had an acephalous fetus attached to the surface of his breast (possibly "A-ke").

Dickinson describes a wonderful child five years old, who, by an extraordinary freak of nature, was an amalgamation of two children. From the body of an otherwise perfectly formed child was a supernumerary head protruding from a broad base attached to the lower lumbar and sacral region. This cephalic mass was covered with hair about four or five inches long, and showed the rudiments of an eye, nose, mouth, and chin. This child was on exhibition when Dickinson saw it. Montare and Reyes were commissioned by the Academy of Medicine of Havana to examine and report on a monstrous girl of seven months, living in Cuba. The girl was healthy and well developed, and from the middle line of her body between the xiphoid cartilage and the umbilicus, attached by a soft pedicle, was an accessory individual, irregular, of ovoid shape, the smaller end, representing the head, being upward. The parasite measured a little over 1 foot in length, 9 inches about the head, and 7 3/4 inches around the neck. The cranial bones were distinctly felt, and the top of the head was covered by a circlet of hair. There were two rudimentary eyebrows; the left eye was represented by a minute perforation encircled with hair; the right eye was traced by one end of a mucous groove which ran down to another transverse groove representing the mouth; the right third of this latter groove showed a primitive tongue and a triangular tooth, which appeared at the fifth month. There was a soft, imperforate nose, and the elements of the vertebral column could be distinguished beneath the skin; there were no legs; apparently no vascular sounds; there was separate sensation, as the parasite could be pinched without attracting the perfect infant's notice. The mouth of the parasite constantly dribbled saliva, but showed no indication of receiving aliment.

Louise L., known as "La dame a quatre jambes," was born in 1869, and had attached to her pelvis another rudimentary pelvis and two atrophied legs of a parasite, weighing 8 kilos. The attachment was effected by means of a pedicle 33 cm. in diameter, having a bony basis, and being fixed without a joint. The attachment almost obliterated the vulva and the perineum was displaced far backward. At the insertion of the parasite were two rudimentary mammae, one larger than the other. No genitalia were seen on the parasite and it exhibited no active movements, the joints of both limbs being ankylosed. The woman could localize sensations in the parasite except those of the feet. She had been married five years, and bore, in the space of three years, two well-formed daughters.

Quite recently there was exhibited in the museums of the United States an individual bearing the name "Laloo," who was born in Oudh, India, and was the second of four children. At the time of examination he was about nineteen years of age. The upper portion of a parasite was firmly attached to the lower right side of the sternum of the individual by a bony pedicle, and lower by a fleshy pedicle, and apparently contained intestines. The anus of the parasite was imperforate; a well-developed penis was found, but no testicles; there was a luxuriant growth of hair on the pubes. The penis of the parasite was said to show signs of erection at times, and urine passed through it without the knowledge of the boy. Perspiration and elevation of temperature seemed to occur simultaneously in both. To pander to the morbid curiosity of the curious, the "Dime Museum" managers at one time shrewdly clothed the parasite in female attire, calling the two brother and sister; but there is no doubt that all the traces of sex were of the male type. An analogous case was that of "A-Ke," a Chinaman, who was exhibited in London early in the century, and of whom and his parasite anatomic models are seen in our museums. Figure 58 represents an epignathus, a peculiar type parasitic monster, in which the parasite is united to the inferior maxillary bone of the autosite.

CLASS IX.—Of "Lusus naturae" none is more curious than that of duplication of the lower extremities. Pare says that on January 9, 1529, there was living in Germany a male infant having four legs and four arms. In Paris, at the Academie des Sciences, on September 6, 1830, there was presented by Madame Hen, a midwife, a living male child with four legs, the anus being nearly below the middle of the third buttock; and the scrotum between the two left thighs, the testicles not yet descended. There was a well-formed and single pelvis, and the supernumerary legs were immovable. Aldrovandus mentions several similar instances, and gives the figure of one born in Rome; he also describes several quadruped birds. Bardsley speaks of a male child with one head, four arms, four legs, and double generative organs. He gives a portrait of the child when it was a little over a year old. Heschl published in Vienna in 1878 a description of a girl of seventeen, who instead of having a duplication of the superior body, as in "Millie-Christine, the two-headed nightingale," had double parts below the second lumbar vertebra. Her head and upper body resembled a comely, delicate girl of twelve.

Wells a describes Mrs. B., aged twenty, still alive and healthy. The duplication in this case begins just above the waist, the spinal column dividing at the third lumbar vertebra, below this point everything being double. Micturition and defecation occur at different times, but menstruation occurs simultaneously. She was married at nineteen, and became pregnant a year later on the left side, but abortion was induced at the fourth month on account of persistent nausea and the expectation of impossible delivery. Whaley, in speaking of this case, said Mrs. B. utilized her outside legs for walking; he also remarks that when he informed her that she was pregnant on the left side she replied, "I think you are mistaken; if it had been on my right side I would come nearer believing it;"—and after further questioning he found, from the patient's observation, that her right genitals were almost invariably used for coitus. Bechlinger of Para, Brazil, describes a woman of twenty-five, a native of Martinique, whose father was French and mother a quadroon, who had a modified duplication of the lower body. There was a third leg attached to a continuation of the processus coceygeus of the sacrum, and in addition to well developed mammae regularly situated, there were two rudimentary ones close together above the pubes. There were two vaginae and two well-developed vulvae, both having equally developed sensations. The sexual appetite was markedly developed, and coitus was practised in both vaginae. A somewhat similar case, possibly the same, is that of Blanche Dumas, born in 1860. She had a very broad pelvis, two imperfectly developed legs, and a supernumerary limb attached to the symphysis, without a joint, but with slight passive movement. There was a duplication of bowel, bladder, and genitalia. At the junction of the rudimentary limb with the body, in front, were two rudimentary mammary glands, each containing a nipple.

Other instances of supernumerary limbs will be found in Chapter VI.

CLASS X.—The instances of diphallic terata, by their intense interest to the natural bent of the curious mind, have always elicited much discussion. To many of these cases have been attributed exaggerated function, notwithstanding the fact that modern observation almost invariably shows that the virile power diminishes in exact proportion to the extent of duplication. Taylor quotes a description of a monster, exhibited in London, with two distinct penises, but with only one distinct testicle on either side. He could exercise the function of either organ.

Schenck, Schurig, Bartholinus, Loder, and Ollsner report instances of diphallic terata; the latter case a was in a soldier of Charles VI, twenty-two years old, who applied to the surgeon for a bubonic affection, and who declared that he passed urine from the orifice of the left glans and also said that he was incapable of true coitus. Valentini mentions an instance in a boy of four, in which the two penises were superimposed. Bucchettoni speaks of a man with two penises placed side by side. There was an anonymous case described of a man of ninety-three with a penis which was for more than half its length divided into two distinct members, the right being somewhat larger than the left. From the middle of the penis up to the symphysis only the lower wall of the urethra was split. Jenisch describes a diphallic infant, the offspring of a woman of twenty-five who had been married five years. Her first child was a well-formed female, and the second, the infant in question, cried much during the night, and several times vomited dark-green matter. In lieu of one penis there were two, situated near each other, the right one of natural size and the left larger, but not furnished with a prepuce. Each penis had its own urethra, from which dribbled urine and some meconium. There was a duplication of each scrotum, but only one testicle in each, and several other minor malformations.

Gore, reported by Velpeau, has seen an infant of eight and one-half months with two penises and three lower extremities. The penises were 4 cm. apart and the scrotum divided, containing one testicle in each side. Each penis was provided with a urethra, urine being discharged from both simultaneously. In a similar case, spoken of by Geoffroy-Saint-Hilaire, the two organs were also separate, but urine and semen escaped sometimes from one, sometimes from both.

The most celebrated of all the diphallic terata was Jean Baptista dos Santos, who when but six months old was spoken of by Acton. His father and mother were healthy and had two well-formed children. He was easily born after an uneventful pregnancy. He was good-looking, well proportioned, and had two distinct penises, each as large as that of a child of six months. Urination proceeded simultaneously from both penises; he had also two scrotums. Behind and between the legs there was another limb, or rather two, united throughout their length. It was connected to the pubis by a short stem 1/2 inch long and as large as the little finger, consisting of separate bones and cartilages. There was a patella in the supernumerary limb on the anal aspect, and a joint freely movable. This compound limb had no power of motion, but was endowed with sensibility. A journal in London, after quoting Acton's description, said that the child had been exhibited in Paris, and that the surgeons advised operation. Fisher, to whom we are indebted for an exhaustive work in Teratology, received a report from Havana in July, 1865, which detailed a description of Santos at twenty-two years of age, and said that he was possessed of extraordinary animal passion, the sight of a female alone being sufficient to excite him. He was said to use both penises, after finishing with one continuing with the other; but this account of him does not agree with later descriptions, in which no excessive sexual ability had been noticed. Hart describes the adult Santos in full, and accompanies his article with an illustration. At this time he was said to have developed double genitals, and possibly a double bladder communicating by an imperfect septum. At adulthood the anus was three inches anterior to the os coceygeus. In the sitting or lying posture the supernumerary limb rested on the front of the inner surface of the lower third of his left thigh. He was in the habit of wearing this limb in a sling, or bound firmly to the right thigh, to prevent its unseemly dangling when erect. The perineum proper was absent, the entire space between the anus and the posterior edge of the scrotum being occupied by the pedicle. Santos' mental and physical functions were developed above normal, and he impressed everybody with his accomplishments. Geoffroy-Saint-Hilaire records an instance in which the conformation was similar to that of Santos. There was a third lower extremity consisting of two limbs fused into one with a single foot containing ten distinct digits. He calls the case one of arrested twin development.

Van Buren and Keyes describe a case in a man of forty-two, of good, healthy appearance. The two distinct penises of normal size were apparently well formed and were placed side by side, each attached at its root to the symphysis. Their covering of skin was common as far as the base of the glans; at this point they seemed distinct and perfect, but the meatus of the left was imperforate. The right meatus was normal, and through it most of the urine passed, though some always dribbled through an opening in the perineum at a point where the root of the scrotum should have been. On lifting the double-barreled penis this opening could be seen and was of sufficient size to admit the finger. On the right side of the aperture was an elongated and rounded prominence similar in outline to a labium majus. This prominence contained a testicle normal in shape and sensibility, but slightly undersized, and surrounded, as was evident from its mobility, by a tunica vaginalis. The left testicle lay on the tendon of the adductor longus in the left groin; it was not fully developed, but the patient had sexual desires, erections, and emissions. Both penises became erect simultaneously, the right more vigorously. The left leg was shorter than the right and congenitally smaller; the mammae were of normal dimensions.

Sangalli speaks of a man of thirty-five who had a supernumerary penis, furnished with a prepuce and capable of erection. At the apex of the glans opened a canal about 12 cm. long, through which escaped monthly a serous fluid. Smith mentions a man who had two penises and two bladders, on one of which lithotomy was performed. According to Ballantyne, Taruffi, the scholarly observer of terata, mentions a child of forty-two months and height of 80 cm. who had two penises, each furnished with a urethra and well-formed scrotal sacs which were inserted in a fold of the groin. There were two testicles felt in the right scrotum and one in the left. Fecal evacuations escaped through two anal orifices. There is also another case mentioned similar to the foregoing in a man of forty; but here there was an osseous projection in the middle line behind the bladder. This patient said that erection was simultaneous in both penises, and that he had not married because of his chagrin over his deformity. Cole speaks of a child with two well-developed male organs, one to the left and the other to the right of the median line, and about 1/4 or 1/2 inch apart at birth. The urethra bifurcated in the perineal region and sent a branch to each penis, and urine passed from each meatus. The scrotum was divided into three compartments by two raphes, and each compartment contained a testicle. The anus at birth was imperforate, but the child was successfully operated on, and at its sixtieth day weighed 17 pounds.

Lange says that an infant was brought to Karg for relief of anal atresia when fourteen days old. It was found to possess duplicate penises, which communicated each to its distinct half of the bladder as defined by a median fold. The scrotum was divided into three portions by two raphes, and each lateral compartment contained a fully formed testicle. This child died because of its anal malformation, which we notice is a frequent associate of malformations or duplicity of the penis. There is an example in an infant described in which there were two penises, each about 1/2 inch long, and a divided scrotal sac 21 inches long. Englisch speaks of a German of forty who possessed a double penis of the bifid type.

Ballantyne and his associates define diphallic terata as individuals provided with two more or less well-formed and more or less separate penises, who may show also other malformations of the adjoining parts and organs (e.g., septate bladder), but who are not possessed of more than two lower limbs. This definition excludes, therefore, the cases in which in addition to a double penis there is a supernumerary lower extremity—such a case, for example, as that of Jean Baptista dos Santos, so frequently described by teratologists. It also excludes the more evident double terata, and, of course, the cases of duplication of the female genital organs (double clitoris, vulva, vagina, and uterus). Although Schurig, Meckel, Himly, Taruffi, and others give bibliographic lists of diphallic terata, even in them erroneous references are common, and there is evidence to show that many cases have been duplicated under different names. Ballantyne and Skirving have consulted all the older original references available and eliminated duplications of reports and, adhering to their original definition, have collected and described individually 20 cases; they offer the following conclusions:—

1. Diphallus, or duplication of the penis in an otherwise apparently single individual, is a very rare anomaly, records of only 20 cases having been found in a fairly exhaustive search through teratologic literature. As a distinct and well-authenticated type it has only quite recently been recognized by teratologists.

2. It does not of itself interfere with intrauterine or extrauterine life; but the associated anomalies (e.g., atresia ani) may be sources of danger. If not noticed at birth, it is not usually discovered till adult life, and even then the discovery is commonly accidental.

3. With regard to the functions of the pelvic viscera, urine may be passed by both penises, by one only, or by neither. In the last instance it finds exit by an aperture in the perineum. There is reason to believe that semen may be passed in the same way; but in most of the recorded cases there has been sterility, if not inability to perform the sexual act.

4. All the degrees of duplication have been met with, from a fissure of the glans penis to the presence of two distinct penises inserted at some distance from each other in the inguinal regions.

5. The two penises are usually somewhat defective as regards prepuce, urethra, etc.; they may lie side by side, or more rarely may be situated anteroposteriorly; they may be equal in size, or less commonly one is distinctly larger than the other; and one or both may be perforate or imperforate.

6. The scrotum may be normal or split; the testicles, commonly two in number, may be normal or atrophic, descended or undescended; the prostate may be normal or imperfectly developed, as may also the vasa deferentia and vesiculae seminales.

7. The commonly associated defects are: More or less completely septate bladder, atresia ani, or more rarely double anus, double urethra, increased breadth of the bony pelvis with defect of the symphysis pubis, and possibly duplication of the lower end of the spine, and hernia of some of the abdominal contents into a perineal pouch. Much more rarely, duplication of the heart, lungs, stomach, and kidneys has been noted, and the lower limbs may be shorter than normal.

CLASS XI.—Cases of fetus in fetu, those strange instances in which one might almost say that a man may be pregnant with his brother or sister, or in which an infant may carry its twin without the fact being apparent, will next be discussed. The older cases were cited as being only a repetition of the process by which Eve was born of Adam. Figure 63 represents an old engraving showing the birth of Eve. Bartholinus, the Ephemerides, Otto, Paullini, Schurig, and Plot speak of instances of fetus in fetu. Ruysch describes a tumor contained in the abdomen of a man which was composed of hair, molar teeth, and other evidences of a fetus. Huxham reported to the Royal Society in 1748 the history of a child which was born with a tumor near the anus larger than the whole body of the child; this tumor contained rudiments of an embryo. Young speaks of a fetus which lay encysted between the laminae of the transverse mesocolon, and Highmore published a report of a fetus in a cyst communicating with the duodenum. Dupuytren gives an example in a boy of thirteen, in whom was found a fetus.

Gaetano-Nocito, cited by Philipeaux, has the history of a taken with a great pain in the right hypochondrium, and from which issued subsequently fetal bones and a mass of macerated embryo. His mother had had several double pregnancies, and from the length of the respective tibiae one of the fetuses seemed to be of two months' and the other of three months' intrauterine life. The man died five years after the abscess had burst spontaneously.

Brodie speaks of a case in which fetal remains were taken from the abdomen of a girl of two and one-half years. Gaither describes a child of two years and nine months, supposed to be affected with ascites, who died three hours after the physician's arrival. In its abdomen was found a fetus weighing almost two pounds and connected to the child by a cord resembling an umbilical cord. This child was healthy for about nine months, and had a precocious longing for ardent spirits, and drank freely an hour before its death.

Blundell says that he knew "a boy who was literally and without evasion with child, for the fetus was contained in a sac communicating with the abdomen and was connected to the side of the cyst by a short umbilical cord; nor did the fetus make its appearance until the boy was eight or ten years old, when after much enlargement of pregnancy and subsequent flooding the boy died." The fetus, removed after death, on the whole not very imperfectly formed, was of the size of about six or seven months' gestation. Bury cites an account of a child that had a second imperfectly developed fetus in its face and scalp. There was a boy by the name of Bissieu who from the earliest age had a pain in one of his left ribs; this rib was larger than the rest and seemed to have a tumor under it. He died of phthisis at fourteen, and after death there was found in a pocket lying against the transverse colon and communicating with it all the evidences of a fetus.

At the Hopital de la Charite in Paris, Velpeau startled an audience of 500 students and many physicians by saying that he expected to find a rudimentary fetus in a scrotal tumor placed in his hands for operation. His diagnosis proved correct, and brought him resounding praise, and all wondered as to his reasons for expecting a fetal tumor. It appears that he had read with care a report by Fatti of an operation on the scrotum of a child which had increased in size as the child grew, and was found to contain the ribs, the vertebral column, the lower extremities as far as the knees, and the two orbits of a fetus; and also an account of a similar operation performed by Wendt of Breslau on a Silesian boy of seven. The left testicle in this case was so swollen that it hung almost to the knee, and the fetal remains removed weighed seven ounces.

Sulikowski relates an instance of congenital fetation in the umbilicus of a girl of fourteen, who recovered after the removal of the anomaly. Aretaeos described to the members of the medical fraternity in Athens the case of a woman of twenty-two, who bore two children after a seven months' pregnancy. One was very rudimentary and only 21 inches long, and the other had an enormous head resembling a case of hydrocephalus. On opening the head of the second fetus, another, three inches long, was found in the medulla oblongata, and in the cranial cavity with it were two additional fetuses, neither of which was perfectly formed.

Broca speaks of a fetal cyst being passed in the urine of a man of sixty- one; the cyst contained remnants of hair, bone, and cartilage. Atlee submits quite a remarkable case of congenital ventral gestation, the subject being a girl of six, who recovered after the discharge of the fetal mass from the abdomen. McIntyre speaks of a child of eleven, playing about and feeling well, but whose abdomen progressively increased in size 1 1/2 inches each day. After ten days there was a large fluctuating mass on the right side; the abdomen was opened and the mass enucleated; it was found to contain a fetal mass weighing nearly five pounds, and in addition ten pounds of fluid were removed. The child made an early recovery. Rogers mentions a fetus that was found in a man's bladder. Bouchacourt reports the successful extirpation of the remains of a fetus from the rectum of a child of six. Miner describes a successful excision of a congenital gestation.

Modern literature is full of examples, and nearly every one of the foregoing instances could be paralleled from other sources. Rodriguez is quoted as reporting that in July, 1891, several newspapers in the city of Mexico published, under the head of "A Man-mother," a wonderful story, accompanied by wood-cuts, of a young man from whose body a great surgeon had extracted a "perfectly developed fetus." One of these wood-cuts represented a tumor at the back of a man opened and containing a crying baby. In commenting upon this, after reviewing several similar cases of endocymian monsters that came under his observation in Mexico, Rodriguez tells what the case which had been so grossly exaggerated by the lay journals really was: An Indian boy, aged twenty-two, presented a tumor in the sacrococcygeal region measuring 53 cm. in circumference at the base, having a vertical diameter of 17 cm. and a transverse diameter of 13 cm. It had no pedicle and was fixed, showing unequal consistency. At birth this tumor was about the size of a pigeon's egg. A diagnosis of dermoid cyst was made and two operations were performed on the boy, death following the second. The skeleton showed interesting conditions; the rectum and pelvic organs were natural, and the contents of the cyst verified the diagnosis.

Quite similar to the cases of fetus in fetu are the instances of dermoid cysts. For many years they have been a mystery to physiologists, and their origin now is little more than hypothetic. At one time the fact of finding such a formation in the ovary of an unmarried woman was presumptive evidence that she was unchaste; but this idea was dissipated as soon as examples were reported in children, and today we have a well-defined difference between congenital and extrauterine pregnancy. Dermoid cysts of the ovary may consist only of a wall of connective tissue lined with epidermis and containing distinctly epidermic scales which, however, may be rolled up in firm masses of a more or less soapy consistency; this variety is called by Orth epidermoid cyst; or, according to Warren, a form of cyst made up of skin containing small and ill-defined papillae, but rich in hair follicles and sebaceous glands. Even the erector pili muscle and the sudoriparous gland are often found. The hair is partly free and rolled up into thick balls or is still attached to the walls. A large mass of sebaceous material is also found in these cysts. Thomson reports a case of dermoid cyst of the bladder containing hair, which cyst he removed. It was a pedunculated growth, and it was undoubtedly vesical and not expelled from some ovarian source through the urinary passage, as sometimes occurs.

The simpler forms of the ordinary dermoid cysts contain bone and teeth. The complicated teratoma of this class may contain, in addition to the previously mentioned structures, cartilage and glands, mucous and serous membrane, muscle, nerves, and cerebral substance, portions of eyes, fingers with nails, mammae, etc. Figure 64 represents a cyst containing long red hair that was removed from a blonde woman aged forty-four years who had given birth to six children. Cullingworth reports the history of a woman in whom both ovaries were apparently involved by dermoids, who had given birth to 12 children and had three miscarriages—the last, three months before the removal of the growths. The accompanying illustration, taken from Baldy, pictures a dermoid cyst of the complicated variety laid open and exposing the contents in situ. Mears of Philadelphia reports a case of ovarian cyst removed from a girl of six and a half by Bradford of Kentucky in 1875. From this age on to adult life many similar cases are recorded. Nearly every medical museum has preserved specimens of dermoid cysts, and almost all physicians are well acquainted with their occurrence. The curious formations and contents and the bizarre shapes are of great variety. Graves mentions a dermoid cyst containing the left side of a human face, an eye, a molar tooth, and various bones. Dermoid cysts are found also in regions of the body quite remote from the ovary. The so-called "orbital wens" are true inclusion of the skin of a congenital origin, as are the nasal dermoids and some of the cysts of the neck.

Weil reported the case of a man of twenty-two years who was born with what was supposed to be a spina bifida in the lower sacral region. According to Senn, the swelling never caused any pain or inconvenience until it inflamed, when it opened spontaneously and suppurated, discharging a large quantity of offensive pus, hair, and sebaceous material, thus proving it to have been a dermoid. The cyst was freely incised, and there were found numerous openings of sweat glands, from which drops of perspiration escaped when the patient was sweating.

Dermoid cysts of the thorax are rare. Bramann reported a case in which a dermoid cyst of small size was situated over the sternum at the junction of the manubrium with the gladiolus, and a similar cyst in the neck near the left cornu of the hyoid bone. Chitten removed a dermoid from the sternum of a female of thirty-nine, the cyst containing 11 ounces of atheromatous material. In the Museum of St. Bartholomew's Hospital in London there is a congenital tumor which was removed from the anterior mediastinum of a woman of twenty one, and contained portions of skin, fat, sebaceous material, and two pieces of bone similar to the superior maxilla, and in which several teeth were found. Dermoids are found in the palate and pharynx, and open dermoids of the conjunctiva are classified by Sutton with the moles. According to Senn, Barker collected sixteen dermoid tumors of the tongue. Bryk successfully removed a tumor of this nature the size of a fist. Wellington Gray removed an enormous lingual dermoid from the mouth of a negro. It contained 40 ounces of atheromatous material. Dermoids of the rectum are reported. Duyse reports the history of a case of labor during which a rectal dermoid was expelled. The dermoid contained a cerebral vesicle, a rudimentary eye, a canine and a molar tooth, and a piece of bone. There is little doubt that many cases of fetus in fetu reported were really dermoids of the scrotum.

Ward reports the successful removal of a dermoid cyst weighing 30 pounds from a woman of thirty-two, the mother of two children aged ten and twelve, respectively. The report is briefly as follows: "The patient has always been in good health until within the last year, during which time she has lost flesh and strength quite rapidly, and when brought to my hospital by her physician, Dr. James of Williamsburg, Kansas, was quite weak, although able to walk about the house. A tumor had been growing for a number of years, but its growth was so gradual that the patient had not considered her condition critical until quite recently. The tumor was diagnosed to be cystoma of the left ovary. Upon opening the sac with the trocar we were confronted by complications entirely unlooked for, and its use had to be abandoned entirely because the thick contents of the cyst would not flow freely, and the presence of sebaceous matter blocked the instrument. As much of the fluid as possible was removed, and the abdominal incision was enlarged to allow of the removal of the large tumor. An ovarian hematoma the size of a large orange was removed from the right side. We washed the intestines quite as one would wash linen, since some of the contents of the cyst had escaped into the abdominal cavity. The abdomen was closed without drainage, and the patient placed in bed without experiencing the least shock. Her recovery was rapid and uneventful. She returned to her home in four weeks after the operation.

"The unusual feature in this case was the nature of the contents of the sac. There was a large quantity of long straight hair growing from the cyst wall and an equal amount of loose hair in short pieces floating through the tumor- contents, a portion of which formed nuclei for what were called 'moth-balls,' of which there were about 1 1/2 gallons. These balls, or marbles, varied from the size of moth-balls, as manufactured and sold by druggists, to that of small walnuts. They seemed to be composed of sebaceous matter, and were evidently formed around the short hairs by the motion of the fluid produced by walking or riding. There was some tissue resembling true skin attached to the inner wall of the sac."

There are several cases of multiple dermoid cysts on record, and they may occur all over the body. Jamieson reports a case in which there were 250, and in Maclaren's case there were 132. According to Crocker, Hebra and Rayer also each had a case. In a case of Sangster, reported by Politzer, although most of the dermoids, as usual, were like fibroma-nodules and therefore the color of normal skin, those over the mastoid processes and clavicle were lemon-yellow, and were generally thought to be xanthoma until they were excised, and Politzer found they were typical dermoid cysts with the usual contents of degenerated epithelium and hair.

Hermaphroditism.—Some writers claim that Adam was the first hermaphrodite and support this by Scriptural evidence. We find in some of the ancient poets traces of an Egyptian legend in which the goddess of the moon was considered to be both male and female. From mythology we learn that Hermaphroditus was the son of Hermes, or Mercury, and Venus Aphrodite, and had the powers both of a father and mother. In speaking of the foregoing Ausonius writes, "Cujus erat facies in qua paterque materque cognosci possint, nomen traxit ab illis." Ovid and Virgil both refer to legendary hermaphrodites, and the knowledge of their existence was prevalent in the olden times. The ancients considered the birth of hermaphrodites bad omens, and the Athenians threw them into the sea, the Romans, into the Tiber. Livy speaks of an hermaphrodite being put to death in Umbria, and another in Etruria. Cicero, Aristotle, Strabonius, and Pliny all speak concerning this subject. Martial and Tertullian noticed this anomaly among the Romans. Aetius and Paulus Aegineta speak of females in Egypt with prolonged clitorides which made them appear like hermaphrodites. Throughout the Middle Ages we frequently find accounts, naturally exaggerated, of double-sexed creatures. Harvey, Bartholinus, Paullini, Schenck, Wolff, Wrisberg, Zacchias, Marcellus Donatus, Haller, Hufeland, de Graff, and many others discuss hermaphroditism. Many classifications have been given, as, e.g., real and apparent;

masculine, feminine, or neuter; horizontal and vertical; unilateral and bilateral, etc. The anomaly in most cases consists of a malformation of the external genitalia. A prolonged clitoris, prolapsed ovaries, grossness of figure, and hirsute appearance have been accountable for many supposed instances of hermaphrodites. On the other hand, a cleft scrotum, an ill-developed penis, perhaps hypospadias or epispadias, rotundity of the mammae, and feminine contour have also provoked accounts of similar instances. Some cases have been proved by dissection to have been true hermaphrodites, portions or even entire genitalia of both sexes having been found.

Numerous accounts, many mythical, but always interesting, are given of these curious persons. They have been accredited with having performed the functions of both father and mother, notwithstanding the statements of some of the best authorities that they are always sterile. Observation has shown that the sexual appetite diminishes in proportion to the imperfections in the genitalia, and certainly many of these persons are sexually indifferent.

We give descriptions of a few of the most famous or interesting instances of hermaphroditism. Pare speaks of a woman who, besides a vulva, from which she menstruated, had a penis, but without prepuce or signs of erectility. Haller alludes to several cases in which prolonged clitorides have been the cause of the anomaly. In commenting on this form of hermaphroditism Albucasiusus describes a necessary operation for the removal of the clitoris.

Columbus relates the history of an Ethiopian woman who was evidently a spurious female hermaphrodite. The poor wretch entreated him to cut off her penis, an enlarged clitoris, which she said was an intolerable hindrance to her in coitus. De Graff and Riolan describe similar cases. There is an old record of a similar creature, supposing herself to be a male, who took a wife, but previously having had connection with a man, the outcome of which was pregnancy, was shortly after marriage delivered of a daughter. There is an account of a person in Germany who, for the first thirty years of life, was regarded as feminine, and being of loose morals became a mother. At a certain period she began to feel a change in her sexual inclinations; she married and became the father of a family. This is doubtless a distortion of the facts of the case of Catherine or Charles Hoffman, born in 1824, and who was considered a female until the age of forty. At puberty she had the instincts of a woman, and cohabitated with a male lover for twenty years. Her breasts were well formed and she menstruated at nineteen. At the age of forty-six her sexual desires changed, and she attempted coitus as a man, with such evident satisfaction that she married a woman soon afterward. Fitch speaks of a house-servant with masculine features and movements, aged twenty-eight, and 5 feet and 9 inches tall, who was arrested by the police for violating the laws governing prostitution. On examination, well-developed male and female organs of generation were found. The labia majora were normal and flattened on the anterior surface. The labia minora and hymen were absent. The vagina was spacious and the woman had a profuse leukorrhea. She stated that several years previously she gave birth to a normal child. In place of a clitoris she had a penis which, in erection, measured 5 1/4 inches long and 3 5/8 inches in circumference. The glans penis and the urethra were perfectly formed. The scrotum contained two testicles, each about an inch long; the mons veneris was sparsely covered with straight, black hair. She claimed functional ability with both sets of genitalia, and said she experienced equal sexual gratification with either. Semen issued from the penis, and every three weeks she had scanty menstruation, which lasted but two days.

Beclard showed Marie-Madeline Lefort, nineteen years of age, 1 1/2 meters in height. Her mammae were well developed, her nipples erectile and surrounded by a brown areola, from which issued several hairs. Her feet were small, her pelvis large, and her thighs like those of a woman. Projecting from the vulva was a body looking like a penis 7 cm. long and slightly erectile at times; it was imperforate and had a mobile prepuce. She had a vulva with two well-shaped labia as shown by the accompanying illustration. She menstruated slightly and had an opening at the root of the clitoris. The parotid region showed signs of a beard and she had hair on her upper lip. On August 20, 1864, a person came into the Hotel-Dieu, asking treatment for chronic pleurisy. He said his age was sixty-five, and he pursued the calling of a mountebank, but remarked that in early life he had been taken for a woman. He had menstruated at eight and had been examined by doctors at sixteen. The menstruation continued until 1848, and at its cessation he experienced the feelings of a male. At this time he presented the venerable appearance of a long-bearded old man. At the autopsy, about two months later, all the essentials of a female were delineated. A Fallopian tube, ovaries, uterus, and round ligaments were found, and a drawing in cross-section of the parts was made. There is no doubt but that this individual was Marie-Madeline Lefort in age.

Worbe speaks of a person who was supposed to be feminine for twenty-two years. At the age of sixteen she loved a farmer's son, but the union was delayed for some reason, and three years later her grace faded and she became masculine in her looks and tastes. It was only after lengthy discussion, in which the court took part, that it was definitely settled that this person was a male.

Adelaide Preville, who was married as a female, and as such lived the last ten years of her life in France, was found on dissection at the Hotel-Dieu to be a man. A man was spoken of in both France and Germany a who passed for many years as a female. He had a cleft scrotum and hypospadias, which caused the deception. Sleeping with another servant for three years, he constantly had sexual congress with her during this period, and finally impregnated her. It was supposed in this case that the posterior wall of the vagina supplied the deficiency of the lower boundary of the urethra, forming a complete channel for the semen to proceed through. Long ago in Scotland a servant was condemned to death by burial alive for impregnating his master's daughter while in the guise and habit of a woman. He had always been considered a woman. We have heard of a recent trustworthy account of a pregnancy and delivery in a girl who had been impregnated by a bedfellow who on examination proved to be a male pseudohermaphrodite.

Fournier speaks of an individual in Lisbon in 1807 who was in the highest degree graceful, the voice feminine, the mammae well developed, The female genitalia were normal except the labia majora, which were rather diminutive. The thighs and the pelvis. were not so wide as those of a woman. There was some beard on the chin, but it was worn close. the male genitalia were of the size and appearance of a male adult and were covered with the usual hair. This person had been twice pregnant and aborted at the third and fifth month. During coitus the penis became erect, etc.

Schrell describes a case in which, independent of the true penis and testicles, which were well formed, there existed a small vulva furnished with labia and nymphae, communicating with a rudimentary uterus provided with round ligaments and imperfectly developed ovaries. Schrell remarks that in this case we must notice that the female genitalia were imperfectly developed, and adds that perfect hermaphroditism is a physical impossibility without great alterations of the natural connections of the bones and other parts of the pelvis. Cooper describes a woman with an enormous development of the clitoris, an imperforate uterus, and absence of vagina; at first sight of the parts they appeared to be those of a man.

In 1859 Hugier succeeded in restoring a vagina to a young girl of twenty who had an hypertrophied clitoris and no signs of a vagina. The accompanying illustrations show the conformation of the parts before operation with all the appearance of ill-developed male genitalia, and the appearance afterward with restitution of the vaginal opening.

Virchow in 1872, Boddaert in 1875, and Marchand in 1883 report cases of duplication of the genitalia, and call their cases true hermaphrodites from an anatomic standpoint. There is a specimen in St. Bartholomew's Hospital in London from a man of forty-four, who died of cerebral hemorrhage. He was well formed and had a beard and a full-sized penis. He was married, and it was stated that his wife had two children. The bladder and the internal organs of generation were those of a man in whom neither testis had descended into the scrotum, and in whom the uterus masculinus and vagina were developed to an unusual degree. The uterus, nearly as large as in the adult female, lay between the bladder and rectum, and was enclosed between two layers of peritoneum, to which, on either side of the uterus, were attached the testes. There was also shown in London the pelvic organs from a case of complex or vertical hermaphroditism occurring in a child of nine months who died from the effects of an operation for the radical cure of a right inguinal hernia. The external organs were those of a male with undescended testes. The bladder was normal and its neck was surrounded by a prostate gland. Projecting backward were a vagina, uterus, and broad ligaments, round ligaments, and Fallopian tubes, with the testes in the position of the ovaries. There were no seminal vesicles. The child died eleven days after the operation. The family history states that the mother had had 14 children and eight miscarriages. Seven of the children were dead and showed no abnormalities. The fifth and sixth children were boys and had the same sexual arrangement.

Barnes, Chalmers, Sippel, and Litten describe cases of spurious hermaphroditism due to elongation of the clitoris. In Litten's case a the clitoris was 3 1/2 inches long, and there was hydrocele of the processus vaginalis on both sides, making tumors in the labium on one side and the inguinal canal on the other, which had been diagnosed as testicles and again as ovaries. There was associate cystic ovarian disease. Plate 4 is taken from a case of false external bilateral hermaphroditism. Phillips mentions four cases of spurious hermaphroditism in one family, and recently Pozzi tells of a family of nine individuals in whom this anomaly was observed. The first was alive and had four children; the second was christened a female but was probably a male; the third, fourth, and fifth were normal but died young; the sixth daughter was choreic and feeble-minded, aged twenty-nine, and had one illegitimate child; the seventh, a boy, was healthy and married; the eighth was christened a female, but when seventeen was declared by the Faculty to be a male; the ninth was christened a female, but at eighteen the genitals were found to be those of a male, though the mammae were well developed.

O'Neill speaks of a case in which the clitoris was five inches long and one inch thick, having a groove in its inferior surface reaching down to an oblique opening in the perineum. The scrotum contained two hard bodies thought to be testicles, and the general appearance was that of hypospadias. Postmortem a complete set of female genitalia was found, although the ovaries were very small. The right round ligament was exceedingly thick and reached down to the bottom of the false scrotum, where it was firmly attached. The hard bodies proved to be on one side an irreducible omental hernia, probably congenital, and on the other a hardened mass having no glandular structure. The patient was an adult. As we have seen, there seems to be a law of evolution in hermaphroditism which prevents perfection. If one set of genitalia are extraordinarily developed, the other set are correspondingly atrophied. In the case of extreme development of the clitoris and approximation to the male type we must expect to find imperfectly developed uterus or ovaries. This would answer for one of the causes of sterility in these cases.

There is a type of hermaphroditism in which the sex cannot be definitely declared, and sometimes dissection does not definitely indicate the predominating sex. Such cases are classed under the head of neuter hermaphrodites, possibly an analogy of the "genus epicoenum" of Quintilian. Marie Dorothee, of the age of twenty-three, was examined and declared a girl by Hufeland and Mursina, while Stark, Raschig, and Martens maintained that she was a boy. This formidable array of talent on both sides provoked much discussion in contemporary publications, and the case attracted much notice. Marc saw her in 1803, at which time she carried contradicting certificates as to her sex. He found an imperforate penis, and on the inferior face near the root an opening for the passage of urine. No traces of nymphae, vagina, testicles, nor beard were seen. The stature was small, the form debilitated, and the voice effeminate. Marc came to the conclusion that it was impossible for any man to determine either one sex or the other. Everard Home dissected a dog with apparent external organs of the female, but discovered that neither sex was sufficiently pronounced to admit of classification. Home also saw at the Royal Marine Hospital at Plymouth, in 1779, a marine who some days after admission was reported to be a girl. On examination Home found him to possess a weak voice, soft skin, voluminous breasts, little beard, and the thighs and legs of a woman. There was fat on the pubis, the penis was short and small and incapable of erection, the testicles of fetal size; he had no venereal desires whatever, and as regards sex was virtually neuter.

The legal aspect of hermaphroditism has always been much discussed. Many interesting questions arise, and extraordinary complications naturally occur. In Rome a hermaphrodite could be a witness to a testament, the exclusive privilege of a man, and the sex was settled by the predominance. If the male aspect and traits together with the generative organs of man were most pronounced, then the individual could call himself a man. "Hermaphroditus an ad testamentum adhiberi possit qualitas sesus incalescentis ostendit."

There is a peculiar case on record in which the question of legal male inheritance was not settled until the individual had lived as a female for fifty-one years. This person was married when twenty-one, but finding coitus impossible, separated after ten years, and though dressing as a female had coitus with other women. She finally lived with her brother, with whom she eventually came to blows. She prosecuted him for assault, and the brother in return charged her with seducing his wife. Examination ensued, and at this ripe age she was declared to be a male.

The literature on hermaphroditism is so extensive that it is impossible to select a proper representation of the interesting cases in this limited space, and the reader is referred to the modern French works on this subject, in which the material is exhaustive and the discussion thoroughly scientific.

CHAPTER VI

MINOR TERATA.

Ancient Ideas Relative to Minor Terata.—The ancients viewed with great interest the minor structural anomalies of man, and held them to be divine signs or warnings in much the same manner as they considered more pronounced monstrosities. In a most interesting and instructive article, Ballantyne quotes Ragozin in saying that the Chaldeo-Babylonians, in addition to their other numerous subdivisions of divination, drew presages and omens for good or evil from the appearance of the liver, bowels, and viscera of animals offered for sacrifice and opened for inspection, and from the natural defects or monstrosities of babies or the young of animals. Ballantyne names this latter subdivision of divination fetomancy or teratoscopy, and thus renders a special chapter as to omens derived from monstrous births, given by Lenormant:—

"The prognostics which the Chaldeans claimed to draw from monstrous births in man and the animals are worthy of forming a class by themselves, insomuch the more as it is the part of their divinatory science with which, up to the present time, we are best acquainted. The development that their astrology had given to 'genethliaque,' or the art of horoscopes of births, had led them early to attribute great importance to all the teratologic facts which were there produced. They claimed that an experience of 470,000 years of observations, all concordant, fully justified their system, and that in nothing was the influence of the stars marked in a more indubitable manner than in the fatal law which determined the destiny of each individual according to the state of the sky at the moment when he came into the world. Cicero, by the very terms which he uses to refute the Chaldeans, shows that the result of these ideas was to consider all infirmities and monstrosities that new-born infants exhibited as the inevitable and irremediable consequence of the action of these astral positions. This being granted, the observation of similar monstrosities gave, as it were, a reflection of the state of the sky; on which depended all terrestrial things; consequently, one might read in them the future with as much certainty as in the stars themselves. For this reason the greatest possible importance was attached to the teratologic auguries which occupy so much space in the fragments of the great treatise on terrestrial presages which have up to the present time been published."

The rendering into English of the account of 62 teratologic cases in the human subject with the prophetic meanings attached to them by Chaldean diviners, after the translation of Opport, is given as follows by Ballantyne, some of the words being untranslatable:—

"When a woman gives birth to an infant—

(1) that has the ears of a lion, there will be a powerful king in the country;

(2) that wants the right ear, the days of the master (king) will be prolonged (reach old age);

(3) that wants both ears, there will be mourning in the country, and the country will be lessened (diminished);

(4) whose right ear is small, the house of the man (in whose house the birth took place) will be destroyed;

(5) whose ears are both small, the house of the man will be built of bricks;

(6) whose right ear is mudissu tehaat (monstrous), there will be an androgyne in the house of the new-born

(7) whose ears are both mudissu (deformed), the country will perish and the enemy rejoice;

(8) whose right ear is round, there will be an androgyne in the house of the new-born;

(9) whose right ear has a wound below, and tur re ut of the man, the house will be estroyed;

(10) that has two ears on the right side and none on the left, the gods will bring about a stable reign, the country will flourish, and it will be a land of repose;

(11) whose ears are both closed, sa a au;

(12) that has a bird's beak, the country will be peaceful;

(13) that has no mouth, the mistress of the house will die;

(14) that has no right nostril, the people of the world will be injured;

(15) whose nostrils are absent, the country will be in affliction, and the house of the man will be ruined;

(16) whose jaws are absent, the days of the master (king) will be prolonged, but the house (where the infant is born) will be ruined.

When a woman gives birth to an infant—

(17) that has no lower jaw, mut ta at mat, the name will not be effaced;

(20) that has no nose, affliction will seize upon the country, and the master of the house will die;

(21) that has neither nose nor virile member (penis), the army of the king will be strong, peace will be in the land, the men of the king will be sheltered from evil influences, and Lilit (a female demon) shall not have power over them;

(22) whose upper lip overrides the lower, the people of the world will rejoice (or good augury for the troops);

(23) that has no lips, affliction will seize upon the land, and the house of the man will be destroyed;

(24) whose tongue is kuri aat, the man will be spared (?);

(25) that has no right hand, the country will be convulsed by an earthquake;

(26) that has no fingers, the town will have no births, the bar shall be lost;

(27) that has no fingers on the right side, the master (king) will not pardon his adversary (or shall be humiliated by his enemies);

(28) that has six fingers on the right side, the man will take the lukunu of the house;

(29) that has six very small toes on both feet, he shall not go to the lukunu;

(30) that has six toes on each foot, the people of the world will be injured (calamity to the troops);

(31) that has the heart open and that has no skin, the country will suffer from calamities;

(32) that has no penis, the master of the house will be enriched by the harvest of his field;

(33) that wants the penis and the umbilicus, there will be ill-will in the house, the woman (wife) will have an overbearing eye (be haughty); but the male descent of the palace will be more extended.

When a woman gives birth to an infant—

(34) that has no well-marked sex, calamity and affliction will seize upon the land; the master of the house shall have no happiness;

(35) whose anus is closed, the country will suffer from want of nourishment;

(36) whose right testicle (?) is absent, the country of the master (king) will perish;

(37) whose right foot is absent, his house will be ruined and there will be abundance in that of the neighbor;

(38) that has no feet, the canals of the country will be cut (intercepted) and the house ruined;

(39) that has the right foot in the form of a fish's tail, the booty of the country of the humble will not be imas sa bir;

(40) whose hands and feet are like four fishes' tails (fins), the master (king) shall perish (?) and his country shall be consumed;

(41) whose feet are moved by his great hunger, the house of the su su shall be destroyed;

(42) whose foot hangs to the tendons of the body, there will be great prosperity in the land;

(43) that has three feet, two in their normal position (attached to the body) and the third between them, there will be great prosperity in the land;

(44) whose legs are male and female, there will be rebellion;

(45) that wants the right heel, the country of the master (king) will be destroyed.

When a woman gives birth to an infant—

(46) that has many white hairs on the head, the days of the king will be prolonged;

(47) that has much ipga on the head, the master of the house will die, the house will be destroyed;

(48) that has much pinde on the head, joy shall go to meet the house (that has a head on the head, the good augury shall enter at its aspect into the house);

(49) that has the head full of hali, there will be ill-will toward him and the master (king) of the town shall die;

(50) that has the head full of siksi the king will repudiate his masters;

(51) that has some pieces of flesh (skin) hanging on the head, there shall be ill-will;

(52) that has some branches (?) (excrescences) of flesh (skin) hanging on the head, there shall be ill-will, the house will perish;

(53) that has some formed fingers (horns ?) on the head, the days of the king will be less and the years lengthened (in the duration of his old age);

(54) that has some kali on the head, there will be a king of the land;

(55) that has a —— of a bird on the head, the master of the house shall not prosper;

(56) that has some teeth already through (cut), the days of the king will arrive at old age, the country will show itself powerful over (against) strange (feeble) lands, but the house where the infant is born will be ruined;

(57) that has the beard come out, there will be abundant rains;

(58) that has some birta on the head, the country will be strengthened (reinforced);

(59) that has on the head the mouth of an old man and that foams (slabbers), there will be great prosperity in the land, the god Bin will give a magnificent harvest (inundate the land with fertility), and abundance shall be in the land;

(60) that has on one side of the head a thickened ear, the first-born of the men shall live a long time (?);

(61) that has on the head two long and thick ears, there will be tranquility and the pacification of litigation (contests);

(62) that has the figure in horn (like a horn ?) . . ."

As ancient and as obscure as are these records, Ballantyne has carefully gone over each, and gives the following lucid explanatory comments:—

"What 'ears like a lion' (No. 1) may have been it is difficult to determine; but doubtless the direction and shape of the auricles were so altered as to give them an animal appearance, and possibly the deformity was that called 'orechio ad ansa' by Lombroso. The absence of one or both ears (Nos. 2 and 3) has been noted in recent times by Virchow (Archiv fur path. Anat. xxx., p. 221), Gradenigo (Taruffi's 'Storia della Teratologia,' vi., p. 552), and others. Generally some cartilaginous remnant is found, but on this point the Chaldean record is silent. Variations in the size of the ears (Nos. 4 and 5) are well known at the present time, and have been discussed at length by Binder (Archiv fur Psychiatrie und Nervenkrankheiten, xx., 1887) and others. The exact malformation indicated in Nos. 6 and 7 is, of course, not to be determined, although further researches in Assyriology may clear up this point. The 'round ear' (No. 8) is one of Binder's types, and that with a 'wound below' (No. 9) probably refers to a case of fistula auris congenita (Toynbee, 'Diseases of the Ear,' 1860). The instance of an infant born with two ears on the right side (No. 10) was doubtless one of cervical auricle or preauricular appendage, whilst closure of the external auditory meatus (No. 11) is a well-known deformity.

"The next thirteen cases (Nos. 12-24) were instances of anomalies of the mouth and nose. The 'bird's beak' (No. 12) may have been a markedly aquiline nose; No. 13 was a case of astoma; and Nos. 14 and 15 were instances of stenosis or atresia of the anterior nares. Fetuses with absence of the maxillae (Nos. 16 and 17) are in modern terminology called agnathous. Deformities like that existing in Nos. 20 and 21 have been observed in paracephalic and cyclopic fetuses. The coincident absence of nose and penis (No. 21) is interesting, especially when taken in conjunction with the popular belief that the size of the former organ varies with that of the latter. Enlargement of the upper lip (No. 22), called epimacrochelia by Taruffi, and absence of the lips (No. 23), known now under the name of brachychelia, have been not unfrequently noticed in recent times. The next six cases (Nos. 25-30) were instances of malformations of the upper limb: Nos. 25, 26. and 27 were probably instances of the so-called spontaneous or intrauterine amputation; and Nos. 28, 29, and 30 were examples of the comparatively common deformity known as polydactyly. No. 31 was probably a case of ectopia cordis.

"Then follow five instances of genital abnormalities (Nos. 32-36), consisting of absence of the penis (epispadias?), absence of penis and umbilicus (epispadias and exomphalos?), hermaphroditism, imperforate anus, and nondescent of one testicle. The nine following cases (Nos. 37-45) were anomalies of the lower limbs: Nos. 37, 38, and 42 may have been spontaneous amputations; Nos. 39 and 40 were doubtless instances of webbed toes (syndactyly), and the deformity indicated in No. 45 was presumably talipes equinus. The infant born with three feet (No. 43) was possibly a case of parasitic monstrosity, several of which have been reported in recent teratologic literature; but what is meant by the statement concerning 'male and female legs' it is not easy to determine.

"Certain of the ten following prodigies (Nos. 46-55) cannot in the present state of our knowledge be identified. The presence of congenital patches of white or gray hair on the scalp, as recorded in No. 46, is not an unknown occurrence at the present time; but what the Chaldeans meant by ipga, pinde, hali riksi, and kali on the head of the new-born infant it is impossible to tell. The guess may be hazarded that cephalhematoma, hydrocephalus, meningocele, nevi, or an excessive amount of vernix caseosa were the conditions indicated, but a wider acquaintance with the meaning of the cuneiform characters is necessary before any certain identification is possible. The 'pieces of skin hanging from the head' (No. 51) may have been fragments of the membranes; but there is nothing in the accompanying prediction to help us to trace the origin of the popular belief in the good luck following the baby born with a caul. If No. 53 was a case of congenital horns on the head, it must be regarded as a unique example, unless, indeed, a form of fetal ichthyosis be indicated.

"The remaining observations (No. 56-62) refer to cases of congenital teeth (No. 56) to deformity of the ears (Nos. 60 and 61), and a horn (No. 62)."

From these early times almost to the present day similar significance has been attached to minor structural anomalies. In the following pages the individual anomalies will be discussed separately and the most interesting examples of each will be cited. It is manifestly evident that the object of this chapter is to mention the most striking instances of abnormism and to give accompanying descriptions of associate points of interest, rather than to offer a scientific exposition of teratology, for which the reader is referred elsewhere.

Congenital defect of the epidermis and true skin is a rarity in pathology. Pastorello speaks of a child which lived for two and a half hours whose hands and feet were entirely destitute of epidermis; the true skin of those parts looked like that of a dead and already putrefying child. Hanks cites the history of a case of antepartum desquamation of the skin in a living fetus. Hochstetter describes a full-term, living male fetus with cutaneous defect on both sides of the abdomen a little above the umbilicus. The placenta and membranes were normal, a fact indicating that the defect was not due to amniotic adhesions; the child had a clubfoot on the left side. The mother had a fall three weeks before labor.

Abnormal Elasticity of the Skin.—In some instances the skin is affixed so loosely to the underlying tissues and is possessed of so great elasticity that it can be stretched almost to the same extent as India rubber. There have been individuals who could take the skin of the forehead and pull it down over the nose, or raise the skin of the neck over the mouth. They also occasionally have an associate muscular development in the subcutaneous tissues similar to the panniculus adiposus of quadrupeds, giving them preternatural motile power over the skin. The man recently exhibited under the title of the "Elastic-Skin Man" was an example of this anomaly. The first of this class of exhibitionists was seen in Buda-Pesth some years since and possessed great elasticity in the skin of his whole body; even his nose could be stretched. Figure 70 represents a photograph of an exhibitionist named Felix Wehrle, who besides having the power to stretch his skin could readily bend his fingers backward and forward. The photograph was taken in January, 1888.

In these congenital cases there is loose attachment of the skin without hypertrophy, to which the term dermatolysis is restricted by Crocker. Job van Meekren, the celebrated Dutch physician of the seventeenth century, states that in 1657 a Spaniard, Georgius Albes, is reported to have been able to draw the skin of the left pectoral region to the left ear, or the skin under the face over the chin to the vertex. The skin over the knee could be extended half a yard, and when it retracted to its normal position it was not in folds. Seiffert examined a case of this nature in a young man of nineteen, and, contrary to Kopp's supposition, found that in some skin from over the left second rib the elastic fibers were quite normal, but there was transformation of the connective tissue of the dermis into an unformed tissue like a myxoma, with total disappearance of the connective-tissue bundles. Laxity of the skin after distention is often seen in multipara, both in the breasts and in the abdominal walls, and also from obesity, but in all such cases the skin falls in folds, and does not have a normal appearance like that of the true "elastic-skin man."

Occasionally abnormal development of the scalp is noticed. McDowall of twenty-two. On each side of the median line of the head there were five deep furrows, more curved and shorter as the distance from the median line increased. In the illustration the hair in the furrows is left longer than that on the rest of the head. The patient was distinctly microcephalic and the right side of the body was markedly wasted. The folds were due to hypertrophy of the muscles and scalp, and the same sort of furrowing is noticed when a dog "pricks his ears." This case may possibly be considered as an example of reversion to inferior types. Cowan records two cases of the foregoing nature in idiots. The first case was a paralytic idiot of thirty-nine, whose cranial development was small in proportion to the size of the face and body; the cranium was oxycephalic; the scalp was lax and redundant and the hair thin; there were 13 furrows, five on each side running anteroposteriorly, and three in the occipital region running transversely. The occipitofrontalis muscle had no action on them. The second case was that of an idiot of forty-four of a more degraded type than the previous one. The cranium was round and bullet-shaped and the hair generally thick. The scalp was not so lax as in the other case, but the furrows were more crooked. By tickling the scalp over the back of the neck the two median furrows involuntarily deepened.

Impervious Skin.—There have been individuals who claimed that their skin was impervious to ordinary puncture, and from time to time these individuals have appeared in some of the larger medical clinics of the world for inspection. According to a recent number of the London Graphic, there is in Berlin a Singhalese who baffles all investigations by physicians by the impenetrability of his skin. The bronzed Easterner, a Hercules in shape, claims to have found an elixir which will render the human skin impervious to any metal point or sharpened edge of a knife or dagger, and calls himself the "Man with Iron Skin." He is now exhibiting himself, and his greatest feat is to pass with his entire body through a hoop the inside of which is hardly big enough to admit his body and is closely set with sharp knife-points, daggers, nails, and similar things. Through this hoop he squeezes his body with absolute impunity. The physicians do not agree as to his immunity, and some of them think that Rhannin, which is his name, is a fakir who has by long practice succeeded in hardening himself against the impressions of metal upon his skin. The professors of the Berlin clinic, however, considered it worth while to lecture about the man's skin, pronouncing it an inexplicable matter. This individual performed at the London Alhambra in the latter part of 1895. Besides climbing with bare feet a ladder whose rungs were sharp-edged swords, and lying on a bed of nail points with four men seated upon him, he curled himself up in a barrel, through whose inner edges nails projected, and was rolled about the stage at a rapid rate. Emerging from thence uninjured, he gracefully bows himself off the stage.

Some individuals claim immunity from burns and show many interesting feats in handling fire. As they are nothing but skilful "fire jugglers" they deserve no mention here. The immunity of the participants in the savage fire ceremonies will be discussed in Chapter IX.

Albinism is characterized by the absolute or relative absence of pigment of the skin, due to an arrest, insufficiency, or retardation of this pigment. Following Trelat and Guinard, we may divide albinism into two classes,— general and partial.

As to the etiology of albinism, there is no known cause of the complete form. Heredity plays no part in the number of cases investigated by the authors. D'Aube, by his observations on white rabbits, believes that the influence of consanguinity is a marked factor in the production of albinism; there are, however, many instances of heredity in this anomaly on record, and this idea is possibly in harmony with the majority of observers. Geoffroy-Saint-Hilaire has noted that albinism can also be a consequence of a pathologic condition having its origin in adverse surroundings, the circumstances of the parents, such as the want of exercise, nourishment, light, etc.

Lesser knew a family in which six out of seven were albinos, and in some tropical countries, such as Loango, Lower Guinea, it is said to be endemic. It is exceptional for the parents to be affected; but in a case of Schlegel, quoted by Crocker, the grandfather was an albino, and Marey describes the case of the Cape May albinos, in which the mother and father were "fair emblems of the African race," and of their children three were black and three were white, born in the following order: two consecutive black boys, two consecutive white girls, one black girl, one white boy. Sym of Edinburgh relates the history of a family of seven children, who were alternately white and black. All but the seventh were living and in good health and mentally without defect. The parents and other relatives were dark. Figure 73 portrays an albino family by the name of Cavalier who exhibited in Minneapolis in 1887.

Examples of the total absence of pigment occur in all races, but particularly is it interesting when seen in negroes who are found absolutely white but preserving all the characteristics of their race, as, for instance, the kinky, woolly hair, flattened nose, thick lips, etc. Rene Claille, in his "Voyage a Tombouctou," says that he saw a white infant, the offspring of a negro and negress. Its hair was white, its eyes blue, and its lashes flaxen. Its pupils were of a reddish color, and its physiognomy that of a Mandingo. He says such cases are not at all uncommon; they are really negro albinos. Thomas Jefferson, in his "History of Virginia," has an excellent description of these negroes, with their tremulous and weak eyes; he remarks that they freckle easily. Buffon speaks of Ethiops with white twins, and says that albinos are quite common in Africa, being generally of delicate constitution, twinkling eyes, and of a low degree of intelligence; they are despised and ill-treated by the other negroes. Prichard, quoted by Sedgwick, speaks of a case of atavic transmission of albinism through the male line of the negro race. The grandfather and the grandchild were albinos, the father being black. There is a case of a brother and sister who were albinos, the parents being of ordinary color but the grandfather an albino. Coinde, quoted by Sedgwick, speaks of a man who, by two different wives, had three albino children.

A description of the ordinary type of albino would be as follows: The skin and hair are deprived of pigment; the eyebrows and eyelashes are of a brilliant white or are yellowish; the iris and the choroid are nearly or entirely deprived of coloring material, and in looking at the eye we see a roseate zone and the ordinary pink pupil; from absence of pigment they necessarily keep their eyes three-quarters closed, being photophobic to a high degree. They are amblyopic, and this is due partially to a high degree of ametropia (caused by crushing of the eyeball in the endeavor to shut out light) and from retinal exhaustion and nystagmus. Many authors have claimed that they have little intelligence, but this opinion is not true. Ordinarily the reproductive functions are normal, and if we exclude the results of the union of two albinos we may say that these individuals are fecund.

Partial albinism is seen. The parts most often affected are the genitals, the hair, the face, the top of the trunk, the nipple, the back of the hands and fingers. Folker reports the history of a case of an albino girl having pink eyes and red hair, the rest of the family having pink eyes and white hair. Partial albinism, necessarily congenital, presenting a piebald appearance, must not be confounded with leukoderma, which is rarely seen in the young and which will be described later.

Albinism is found in the lower animals, and is exemplified ordinarily by rats, mice, crows, robins, etc. In the Zoologic Garden at Baltimore two years ago was a pair of pure albino opossums. The white elephant is celebrated in the religious history of Oriental nations, and is an object of veneration and worship in Siam. White monkeys and white roosters are also worshiped. In the Natural History Museum in London there are stuffed examples of albinism and melanism in the lower animals.

Melanism is an anomaly, the exact contrary of the preceding. It is characterized by the presence in the tissues and skin of an excessive amount of pigment. True total melanism is unknown in man, in whom is only observed partial melanism, characterized simply by a pronounced coloration of part of the integument.

Some curious instances have been related of an infant with a two-colored face, and of others with one side of the face white and the other black; whether they were cases of partial albinism or partial melanism cannot be ascertained from the descriptions.

Such epidermic anomalies as ichthyosis, scleroderma, and molluscum simplex, sometimes appearing shortly after birth, but generally seen later in life, will be spoken of in the chapter on Anomalous Skin Diseases.

Human horns are anomalous outgrowths from the skin and are far more frequent than ordinarily supposed. Nearly all the older writers cite examples. Aldrovandus, Amatus Lusitanus, Boerhaave, Dupre, Schenck, Riverius, Vallisneri, and many others mention horns on the head. In the ancient times horns were symbolic of wisdom and power. Michael Angelo in his famous sculpture of Moses has given the patriarch a pair of horns. Rhodius observed a Benedictine monk who had a pair of horns and who was addicted to rumination. Fabricius saw a man with horns on his head, whose son ruminated; the son considered that by virtue of his ruminating characteristics his father had transmitted to him the peculiar anomaly of the family. Fabricius Hildanus saw a patient with horns all over the body and another with horns on the forehead. Gastaher speaks of a horn from the left temple; Zacutus Lusitanus saw a horn from the heel; Wroe, one of considerable length from the scapula; Cosnard, one from the bregma; the Ephemerides, from the foot; Borellus, from the face and foot, and Ash, horns all over the body. Home, Cooper, and Treves have collected examples of horns, and there is one 11 inches long and 2 1/2 in circumference in a London museum. Lozes collected reports of 71 cases of horns,—37 in females, 31 in males, and three in infants. Of this number, 15 were on the head, eight on the face, 18 on the lower extremities, eight on the trunk, and three on the glans penis. Wilson collected reports of 90 cases,—44 females, 39 males, the sex not being mentioned in the remainder. Of these 48 were on the head, four on the face, four on the nose, 11 on the thigh, three on the leg and foot, six on the back, five on the glans penis, and nine on the trunk. Lebert's collection numbered 109 cases of cutaneous horns. The greater frequency among females is admitted by all authors. Old age is a predisposing cause. Several patients over seventy have been seen and one of ninety-seven.

Instances of cutaneous horns, when seen and reported by the laity, give rise to most amusing exaggerations and descriptions. The following account is given in New South Wales, obviously embellished with apocryphal details by some facetious journalist: The child, five weeks old, was born with hair two inches long all over the body; his features were fiendish and his eyes shone like beads beneath his shaggy brows. He had a tail 18 inches long, horns from the skull, a full set of teeth, and claw-like hands; he snapped like a dog and crawled on all fours, and refused the natural sustenance of a normal child. The mother almost became an imbecile after the birth of the monster. The country people about Bomballa considered this devil-child a punishment for a rebuff that the mother gave to a Jewish peddler selling Crucifixion-pictures. Vexed by his persistence, she said she would sooner have a devil in her house than his picture.

Lamprey has made a minute examination of the much-spoken-of "Horned Men of Africa." He found that this anomaly was caused by a congenital malformation and remarkable development of the infraorbital ridge of the maxillary bone. He described several cases, and through an interpreter found that they were congenital, followed no history of traumatism, caused little inconvenience, and were unassociated with disturbance of the sense of smell. He also learned that the deformity was quite rare in the Cape Coast region, and received no information tending to prove the conjecture that the tribes in West Africa used artificial means to produce the anomaly, although such custom is prevalent among many aborigines.

Probably the most remarkable case of a horn was that of Paul Rodrigues, a Mexican porter, who, from the upper and lateral part of his head, had a horn 14 inches in circumference and divided into three shafts, which he concealed by constantly wearing a peculiarly shaped red cap. There is in Paris a wax model of a horn, eight or nine inches in length, removed from an old woman by the celebrated Souberbielle. Figure 75 is from a wax model supposed to have been taken from life, showing an enormous grayish-black horn proceeding from the forehead. Warren mentions a case under the care of Dubois, in a woman from whose forehead grew a horn six inches in diameter and six inches in height. It was hard at the summit and had a fetid odor. In 1696 there was an old woman in France who constantly shed long horns from her forehead, one of which was presented to the King. Bartholinus mentions a horn 12 inches long. Voigte cites the case of an old woman who had a horn branching into three portions, coming from her forehead. Sands speaks of a woman who had a horn 6 3/4 inches long, growing from her head. There is an account of the extirpation of a horn nearly ten inches in length from the forehead of a woman of eighty-two. Bejau describes a woman of forty from whom he excised an excrescence resembling a ram's horn, growing from the left parietal region. It curved forward and nearly reached the corresponding tuberosity. It was eight cm. long, two cm. broad at the base, and 1 1/2 cm. at the apex, and was quite mobile. It began to grow at the age of eleven and had constantly increased. Vidal presented before the Academie de Medecine in 1886 a twisted horn from the head of a woman. This excrescence was ten inches long, and at the time of presentation reproduction of it was taking place in the woman. Figure 76 shows a case of ichthyosis cornea pictured in the Lancet, 1850.

There was a woman of seventy-five, living near York, who had a horny growth from the face which she broke off and which began to reproduce, the illustration representing the growth during twelve months. Lall mentions a horn from the cheek; Gregory reports one that measured 7 1/2 inches long that was removed from the temple of a woman in Edinburgh; Chariere of Barnstaple saw a horn that measured seven inches growing from the nape of a woman's neck; Kameya Iwa speaks of a dermal horn of the auricle; Saxton of New York has excised several horns from the tympanic membrane of the ear; Noyes speaks of one from the eyelid; Bigelow mentions one from the chin; Minot speaks of a horn from the lower lip, and Doran of one from the neck.

Gould cites the instance of a horn growing from an epitheliomatous penis. The patient was fifty-two years of age and the victim of congenital phimosis. He was circumcised four years previously, and shortly after the wound healed there appeared a small wart, followed by a horn about the size of a marble. Jewett speaks of a penile horn 3 1/2 inches long and 3 3/4 inches in diameter; Pick mentions one 2 1/2 inches long. There is an account of a Russian peasant boy who had a horn on his penis from his earliest childhood. Johnson mentions a case of a horn from the scrotum, which was of sebaceous origin and was subsequently supplanted by an epithelioma.

Ash reported the case of a girl named Annie Jackson, living in Waterford, Ireland, who had horny excrescences from her joints, arms, axillae, nipples, ears, and forehead. Locke speaks of a boy at the Hopital de la Charite in Paris, who had horny excrescences four inches long and 11 inches in circumference growing from his fingers and toes.

Wagstaffe presents a horn which grew from the middle of the leg six inches below the knee in a woman of eighty. It was a flattened spiral of more than two turns, and during forty years' growth had reached the length of 14.3 inches. Its height was 3.8 inches, its skin-attachment 1.5 inches in diameter, and it ended in a blunt extremity of 0.5 inch in diameter. Stephens mentions a dermal horn on the buttocks at the seat of a carcinomatous cicatrix. Harris and Domonceau speak of horns from the leg. Cruveilhier saw a Mexican Indian who had a horn four inches long and eight inches in circumference growing from the left lumbar region. It had been sawed off twice by the patient's son and was finally extirpated by Faget. The length of the pieces was 12 inches. Bellamy saw a horn on the clitoris about the size of a tiger's claw in a its origin from beneath the preputium clitoridis.

Horns are generally solitary but cases of multiple formation are known Lewin and Heller record a syphilitic case with eight cutaneous horns on the palms and soles. A female patient of Manzuroff had as many as 185 horns.

Pancoast reports the case of a man whose nose, cheeks, forehead, and lips were covered with horny growths, which had apparently undergone epitheliomatous degeneration. The patient was a sea-captain of seventy-eight, and had been exposed to the winds all his life. He had suffered three attacks of erysipelas from prolonged exposure. When he consulted Pancoast the horns had nearly all fallen off and were brought to the physician for inspection; and the photograph was taken after the patient had tied the horns in situ on his face.

Anomalies of the Hair.—Congenital alopecia is quite rare, and it is seldom that we see instances of individuals who have been totally destitute of hair from birth. Danz knew of two adult sons of a Jewish family who never had hair or teeth. Sedgwick quotes the case of a man of fifty-eight who ever since birth was totally devoid of hair and in whom sensible perspiration and tears were absent. A cousin on his mother's side, born a year before him, had precisely the same peculiarity. Buffon says that the Turks and some other people practised depilatory customs by the aid of ointments and pomades, principally about the genitals. Atkinson exhibited in Philadelphia a man of forty who never had any distinct growth of hair since birth, was edentulous, and destitute of the sense of smell and almost of that of taste. He had no apparent perspiration, and when working actively he was obliged to wet his clothes in order to moderate the heat of his body. He could sleep in wet clothes in a damp cellar without catching cold. There was some hair in the axillae and on the pubes, but only the slightest down on the scalp, and even that was absent on the skin. His maternal grandmother and uncle were similarly affected; he was the youngest of 21 children, had never been sick, and though not able to chew food in the ordinary manner, he had never suffered from dyspepsia in any form. He was married and had eight children. Of these, two girls lacked a number of teeth, but had the ordinary quantity of hair. Hill speaks of an aboriginal man in Queensland who was entirely devoid of hair on the head, face, and every part of the body. He had a sister, since dead, who was similarly hairless. Hill mentions the accounts given of another black tribe, about 500 miles west of Brisbane, that contained hairless members. This is very strange, as the Australian aboriginals are a very hairy race of people.

Hutchinson mentions a boy of three and a half in whom there was congenital absence of hair and an atrophic condition of the skin and appendages. His mother was bald from the age of six, after alopecia areata. Schede reports two cases of congenitally bald children of a peasant woman (a boy of thirteen and a girl of six months). They had both been born quite bald, and had remained so. In addition there were neither eyebrows nor eyelashes and nowhere a trace of lanugo. The children were otherwise healthy and well formed. The parents and brothers were healthy and possessed a full growth of hair. Thurman reports a case of a man of fifty-eight, who was almost devoid of hair all his life and possessed only four teeth. His skin was very delicate and there was absence of sensible perspiration and tears. The skin was peculiar in thinness, softness, and absence of pigmentation. The hair on the crown of the head and back was very fine, short, and soft, and not more in quantity than that of an infant of three months. There was a similar peculiarity in his cousin-german. Williams mentions the case of a young lady of fifteen with scarcely any hair on the eyebrows or head and no eyelashes. She was edentulous and had never sensibly perspired. She improved under tonic treatment.

Rayer quotes the case of Beauvais, who was a patient in the Hopital de la Charite in 1827. The skin of this man's cranium was apparently completely naked, although in examining it narrowly it was found to be beset with a quantity of very white and silky hair, similar to the down that covers the scalp of infants; here and there on the temples there were a few black specks, occasioned by the stumps of several hairs which the patient had shaved off. The eyebrows were merely indicated by a few fine and very short hairs; the free edges of the eyelids were without cilia, but the bulb of each of these was indicated by a small, whitish point. The beard was so thin and weak that Beauvais clipped it off only every three weeks. A few straggling hairs were observed on the breast and pubic region, as in young people on the approach of puberty. There was scarcely any under the axillae. It was rather more abundant on the inner parts of the legs. The voice was like that of a full-grown and well-constituted man. Beauvais was of an amorous disposition and had had syphilis twice. His mother and both sisters had good heads of hair, but his father presented the same defects as Beauvais.

Instances are on record of women devoid of hair about the genital region. Riolan says that he examined the body of a female libertine who was totally hairless from the umbilical region down.

Congenital alopecia is seen in animals. There is a species of dog, a native of China but now bred in Mexico and in the United States, which is distinguished for its congenital alopecia. The same fact has been observed occasionally in horses, cattle, and dogs. Heusner has seen a pigeon destitute of feathers, and which engendered a female which in her turn transmitted the same characteristic to two of her young.

Sexualism and Hair Growth.—The growth or development of the hair may be accelerated by the state of the organs of generation. This is peculiarly noticeable in the pubic hairs and the beard, and is fully exemplified in the section on precocious development (Chapter VII); however, Moreau de la Sarthe showed a child to the Medical Faculty of Paris in whom precocious development of the testicles had influenced that of the hair to such a degree that, at the age of six, the chest of this boy was as thickly set with hair as is usually seen in adults. It is well known that eunuchs often lose a great part of their beards, and after removal of the ovaries women are seen to develop an extra quantity of hair. Gerberon tells of an infant with a beard, and Paullini and the Ephemerides mention similar instances.

Bearded women are not at all infrequent. Hippocrates mentions a female who grew a beard shortly after menstruation had ceased. It is a well-recognized fact that after the menopause women become more hirsute, the same being the case after removal of any of the functional generative apparatus. Vicat saw a virgin who had a beard, and Joch speaks of "foeminis barbati." Leblond says that certain women of Ethiopia and South America have beards and little or no menstruation. He also says that sterility and excessive chastity are causes of female beards, and cites the case of Schott of a young widow who secluded herself in a cloister, and soon had a beard.

Barbara Urster, who lived in the 16th century, had a beard to her girdle. The most celebrated "bearded woman" was Rosine-Marguerite Muller, who died in a hospital in Dresden in 1732, with a thick beard and heavy mustache. Julia Pastrana had her face covered with thick hair and had a full beard and mustache. She exhibited defective dentition in both jaws, and the teeth present were arranged in an irregular fashion. She had pronounced prognathism, which gave her a simian appearance. Ecker examined in 1876 a woman who died at Fribourg, whose face contained a full beard and a luxuriant mustache.

Harris reports several cases of bearded women, inmates of the Coton Hill Lunatic Asylum. One of the patients was eighty-three years of age and had been insane forty-four years following a puerperal period. She would not permit the hair on her face to be cut, and the curly white hairs had attained a length of from eight to ten inches on the chin, while on the upper lip the hairs were scarcely an inch. This patient was quite womanly in all her sentiments. The second case was a woman of thirty-six, insane from emotional melancholia. She had tufts of thick, curly hair on the chin two inches long, light yellowish in color, and a few straggling hairs on the upper lip. The third case was that of a woman of sixty-four, who exhibited a strong passion for the male sex. Her menstruation had been regular until the menopause. She plaited her beard, and it was seven or eight inches long on the chin and one inch on the lip. This woman had extremely hairy legs. Another case was that of a woman of sixty-two, who, though bald, developed a beard before the climacteric. Her structural proportions were feminine in character, and it is said that her mother, who was sane, had a beard also. A curious case was that of a woman of twenty-three (Mrs. Viola M.), who from the age of three had a considerable quantity of hair on the side of the cheek which eventually became a full beard. She was quite feminine was free from excessive hair elsewhere, her nose and forehead being singularly bare. Her voice was very sweet; she was married at seventeen and a half, having two normal children, and nursed each for one month. "The bearded woman" of every circus side-show is an evidence of the curious interest in which these women are held. The accompanying illustration is a representation of a "bearded woman" born in Bracken County, Ky. Her beard measured 15 inches in length.

There is a class of anomalies in which there is an exaggerated development of hair. We would naturally expect to find the primitive peoples, who are not provided with artificial protection against the wind, supplied with an extra quantity of hair or having a hairy coat like animals; but this is sometimes found among civilized people. This abnormal presence of hair on the human body has been known for many years; the description of Esau in the Bible is an early instance. Aldrovandus says that in the sixteenth century there came to the Canary Islands a family consisting of a father, son, and two daughters, who were covered all over their bodies by long hair, and their portrait, certainly reproduced from life, resembles the modern instances of "dog men."

In 1883 there was shown in England and France, afterward in America, a girl of seven named "Krao," a native of Indo-China. The whole body of this child was covered with black hair. Her face was of the prognathic type, and this, with her extraordinary prehensile powers of feet and lips, gave her the title of "Darwin's missing link." In 1875 there was exhibited in Paris, under the name of "l'homme-chien" Adrien Jeftichew, a Russian peasant of fifty-five, whose face, head, back, and limbs were covered with a brown hairy coat looking like wool and several centimeters long. The other parts of the body were also covered with hair, but less abundantly. This individual had a son of three, Theodore, who was hairy like himself.

A family living in Burmah (Shive-Maon, whose history is told by Crawford and Yule), consisting of a father, a daughter, and a granddaughter, were nearly covered with hair. Figure 84 represents a somewhat similar family who were exhibited in this country.

Teresa Gambardella, a young girl of twelve, mentioned by Lombroso, was covered all over the body, with the exception of the hands and feet, by thick, bushy hair. This hypertrichosis was exemplified in this country only a few months since by a person who went the rounds of the dime museums under the euphonious name of "Jo-Jo, the dog-face boy." His face was truly that of a skye-terrier.

Sometimes the hairy anomalies are but instances of naevus pilosus. The Indian ourang-outang woman examined at the office of the Lancet was an example of this kind. Hebra, Hildebrandt, Jablokoff, and Klein describe similar cases. Many of the older "wild men" were individuals bearing extensive hairy moles.

Rayer remarks that he has seen a young man of sixteen who exhibited himself to the public under the name of a new species of wild man whose breast and back were covered with light brown hair of considerable length.

The surface upon which it grew was of a brownish hue, different from the color of the surrounding integument. Almost the whole of the right arm was covered in the same manner. On the lower extremity several tufts of hair were observed implanted upon brown spots from seven to eight lines in diameter symmetrically disposed upon both legs. The hair was brown, of the same color as that of the head. Bichat informs us that he saw at Paris an unfortunate man who from his birth was afflicted with a hairy covering of his face like that of a wild boar, and he adds that the stories which were current among the vulgar of individuals with a boar's head, wolf's head, etc., undoubtedly referred to cases in which the face was covered to a greater or less degree with hair. Villerme saw a child of six at Poitiers in 1808 whose body, except the feet and hands, was covered with a great number of prominent brown spots of different dimensions, beset with hair shorter and not so strong as that of a boar, but bearing a certain resemblance to the bristles of that animal. These spots occupied about one-fifth of the surface of this child's skin. Campaignac in the early part of this century exhibited a case in which there was a large tuft of long black hair growing from the shoulder. Dufour has detailed a case of a young man of twenty whose sacral region contained a tuft of hair as long and black, thick and pliant, as that of the head, and, particularly remarkable in this case, the skin from which it grew was as fine and white as the integument of the rest of the body. There was a woman exhibited recently, under the advertisement of "the lady with a mane," who had growing from the center of her back between the shoulders a veritable mane of long, black hair, which doubtless proceeded from a form of naevus.

Duyse reports a case of extensive hypertrichosis of the back in a girl aged nine years; her teeth were normal; there was pigmentation of the back and numerous pigmentary nevi on the face. Below each scapula there were tumors of the nature of fibroma molluscum. In addition to hairy nevi on the other parts of the body there was localized ichthyosis.

Ziemssen figures an interesting case of naevus pilosus resembling "bathing tights". There were also present several benign tumors (fibroma molluscum) and numerous smaller nevi over the body. Schulz first observed the patient in 1878. This individual's name was Blake, and he stated that he was born with a large naevus spreading over the upper parts of the thighs and lower parts of the trunk, like bathing-tights, and resembling the pelt of an animal. The same was true of the small hairy parts and the larger and smaller tumors. Subsequently the altered portions of the skin had gradually become somewhat larger. The skin of the large hairy naevus, as well as that of the smaller ones, was stated by Schulz to have been in the main thickened, in part uneven, verrucose, from very light to intensely dark brown in color; the consistency of the larger mammiform and smaller tumors soft, doughy, and elastic. The case was really one of large congenital naevus pilosus and fibroma molluscum combined.

A Peruvian boy was shown at the Westminster Aquarium with a dark, hairy mole situated in the lower part of the trunk and on the thighs in the position of bathing tights. Nevins Hyde records two similar cases with dermatolytic growths. A sister of the Peruvian boy referred to had a still larger growth, extending from the nucha all over the back. Both she and her brother had hundreds of smaller hairy growths of all sizes scattered irregularly over the face, trunk, and limbs. According to

Crocker, a still more extraordinary case, with extensive dermatolytic growths all over the back and nevi of all sizes elsewhere, is described and engraved in "Lavater's Physiognomy," 1848. Baker describes an operation in which a large mole occupying half the forehead was removed by the knife.

In some instances the hair and beard is of an enormous length. Erasmus Wilson of London saw a female of thirty-eight, whose hair measured 1.65 meters long. Leonard of Philadelphia speaks of a man in the interior of this country whose beard trailed on the ground when he stood upright, and measured 2.24 meters long. Not long ago there appeared the famous so-called "Seven Sutherland Sisters," whose hair touched the ground, and with whom nearly every one is familiar through a hair tonic which they extensively advertised. In Nature, January 9, 1892, is an account of a Percheron horse whose mane measured 13 feet and whose tail measured almost ten feet, probably the greatest example of excessive mane development on record. Figure 88 represents Miss Owens, an exhibitionist, whose hair measured eight feet three inches. In Leslie's Weekly, January 2, 1896, there is a portrait of an old negress named Nancy Garrison whose woolly hair was equally as long.

The Ephemerides contains the account of a woman who had hair from the mons veneris which hung to the knees; it was affected with plica polonica, as was also the other hair of the body.

Rayer saw a Piedmontese of twenty-eight, with an athletic build, who had but little beard or hair on the trunk, but whose scalp was covered with a most extraordinary crop. It was extremely fine and silky, was artificially frizzled, dark brown in color, and formed a mass nearly five feet in circumference.

Certain pathologic conditions may give rise to accidental growths of hair. Boyer was accustomed to quote in his lectures the case of a man who, having an inflamed tumor in the thigh, perceived this part becoming covered in a short time with numerous long hairs. Rayer speaks of several instances of this kind. In one the part affected by a blister in a child of two became covered with hair. Another instance was that of a student of medicine, who after bathing in the sea for a length of time, and exposing himself to the hot sun, became affected with coppery patches, from which there sprang a growth of hair. Bricheteau, quoted by the same authority, speaks of a woman of twenty-four, having white skin and hair of deep black, who after a long illness occasioned by an affection analogous to marasmus became covered, especially on the back, breast, and abdomen, with a multitude of small elevations similar to those which appear on exposure to cold. These little elevations became brownish at the end of a few days, and short, fair, silky hair was observed on the summit of each, which grew so rapidly that the whole surface of the body with the exception of the hands and face became velvety. The hair thus evolved was afterward thrown out spontaneously and was not afterward reproduced.

Anomalies of the Color of the Hair.—New-born infants sometimes have tufts of hair on their heads which are perfectly white in color. Schenck speaks of a young man whose beard from its first appearance grew white. Young men from eighteen to twenty occasionally become gray; and according to Rayer, paroxysms of rage, unexpected and unwelcome news, diseases of the scalp such as favus, wounds of the head, habitual headache, over-indulgence of the sexual appetite, mercurial courses too frequently repeated, too great anxiety, etc., have been known to blanch the hair prematurely.

The well-accepted fact of the sudden changing of the color of the hair from violent emotions or other causes has always excited great interest, and many ingenious explanations have been devised to account for it. There is a record in the time of Charles V of a young man who was committed to prison in 1546 for seducing his girl companion, and while there was in great fear and grief, expecting a death-sentence from the Emperor the next day. When brought before his judge, his face was wan and pale and his hair and beard gray, the change having taken place in the night. His beard was filthy with drivel, and the Emperor, moved by his pitiful condition, pardoned him. There was a clergyman of Nottingham whose daughter at the age of thirteen experienced a change from jet-blackness of the hair to white in a single night, but this was confined to a spot on the back of the head 1 1/2 inches in length. Her hair soon became striped, and in seven years was totally white. The same article speaks of a girl in Bedfordshire, Maria Seeley, aged eight, whose face was swarthy, and whose hair was long and dark on one side and light and short on the other. One side of her body was also brown, while the other side was light and fair. She was seen by the faculty in London, but no cause could be established.

Voigtel mentions the occurrence of canities almost suddenly. Bichat had a personal acquaintance whose hair became almost entirely gray in consequence of some distressing news that reached him. Cassan records a similar case. According to Rayer, a woman by the name of Perat, summoned before the Chamber of Peers to give evidence in the trial of the assassin Louvel, was so much affected that her hair became entirely white in a single night Byron makes mention of this peculiar anomaly in the opening stanzas of the "Prisoner of Chillon:"—

"My hair is gray, but not with years,
Nor grew it white
In a single night.
As men's have grown from sudden fears."

The commentators say that Byron had reference to Ludovico Sforza and others. The fact of the change is asserted of Marie Antoinette, the wife of Louis XVI, though in not quite so short a period, grief and not fear being the cause. Ziemssen cites Landois' case of a compositor of thirty-four who was admitted to a hospital July 9th with symptoms of delirium tremens; until improvement began to set in (July 13th) he was continually tormented by terrifying pictures of the imagination. In the night preceding the day last mentioned the hair of the head and beard of the patient, formerly blond, became gray. Accurate examination by Landois showed the pigment contents of the hair to be unchanged, and led him to believe that the white color was solely due to the excessive development of air-bubbles in the hair shaft. Popular belief brings the premature and especially the sudden whitening into connection with depressing mental emotions. We might quote the German expression—"Sich graue Haare etwas wachsen lassen" ("To worry one's self gray"). Brown-Sequard observed on several occasions in his own dark beard hairs which had turned white in a night and which he epileptoid. He closes his brief communication on the subject with the belief that it is quite possible for black hair to turn white in one night or even in a less time, although Hebra and Kaposi discredit sudden canities (Duhring). Raymond and Vulpian observed a lady of neurotic type whose hair during a severe paroxysm of neuralgia following a mental strain changed color in five hours over the entire scalp except on the back and sides; most of the hair changed from black to red, but some to quite white, and in two days all the red hair became white and a quantity fell off. The patient recovered her general health, but with almost total loss of hair, only a few red, white, and black hairs remaining on the occipital and temporal regions. Crocker cites the case of a Spanish cock which was nearly killed by some pigs. The morning after the adventure the feathers of the head had become completely white, and about half of those on the back of the neck were also changed.

Dewees reports a case of puerperal convulsions in a patient under his care which was attended with sudden canities. From 10 A.M. to 4 P.M. 50 ounces of blood were taken. Between the time of Dr. Dewees' visits, not more than an hour, the hair anterior to the coronal suture turned white. The next day it was less light, and in four or five days was nearly its natural color. He also mentions two cases of sudden blanching from fright.

Fowler mentions the case of a healthy girl of sixteen who found one morning while combing her hair, which was black, that a strip the whole length of the back hair was white, starting from a surface about two inches square around the occipital protuberance. Two weeks later she had patches of ephelis over the whole body.

Prentiss, in Science, October 3, 1890, has collected numerous instances of sudden canities, several of which will be given:—

"In the Canada Journal of Medical Science, 1882, p. 113, is reported a case of sudden canities due to business-worry. The microscope showed a great many air-vesicles both in the medullary substance and between the medullary and cortical substance.

"In the Boston Medical and Surgical Journal, 1851, is reported a case of a man thirty years old, whose hair 'was scared' white in a day by a grizzly bear. He was sick in a mining camp, was left alone, and fell asleep. On waking he found a grizzly bear standing over him.

"A second case is that of a man of twenty-three years who was gambling in California. He placed his entire savings of $1100 on the turn of a card. He was under tremendous nervous excitement while the cards were being dealt. The next day his hair was perfectly white.

"In the same article is the statement that the jet-black hair of the Pacific Islanders does not turn gray gradually, but when it does turn it is sudden, usually the result of fright or sudden emotions."

D'Alben, quoted by Fournier, describes a young man of twenty-four, an officer in the regiment of Touraine in 1781, who spent the night in carnal dissipation with a mulatto, after which he had violent spasms, rendering flexion of the body impossible. His beard and hair on the right side of the body was found as white as snow, the left side being unchanged. He appeared before the Faculte de Montpelier, and though cured of his nervous symptoms his hair was still white, and no suggestion of relief was offered him.

Louis of Bavaria, who died in 1294, on learning of the innocence of his wife, whom he had put to death on a suspicion of her infidelity, had a change of color in his hair, which became white almost immediately. Vauvilliers, the celebrated Hellenist, became white-haired almost immediately after a terrible dream, and Brizard, the comedian, experienced the same change after a narrow escape from drowning in the Rhone. The beard and the hair of the Duke of Brunswick whitened in twenty-four hours after hearing that his father had been mortally wounded at the battle of Auerstadt.

De Schweinitz speaks of a well-formed and healthy brunette of eighteen in whom the middle portion of the cilia of the right upper eyelid and a number of the hairs of the lower lid turned white in a week. Both eyes were myopic, but no other cause could be assigned. Another similar case is cited by Hirshberg, and the authors have seen similar cases. Thornton of Margate records the case of a lady in whom the hair of the left eyebrow and eyelashes began to turn white after a fortnight of sudden grief, and within a week all the hair of these regions was quite white and remained so. No other part was affected nor was there any other symptom. After a traumatic ophthalmitis of the left and sympathetic inflammation of the right eye in a boy of nine, Schenck observed that a group of cilia of the right upper lid and nearly all the lashes of the upper lid of the left eye, which had been enucleated, turned silvery-white in a short time. Ludwig has known the eyelashes to become white after small-pox. Communications are also on record of local decolorization of the eyebrows and lashes in neuralgias of isolated branches of the trigeminus, especially of the supraorbital nerve.

Temporary and Partial Canities.—Of special interest are those cases in which whiteness of the hair is only temporary. Thus, Compagne mentions a case in which the black hair of a woman of thirty-six began to fade on the twenty-third day of a malignant fever, and on the sixth day following was perfectly white, but on the seventh day the hairs became darker again, and on the fourteenth day after the change they had become as black as they were originally. Wilson records a case in which the hair lost its color in winter and regained it in summer. Sir John Forbes, according to Crocker, had gray hair for a long time, then suddenly it all turned white, and after remaining so for a year it returned to its original gray.

Grayness of the hair is sometimes only partial. According to Crocker an adult whose hair was generally brown had a tuft of white hair over the temple, and several like cases are on record. Lorry tells us that grayness of one side only is sometimes occasioned by severe headache. Hagedorn has known the beard to be black in one place and white in another. Brandis mentions the hair becoming white on one side of the face while it continued of its former color on the other. Rayer quotes cases of canities of the whole of one side of the body.

Richelot observed white mottling of hair in a girl sick with chlorosis. The whitening extended from the roots to a distance of two inches. The probable cause was a temporary alteration of the pigment-forming function. When the chlorosis was cured the natural color returned. Paullini and Riedlin, as well as the Ephemerides, speak of different colored hair in the same head, and it is not at all rare to see individuals with an anomalously colored patch of hair on the head. The members of the ancient house of Rohan were said to possess a tuft of white hair on the front of their heads.

Michelson of Konigsberg describes a curious case in a barrister of twenty-three affected with partial canities. In the family of both parents there was stated to be congenital premature canities, and some white hairs had been observed even in childhood. In the fifteenth year, after a grave attack of scarlet fever, the hair to a great extent fell out. The succeeding growth of hair was stated to have been throughout lighter in tissue and color and fissured at the points. Soon after bunches of white hair appeared on the occiput, and in the succeeding years small patches of decolored hairs were observed also on the anterior and lateral portions of the scalp. In the spring of 1880 the patient exhibited signs of infiltration of the apex of the right lung, and afterward a violent headache came on. At the time of the report the patient presented the appearance shown in Figure 89. The complexion was delicate throughout, the eyelashes and eyelids dark brown, the moustache and whiskers blond, and in the latter were a few groups of white hair. The white patches were chiefly on the left side of the head. The hairs growing on them were unpigmented, but otherwise normal. The patient stated that his head never sweated. He was stout and exhibited no signs of internal disease, except at the apex of the right lung.

Anomalous Color Changes of the Hair.—The hair is liable to undergo certain changes of color connected with some modification of that part of the bulb secreting its coloring-matter. Alibert, quoted by Rayer, gives us a report of the case of a young lady who, after a severe fever which followed a very difficult labor, lost a fine head of hair during a discharge of viscid fluid, which inundated the head in every part. He tells us, further, that the hair grew again of a deep black color after the recovery of the patient. The same writer tells of the case of James B—, born with brown hair, who, having lost it all during the course of a sickness, had it replaced with a crop of the brightest red. White and gray hair has also, under peculiar circumstances, been replaced by hair of the same color as the individual had in youth. We are even assured by Bruley that in 1798 the white hair of a woman sixty years of age changed to black a few days before her death. The bulbs in this case were found of great size, and appeared gorged with a substance from which the hair derived its color. The white hairs that remained, on the contrary, grew from shriveled bulbs much smaller than those producing the black. This patient died of phthisis.

A very singular case, published early in the century, was that of a woman whose hair, naturally fair, assumed a tawny red color as often as she was affected with a certain fever, and returned to its natural hue as soon as the symptoms abated. Villerme alludes to the case of a young lady, sixteen years of age, who had never suffered except from trifling headaches, and who, in the winter of 1817, perceived that the hair began to fall out from several parts of her head, so that before six months were over she became entirely bald. In the beginning of January, 1819, her head became covered with a kind of black wool over those places that were first denuded, and light brown hair began to develop from the rest of the scalp. Some of this fell out again when it had grown from three to four inches; the rest changed color at different distances from its end and grew of a chestnut color from the roots. The hair, half black, half chestnut, had a very singular appearance.

Alibert and Beigel relate cases of women with blond hair which all came off after a severe fever (typhus in one case), and when it grew again it was quite black. Alibert also saw a young man who lost his brown hair after an illness, and after restoration it became red. According to Crocker, in an idiotic girl of epileptic type (in an asylum at Edinburgh), with alternating phases of stupidity and excitement, the hair in the stupid phase was blond and in the excited condition red. The change of color took place in the course of two or three days, beginning first at the free ends, and remaining of the same tint for seven or eight days. The pale hairs had more air-spaces than the darker ones. There was much structural change in the brain and spinal cord. Smyly of Dublin reported a case of suppurative disease of the temporal bone, in which the hair changed from a mouse-color to a reddish-brown; and Squire records a congenital case in a deaf mute, in whom the hair on the left side was in light patches of true auburn and dark patches of dark brown like a tortoise-shell cap; on the other side the hair was a dark brown. Crocker mentions the changes which have occurred in rare instances after death from dark brown to red.

Chemic colorations of various tints occur. Blue hair is seen in workers in cobalt mines and indigo works; green hair in copper smelters; deep red-brown hair in handlers of crude anilin; and the hair is dyed a purplish-brown whenever chrysarobin applications used on a scalp come in contact with an alkali, as when washed with soap. Among such cases in older literature Blanchard and Marcellus Donatus speak of green hair; Rosse saw two instances of the same, for one of which he could find no cause; the other patient worked in a brass foundry.

Many curious causes are given for alopecia. Gilibert and Merlet mention sexual excess; Marcellus Donatus gives fear; the Ephemerides speaks of baldness from fright; and Leo Africanus, in his description of Barbary, describes endemic baldness. Neyronis makes the following observation: A man of seventy-three, convalescent from a fever, one morning, about six months after recovery perceived that he had lost all his hair, even his eyelashes, eyebrows, nostril-hairs, etc. Although his health continued good, the hair was never renewed.

The principal anomalies of the nails observed are absence, hypertrophy, and displacement of these organs. Some persons are born with finger-nails and toe-nails either very rudimentary or entirely absent; in others they are of great length and thickness. The Chinese nobility allow their finger-nails to grow to a great length and spend much time in the care of these nails. Some savage tribes have long and thick nails resembling the claws of beasts, and use them in the same way as the lower animals. There is a description of a person with finger-nails that resembled the horns of a goat.

Neuhof, in his books on Tartary and China, says that many Chinamen have two nails on the little toe, and other instances of double nails have been reported.

The nails may be reversed or arise from anomalous positions. Bartholinus speaks of nails from the inner side of the digits; in another case, in which the fingers were wanting, he found the nails implanted on the stumps. Tulpius says he knew of a case in which nails came from the articulations of three digits; and many other curious arrangements of nails are to be found.

Rouhuot sent a description and drawing of some monstrous nails to the Academie des Sciences de Paris. The largest of these was the left great toe-nail, which, from its extremity to its root, measured 4 3/4 inches; the laminae of which it consisted were placed one over the other, like the tiles on a roof, only reversed. This nail and several of the others were of unequal thickness and were variously curved, probably on account of the pressure of the shoe or the neighboring digits. Rayer mentions two nails sent to him by Bricheteau, physician of the Hopital Necker, belonging to an old woman who had lived in the Salpetriere. They were very thick and spirally twisted, like the horns of a ram. Saviard informs us that he saw a patient at the Hotel Dieu who had a horn like that of a ram, instead of a nail, on each great toe, the extremities of which were turned to the metatarsus and overlapped the whole of the other toes of each foot. The skeleton of Simore, preserved in Paris, is remarkable for the ankylosis of all the articulations and the considerable size of all the nails. The fingers and toes, spread out and ankylosed, ended in nails of great length and nearly of equal thickness. A woman by the name of Melin, living in the last century in Paris, was surnamed "the woman with nails;" according to the description given by Saillant in 1776 she presented another and not less curious instance of the excessive growth of the nails.

Musaeus gives an account of the nails of a girl of twenty, which grew to such a size that some of those of the fingers were five inches in length. They were composed of several layers, whitish interiorly, reddish-gray on the exterior, and full of black points. These nails fell off at the end of four months and were succeeded by others. There were also horny laminae on the knees and shoulders and elbows which bore a resemblance to nails, or rather talons. They were sensitive only at the point of insertion into the skin. Various other parts of the body, particularly the backs of the hands, presented these horny productions. One of them was four inches in length. This horny growth appeared after small-pox. Ash, in the Philosophical Transactions, records a somewhat similar case in a girl of twelve.

Anomalies of the Teeth.—Pliny, Colombus, van Swieten, Haller, Marcellus Donatus, Baudelocque, Soemmering, and Gardien all cite instances in which children have come into the world with several teeth already erupted. Haller has collected 19 cases of children born with teeth. Polydorus Virgilus describes an infant who was born with six teeth. Some celebrated men are supposed to have been born with teeth; Louis XIV was accredited with having two teeth at birth. Bigot, a physician and philosopher of the sixteenth century; Boyd, the poet; Valerian, Richard III, as well as some of the ancient Greeks and Romans, were reputed to have had this anomaly. The significance of the natal eruption of teeth is not always that of vigor, as many of the subjects succumb early in life. There were two cases typical of fetal dentition shown before the Academie de Medecine de Paris. One of the subjects had two middle incisors in the lower jaw and the other had one tooth well through. Levison saw a female born with two central incisors in the lower jaw.

Thomas mentions a case of antenatal development of nine teeth. Puech, Mattei, Dumas, Belluzi, and others report the eruption of teeth in the newborn. In Dumas' case the teeth had to be extracted on account of ulceration of the tongue. Instances of triple dentition late in life are quite numerous, many occurring after a hundred years. Mentzelius speaks of a man of one hundred and ten who had nine new teeth. Lord Bacon cites the case of a Countess Desmond, who when over a century old had two new teeth; Hufeland saw an instance of dentition at one hundred and sixteen; Nitzsch speaks of one at one hundred, and the Ephemerides contain an account of a triple dentition at one hundred and twenty. There is an account of a country laborer who lost all his teeth by the time he arrived at his sixtieth year of age, but about a half year afterward a new set made their appearance. Bisset mentions an account of an old woman who acquired twelve molar teeth at the age of ninety-eight. Carre notes a case of dental eruption in an individual of eighty-five. Mazzoti speaks of a third dentition, and

Ysabeau writes of dentition of a molar at the age of ninety-two. There is a record of a physician of the name of Slave who retained all his second teeth until the age of eighty, when they fell out; after five years another set appeared, which he retained until his death at one hundred. In the same report there is mentioned an old Scotchman who died at one hundred and ten, whose teeth were renewed at an advanced age after he had lost his second teeth. One of the older journals speaks of dentition at seventy, eighty-four, ninety, and one hundred and fourteen. The Philosophical Transactions of London contain accounts of dentition at seventy-five and eighty-one. Bassett tells of an old woman who had twelve molar teeth at the age of eighty-eight. In France there is recorded dentition at eighty-five and an account of an old man of seventy-three who had six new teeth. Von Helmont relates an instance of triple dentition at the same age. There is recorded in Germany an account of a woman of ninety who had dentition at forty-seven and sixty-seven, each time a new set of teeth appearing; Hunter and Petrequin have observed similar cases. Carter describes an example of third dentition. Lison makes a curious observation of a sixth dentition.

Edentulousness.—We have already noticed the association of congenital alopecia with edentulousness, but, strange to say, Magitot has remarked that "l'homme-chien," was the subject of defective dentition. Borellus found atrophy of all the dental follicles in a woman of sixty who never had possessed any teeth. Fanton-Touvet saw a boy of nine who had never had teeth, and Fox a woman who had but four in both jaws; Tomes cites several similar instances. Hutchinson speaks of a child who was perfectly edentulous as to temporary teeth, but who had the permanent teeth duly and fully erupted. Guilford describes a man of forty-eight, who was edentulous from birth, who also totally lacked the sense of smell, and was almost without the sense of taste; the surface of his body was covered with fine hairs and he had never had visible perspiration. This is probably the same case quoted in the foregoing paragraph in regard to the anomalies of hair. Otto, quoted by Sedgwick, speaks of two brothers who were both totally edentulous. It might be interesting in this connection to note that Oudet found in a fetus at term all the dental follicles in a process of suppuration, leaving no doubt that, if the fetus had been born viable, it would have been edentulous. Giraldes mentions the absence of teeth in an infant of sixteen months. Bronzet describes a child of twelve, with only half its teeth, in whom the alveolar borders receded as in age. Baumes remarks that he had seen a man who never had any teeth.

The anomalies of excessive dentition are of several varieties, those of simple supernumerary teeth, double or triple rows, and those in anomalous positions. Ibbetson saw a child with five incisors in the inferior maxillary bone, and Fanton-Touvet describes a young lady who possessed five large incisors of the first dentition in the superior maxilla. Rayer notes a case of dentition of four canines, which first made their appearance after pain for eight days in the jaws and associated with convulsions. In an Ethiopian Soemmering has seen one molar too many on each side and in each jaw. Ploucquet and Tesmer have seen five incisors and Fanchard six. Many persons have the supernumerary teeth parallel with their neighbors, anteriorly or posteriorly. Costa reports a case in which there were five canine teeth in the upper jaw, two placed laterally on either side, and one on the right side behind the other two. The patient was twenty-six years of age, well formed and in good health.

In some cases there is fusion of the teeth. Pliny, Bartholinus, and Melanthon pretend to have seen the union of all the teeth, making a continuous mass. In the "Musee de l'ecole dentaire de Paris" there are several milk-teeth, both of the superior and inferior maxilla, which are fused together. Bloch cites a case in which there were two rows of teeth in the superior maxilla. Hellwig has observed three rows of teeth, and the Ephemerides contain an account of a similar anomaly.

Extraoral Dentition.—Probably the most curious anomaly of teeth is that in which they are found in other than normal positions. Albinus speaks of teeth in the nose and orbit; Borellus, in the palate; Fabricius Hildanus, under the tongue; Schenck, from the palate; and there are many similar modern records. Heister in 1743 wrote a dissertation on extraoral teeth. The following is a recent quotation:

"In the Norsk Magazin fur Laegevidenskaben, January, 1895, it is reported that Dr. Dave, at a meeting of the Medical Society in Christiania, showed a tooth removed from the nose of a woman aged fifty-three. The patient had consulted him for ear-trouble, and the tooth was found accidentally during the routine examination. It was easily removed, having been situated in a small depression at the junction of the floor and external wall of the nasal cavity, 22 mm. from the external nares. This patient had all her teeth; they were placed somewhat far from each other. The tooth resembled a milk canine; the end of the imperfect root was covered with a fold of mucous membrane, with stratified epithelium. The speaker suggested that part of the mucous membrane of the mouth with its tooth-germ had become impacted between the superior and premaxillary bones and thus cut off from the cavity of the mouth. Another speaker criticised this fetal dislocation and believed it to be due to an inversion—a development in the wrong direction—by which the tooth had grown upward into the nose. The same speaker also pointed out that the stratified epithelium of the mucous membrane did not prove a connection with the cavity of the mouth, as it is known that cylindric epithelium-cells after irritative processes are replaced by flat ones."

Delpech saw a young man in 1829 who had an opening in the palatine vault occasioned by the extraction of a tooth. This opening communicated with the nasal fossa by a fracture of the palatine and maxillary bones; the employment of an obturator was necessary. It is not rare to see teeth, generally canine, make their eruption from the vault of the palate; and these teeth are not generally supernumerary, but examples of vice and deviation of position. Fanton-Touvet, however, gives an example of a supernumerary tooth implanted in the palatine arch. Branch a describes a little negro boy who had two large teeth in the nose; his dentition was otherwise normal, but a portion of the nose was destroyed by ulceration. Roy describes a Hindoo lad of fourteen who had a tooth in the nose, supposed to have been a tumor. It was of the canine type, and was covered with enamel to the junction with the root, which was deeply imbedded in the side and upper part of the antrum. The boy had a perfect set of permanent teeth and no deformity, swelling, or cystic formation of the jaw. This was clearly a case of extrafollicular development and eruption of the tooth in an anomalous position, the peculiarity being that while in other similar cases the crown of the tooth shows itself at the floor of the nasal cavity from below upward, in this instance the dental follicle was transposed, the eruption being from above downward. Hall cites an instance in which the right upper canine of a girl erupted in the nose. The subject showed marked evidence of hereditary syphilis. Carver describes a child who had a tooth growing from the lower right eyelid. The number of deciduous teeth was perfect; although this tooth was canine it had a somewhat bulbulous fang.

Of anomalies of the head the first to be considered will be the anencephalous monsters who, strange to say, have been known to survive birth. Clericus cites an example of life for five days in a child without a cerebrum. Heysham records the birth of a child without a cerebrum and remarks that it was kept alive for six days. There was a child born alive in Italy in 1831 without a brain or a cerebellum—in fact, no cranial cavity—and yet it lived eleven hours. A somewhat similar case is recorded in the last century. In the Philosophical Transactions there is mentioned a child virtually born without a head who lived four days; and Le Duc records a case of a child born without brain, cerebellum, or medulla oblongata, and who lived half an hour. Brunet describes an anencephalous boy born at term who survived his birth. Saviard delivered an anencephalous child at term which died in thirty-six hours. Lawrence mentions a child with brain and cranium deficient that lived five days. Putnam speaks of a female nosencephalous monster that lived twenty-nine hours. Angell and Elsner in March, 1895, reported a case of anencephaly, or rather pseudencephaly, associated with double divergent strabismus and limbs in a state of constant spastic contraction. The infant lived eight days. Geoffroy-Saint-Hilaire cites an example of anencephaly which lived a quarter of an hour. Fauvel mentioned one that lived two hours, and Sue describes a similar instance in which life persisted for seven hours and distinct motions were noticed. Malacarne saw life in one for twelve hours, and Mery has given a description of a child born without brain that lived almost a full day and took nourishment. In the Hotel-Dieu in Paris in 1812 Serres saw a monster of this type which lived three days, and was fed on milk and sugared water, as no nurse could be found who was willing to suckle it.

Fraser mentions a brother and sister, aged twenty and thirty, respectively, who from birth had exhibited signs of defective development of the cerebellum. They lacked power of coordination and walked with a drunken, staggering gait; they could not touch the nose with the finger when their eyes were shut, etc. The parents of these unfortunate persons were perfectly healthy, as were the rest of their family. Cruveilhier cites a case of a girl of eleven who had absolutely no cerebellum, with the same symptoms which are characteristic in such cases. There is also recorded the history of a man who was deficient in the corpus callosum; at the age of sixty-two, though of feeble intelligence, he presented no signs of nervous disorder. Claude Bernard made an autopsy on a woman who had no trace of olfactory lobes, and after a minute inquiry into her life he found that her sense of smell had been good despite her deficiency.

Buhring relates the history of a case somewhat analogous to viability of anencephalous monsters. It was a bicephalous child that lived thirty-two hours after he had ligated one of its heads.

{footnote} The argument that the brain is not the sole organ of the mind is in a measure substantiated by a wonderful case of a decapitated rooster, reported from Michigan. A stroke of the knife bad severed the larynx and removed the whole mass of the cerebrum, leaving the inner aspect and base of the skull exposed. The cerebrum was partly removed; the external auditory meatus was preserved. Immediately after the decapitation the rooster was left to its supposed death struggles, but it ran headless to the barn, where it was secured and subsequently fed by pushing corn down its esophagus, and allowing water to trickle into this tube from the spout of an oil-can. The phenomena exhibited by the rooster were quite interesting. It made all the motions of pecking, strutted about, flapped its wings, attempted to crow, but, of course, without making any sound. It exhibited no signs of incoordination, but did not seem to hear. A ludicrous exhibition was the absurd, sidelong pas seul made toward the hens.

Ward mentions an instance of congenital absence of the corpora callosum. Paget and Henry mention cases in which the corpora callosum, the fornix, and septum lucidum were imperfectly formed. Maunoir reports congenital malformation of the brain, consisting of almost complete absence of the occipital lobe. The patient died at the twenty-eighth month. Combettes reports the case of a girl who died at the age of eleven who had complete absence of the cerebellum in addition to other minor structural defects; this was probably the case mentioned by Cruveilhier.

Diminution in volume of the head is called microcephaly. Probably the most remarkable case on record is that mentioned by Lombroso. The individual was called "l'homme-oiseau," or the human bird, and his cranial capacity was only 390 c.c. Lombroso speaks of another individual called "l'homme-lapin," or man-rabbit, whose cranium was only slightly larger than that of the other, measuring 490 mm. in circumference. Castelli alludes to endemic microcephaly among some of the peoples of Asia. We also find it in the Caribbean Islands, and from the skulls and portraits of the ancient Aztecs we are led to believe that they were also microcephalic.

Two creatures of celebrity were Maximo and Bartola, who for twenty-five years have been shown in America and in Europe under the name of the "Aztecs" or the "Aztec children". They were male and female and very short, with heads resembling closely the bas-reliefs on the ancient Aztec temples of Mexico. Their facial angle was about 45 degrees, and they had jutting lips and little or no chin. They wore their hair in an enormous bunch to magnify the deformity. These curiosities were born in Central America and were possibly half Indian and Negro. They were little better than idiots in point of intelligence.

Figure 92 represents a microcephalic youth known as the "Mexican wild boy," who was shown with the Wallace circus.

Virchow exhibited a girl of fourteen whose face was no larger than that of a newborn child, and whose head was scarcely as large as a man's fist. Magitot reported a case of a microcephalic woman of thirty who weighed 70 pounds.

Hippocrates and Strabonius both speak of head-binding as a custom inducing artificial microcephaly, and some tribes of North American Indians still retain this custom.

As a rule, microcephaly is attended with associate idiocy and arrested development of the rest of the body. Ossification of the fontanelles in a mature infant would necessarily prevent full development of the brain. Osiander and others have noticed this anomaly. There are cases on record in which the fontanelles have remained open until adulthood.

Augmentation of the volume of the head is called macrocephaly, and there are a number of curious examples related. Benvenuti describes an individual, otherwise well formed, whose head began to enlarge at seven. At twenty-seven it measured over 37 inches in circumference and the man's face was 15 inches in height; no other portion of his body increased abnormally; his voice was normal and he was very intelligent. He died of apoplexy at the age of thirty.

Fournier speaks of a cranium in the cabinet of the Natural History Museum of Marseilles of a man by the name of Borghini, who died in 1616. At the time he was described he was fifty years old, four feet in height; his head measured three feet in circumference and one foot in height. There was a proverb in Marseilles, "Apas mai de sen que Borghini," meaning in the local dialect, "Thou hast no more wit than Borghini." This man, whose fame became known all over France, was not able, as he grew older, to maintain the weight of his head, but carried a cushion on each shoulder to prop it up. Fournier also quotes the history of a man who died in the same city in 1807 at the age of sixty-seven. His head was enormous, and he never lay on a bed for thirty years, passing his nights in a chair, generally reading or writing. He only ate once in twenty-four or thirty hours, never warmed himself, and never used warm water. His knowledge was said to have been great and encyclopedic, and he pretended never to have heard the proverb of Borghini. There is related the account of a Moor, who was seen in Tunis early in this century, thirty-one years of age, of middle height, with a head so prodigious in dimensions that crowds flocked after him in the streets. His nose was quite long, and his mouth so large that he could eat a melon as others would an apple. He was an imbecile. William Thomas Andrews was a dwarf seventeen years old, whose head measured in circumference 35 inches; from one external auditory meatus to another, 27 1/4 inches; from the chin over the cranial summit to the suboccipital protuberance, 37 1/2 inches; the distance from the chin to the pubes was 20 inches; and from the pubes to the soles of the feet, 16; he was a monorchid. James Cardinal, who died in Guy's Hospital in 1825, and who was so celebrated for the size of his head, only measured 32 1/2 inches in head-circumference.

The largest healthy brains on record, that is, of men of prominence, are those of Cuvier, weighing 64 1/3 ounces; of Daniel Webster, weighing 63 3/4 ounces (the circumference of whose head was 23 3/4 inches); of Abercrombie, weighing 63 ounces, and of Spurzheim, weighing 55 1/16 ounces. Byron and Cromwell had abnormally heavy brains, showing marked evidence of disease.

A curious instance in this connection is that quoted by Pigne, who gives an account of a double brain found in an infant. Keen reports finding a fornix which, instead of being solid from side to side, consisted of two lateral halves with a triangular space between them.

When the augmentation of the volume of the cranium is caused by an abundant quantity of serous fluid the anomaly is known as hydrocephaly. In this condition there is usually no change in the size of the brain-structure itself, but often the cranial bones are rent far asunder. Minot speaks of a hydrocephalic infant whose head measured 27 1/2 inches in circumference; Bright describes one whose head measured 32 inches; and Klein, one 43 inches. Figure 93 represents a child of six whose head circumference was 36 inches. Figure 94 shows a hydrocephalic adult who was exhibited through this country.

There is a record of a curious monster born of healthy half-caste African parents. The deformity was caused by a deficiency of osseous material of the bones of the head. There was considerable arrest of development of the parietal, temporal, and superior maxillary bones, in consequence of which a very small amount of the cerebral substance could be protected by the membranous expansion of the cranial centers. The inferior maxilla and the frontal bone were both perfect; the ears were well developed and the tongue strong and active; the nostrils were imperforate and there was no roof to the mouth nor floor to the nares. The eyes were curiously free from eyelashes, eyelids, or brows. The cornea threatened to slough. There was double harelip on the left side; the second and third fingers of both hands were webbed for their whole length; the right foot wanted the distal phalanx of the great toe and the left foot was clubbed and drawn inward. The child swallowed when fed from a spoon, appeared to hear, but exhibited no sense of light. It died shortly after the accompanying sketch was made.

Occasionally a deficiency in the osseous material of the cranium or an abnormal dilatation of the fontanelles gives rise to a hernia of the meninges, which, if accompanied by cerebrospinal fluid in any quantity, causes a large and peculiarly shaped tumor called meningocele. If there is a protrusion of brain-substance itself, a condition known as hernia cerebri results.

Complete absence of the inferior maxilla is much rarer in man than in animals. Nicolas and Prenant have described a curious case of this anomaly in a sheep. Gurlt has named subjects presenting the total or partial absence of the inferior maxilla, agnathes or hemiagnathes. Simple atrophy of the inferior maxilla has been seen in man as well as in the lower animals, but is much less frequent than atrophy of the superior maxilla. Langenbeck reports the case of a young man who had the inferior maxilla so atrophied that in infancy it was impossible for him to take milk from the breast. He had also almost complete immobility of the jaws.

Boullard reports a deformity of the visage, resulting in a deficiency of the condyles of the lower jaw. Maurice made an observation on a vice of conformation of the lower jaw which rendered lactation impossible, probably causing the death of the infant on this account. Tomes gives a description of a lower jaw the development of the left ramus of which had been arrested. Canton mentions arrest of development of the left perpendicular ramus of the lower jaw combined with malformation of the external ear.

Exaggerated prominence of the maxillaries is called prognathism; that of the superior maxilla is seen in the North American Indians. Inferior prognathism is observed in man as well as in animals. The bull-dog, for example, displays this, but in this instance the deformity is really superior brachygnathism, the superior maxilla being arrested in development.

Congenital absence of the nose is a very rare anomaly. Maisonneuve has seen an example in an individual in which, in place of the nasal appendix, there was a plane surface perforated by two small openings a little less than one mm. in diameter and three mm. apart.

Exaggeration in volume of the nose is quite frequent. Ballonius speaks of a nose six times larger than ordinary. Viewing the Roman celebrities, we find that Numa, to whom was given the surname Pompilius, had a nose which measured six inches. Plutarch, Lyourgus, and Solon had a similar enlargement, as had all the kings of Italy except Tarquin the Superb.

Early in the last century a man, Thomas Wedders (or Wadhouse), with a nose 7 1/2 inches long, was exhibited throughout Yorkshire. This man expired as he had lived, in a condition of mind best described as the most abject idiocy. The accompanying illustration is taken from a reproduction of an old print and is supposed to be a true likeness of this unfortunate individual.

There are curious pathologic formations about the nose which increase its volume so enormously as to interfere with respiration and even with alimentation; but these will be spoken of in another chapter.

There have been some celebrities whose noses were undersized. The Duc de Guise, the Dauphin d'Auvergne, and William of Orange, celebrated in the romances of chivalry, had extremely short noses.

There are a few recorded cases of congenital division of the nose. Bartholinus, Borellus, and the Ephemerides speak of duplex noses. Thomas of Tours has observed congenital fissure of the nose. Rikere reports the case of an infant of three weeks who possessed a supernumerary nose on the right nasal bone near the inner canthus of the eye. It was pear-shaped, with its base down, and was the size of the natural nose of an infant of that age, and air passed through it. Hubbell, Ronaldson, and Luscha speak of congenital occlusion of the posterior nares. Smith and Jarvis record cases of congenital occlusion of the anterior nares.

Anomalies in size of the mouth are not uncommon. Fournier quotes the history of a man who had a mouth so large that when he opened it all his back teeth could be seen. There is a history of a boy of seventeen who had a preternaturally-sized mouth, the transverse diameter being 6 1/2 inches. The mother claimed that the boy was born with his foot in his mouth and to this fact attributed his deformity. The negro races are noted for their large mouths and thick lips. A negro called "Black Diamond," recently exhibited in Philadelphia, could put both his fists in his mouth.

Morgan reports two cases of congenital macrostoma accompanied by malformation of the auricles and by auricular appendages. Van Duyse mentions congenital macrostoma with preauricular tumors and a dermoid of the eye. Macrostoma is sometimes produced by lateral fissures. In other cases this malformation is unilateral and the fissure ascends, in which instance the fissure may be accompanied by a fistula of the duct of Stensen. Sometimes there is associated with these anomalies curious terminations of the salivary ducts, either through the cheek by means of a fistula or on the anterior part of the neck.

Microstoma.—There are a few cases on record in which the mouth has been so small or ill-defined as not to admit of alimentation. Molliere knew an individual of forty whose mouth was the exact size of a ten-centime piece.

Buchnerus records a case of congenital atresia of the mouth. Cayley, Smith, Sourrouille, and Stankiewiez of Warsaw discuss atresia of the mouth. Cancrum oris, scarlet fever, burns, scurvy, etc., are occasional causes that have been mentioned, the atresia in these instances taking place at any time of life.

Anomalies of the Lips.—The aboriginal tribes are particularly noted for their large and thick lips, some of which people consider enormous lips signs of adornment. Elephantiasis or other pathologic hypertrophy of the labial tissues can produce revolting deformity, such as is seen in Figure 100, representing an individual who was exhibited several years ago in Philadelphia. We have in English the expression, "pulling a long lip." Its origin is said to date back to a semimythical hero of King Arthur's time, who, "when sad at heart and melancholic," would let one of his lips drop below his waist, while he turned the other up like a cap on his head.

Blot records a case of monstrous congenital hypertrophy of the superior lip in an infant of eight months. Buck successfully treated by surgical operations a case of congenital hypertrophy of the under lip, and Detmold mentions a similar result in a young lady with hypertrophy of the lip and lower part of the nose. Murray reports an undescribed malformation of the lower lip occurring in one family.

Hare-lip may be unilateral or double, and may or may not include the palatine arch. In the worst cases it extends in fissures on both sides to the orbit. In other cases the minimum degree of this deformity is seen.

Congenital absence of the tongue does not necessarily make speech, taste, or deglutition impossible. Jussieu cites the case of a girl who was born without a tongue but who spoke very distinctly. Berdot describes a case in which the tongue was deficient, without apparent disturbance of any of the functions. Riolan mentions speech after loss of the tongue from small-pox.

Boddington gives an account of Margaret Cutting, who spoke readily and intelligibly, although she had lost her tongue. Saulquin has an observation of a girl without a tongue who spoke, sang, and swallowed normally. Aurran, Bartholinus, Louis, Parsons, Tulpius, and others mention speech without the presence of a tongue.

Philib reports a case in which mutism, almost simulating that of one congenitally deaf, was due to congenital adhesions of the tongue to the floor of the buccal cavity. Speech was established after removal of the abnormal adhesion. Routier speaks of ankylosis of the tongue of seventeen years' duration.

Jurist records such abnormal mobility of the tongue that the patient was able to project the tongue into the nasopharynx. Wherry and Winslow record similar instances.

There have been individuals with bifid tongues, after the normal type of serpents and saurians, and others who possessed a supernumerary tongue. Rev. Henry Wharton, Chaplain to Archbishop Sancroft, in his journal, written in the seventeenth century, says that he was born with two tongues and passed through life so, one, however, gradually atrophying. In the polyclinic of Schnitzer in Vienna in 1892 Hajek observed in a lad of twelve an accessory tongue 2.4 cm. in length and eight mm. in breadth, forming a tumor at the base of the normal tongue. It was removed by scissors, and on histologic examination proved to be a true tongue with the typical tissues and constituents. Borellus, Ephemerides, Eschenbach, Mortimer, Penada, and Schenck speak of double tongues, and Avicenna and Schenck have seen fissured tongues. Dolaeus records an instance of double tongue in a paper entitled "De puella bilingui," and Beaudry and Brothers speak of cleft tongue. Braine records a case in which there was a large hypertrophied fold of membrane coming from each side of the upper lip.

In some cases there is marked augmentation of the volume of the tongue. Fournier has seen a juggler with a tongue so long that he could extrude it six inches from his mouth. He also refers to a woman in Berlin with a long tongue, but it was thinner than that of a cat. When she laughed it hung over her teeth like a curtain, and was always extremely cold to the touch. In the same article there is a description of a man with a very long neck who could touch his tongue to his chest without reclining his head. Congenital and acquired hypertrophy of the tongue will be discussed later.

Amatus Lusitanus and Portal refer to the presence of hair on the tongue, and later there was an account of a medical student who complained of dyspepsia and a sticky sensation in the mouth. On examination a considerable growth of hair was found on the surface of the tongue. The hairs would be detached in vomiting but would grow again, and when he was last seen they were one inch long. Such are possibly nevoid in formation.

The ordinary anomalies of the palate are the fissures, unilateral, bilateral, median, etc.: they are generally associated with hare-lip. The median fissure commencing between the middle incisors is quite rare.

Many curious forms of obturator or artificial palate are employed to remedy congenital defects. Sercombe mentions a case in which destruction of the entire palate was successfully relieved by mechanical means. In some instances among the lower classes these obturators are simple pieces of wood, so fashioned as to fit into the palatine cleft, and not infrequently the obturator has been swallowed, causing obstruction of the air-passages or occluding the esophagus.

Abnormalism of the Uvula.—Examples of double uvula are found in the older writers, and Hagendorn speaks of a man who was born without a uvula. The Ephemerides and Salmuth describe uvulae so defective as to be hardly noticeable. Bolster, Delius, Hodges, Mackenzie of Baltimore, Orr, Riedel, Schufeldt, and Tidyman are among observers reporting bifurcated and double uvula, and they are quite common. Ogle records instances of congenital absence of the uvula.

Anomalies of the Epiglottis.—Morgagni mentions a man without an epiglottis who ate and spoke without difficulty. He thought the arytenoids were so strongly developed that they replaced the functions of the missing organ. Enos of Brooklyn in 1854 reported absence of the epiglottis without interference with deglutition. Manifold speaks of a case of bifurcated epiglottis. Debloisi records an instance of congenital web of the vocal bands. Mackenzie removed a congenital papillomatous web which had united the vocal cords until the age of twenty-three, thus establishing the voice. Poore also recorded a case of congenital web in the larynx. Elsberg and Scheff mention occlusion of the rima glottidis by a membrane.

Instances of duplication of the epiglottis attended with a species of double voice possess great interest. French described a man of thirty, by occupation a singer and contortionist, who became possessed of an extra voice when he was sixteen. In high and falsetto tones he could run the scale from A to F in an upper and lower range. The compass of the low voice was so small that he could not reach the high notes of any song with it, and in singing he only used it to break in on the falsetto and produce a sensation. He was supposed to possess a double epiglottis.

Roe describes a young lady who could whistle at will with the lower part of her throat and without the aid of her lips. Laryngeal examination showed that the fundamental tones were produced by vibrations of the edges of the vocal cords, and the modifications were effected by a minute adjustment of the ventricular bands, which regulated the laryngeal opening above the cord, and pressing firmly down closed the ventricle and acted as a damper preventing the vibrations of the cords except in their middle third. Morgan in the same journal mentions the case of a boy of nineteen, who seemed to be affected with laryngeal catarrh, and who exhibited distinct diphthongia. He was seen to have two glottic orifices with associate bands. The treatment was directed to the catarrh and consequent paresis of the posterior bands, and he soon lost his evidences of double voice.

{footnote} The following is a description of the laryngeal formation of a singer who has recently acquired considerable notice by her ability to sing notes of the highest tones and to display the greatest compass of voice. It is extracted from a Cleveland, Ohio, newspaper: "She has unusual development of the larynx, which enables her to throw into vibration and with different degrees of rapidity the entire length of the vocal cords or only a part thereof. But of greatest interest is her remarkable control over the muscles which regulate the division and modification of the resonant cavities, the laryngeal, pharyngeal, oral, and nasal, and upon this depends the quality of her voice. The uvula is bifurcated, and the two divisions sometimes act independently. The epiglottis during the production of the highest notes rises upward and backward against the posterior pharyngeal wall in such a way as almost entirely to separate the pharyngeal cavities, at the same time that it gives an unusual conformation to those resonant chambers."

Complete absence of the eyes is a very rare anomaly. Wordsworth describes a baby of seven weeks, otherwise well formed and healthy, which had congenital absence of both eyes. The parents of this child were in every respect healthy. There are some cases of monstrosities with closed, adherent eyelids and absence of eyes. Holmes reports a case of congenital absence of both eyes, the child otherwise being strong and perfect. The child died of cholera infantum. He also reports a case very similar in a female child of American parents. In a girl of eight, of German parents, he reports deficiency of the external walls of each orbit, in addition to great deformity of the side of the head. He also gives an instance of congenital paralysis of the levator palpebrae muscles in a child whose vision was perfect and who was otherwise perfect. Holmes also reports a case of enormous congenital exophthalmos, in which the right eye protruded from the orbit and was no longer covered by the cornea. Kinney has an account of a child born without eyeballs. The delivery was normal, and there was no history of any maternal impression; the child was otherwise healthy and well formed.

Landes reports the case of an infant in which both eyes were absent. There were six fingers on each hand and six toes on each foot. The child lived a few weeks. In some instances of supposed absence of the eyeball the eye is present but diminutive and in the posterior portion of the orbit. There are instances of a single orbit with no eyes and also a single orbit containing two eyes. Again we may have two orbits with an absence of eyes but the presence of the lacrimal glands, or the eyes may be present or very imperfectly developed. Mackenzie mentions cases in which the orbit was more or less completely wanting and a mass of cellular tissue in each eye.

Cases of living cyclopia, or individuals with one eye in the center of the forehead after the manner of the mythical Cyclops, are quite rare. Vallentini in 1884 reports a case of a male cyclopic infant which lived for seventy-three hours. There were median fissures of the upper lip, preauricular appendages, oral deformity, and absence of the olfactory proboscis The fetus was therefore a cyclops arrhynchus, or cyclocephalus. Blok describes a new-born infant which lived for six or seven hours, having but one eye and an extremely small mouth.

The "Four-eyed Man of Cricklade" was a celebrated English monstrosity of whom little reliable information is obtainable. He was visited by W. Drury, who is accredited with reporting the following—

" 'So wondrous a thing, such a lusus naturae, such a scorn and spite of nature I have never seen. It was a dreadful and shocking sight.' This unfortunate had four eyes placed in pairs, 'one eye above the other and all four of a dull brown, encircled with red, the pupils enormously large.' The vision in each organ appeared to be perfect. 'He could shut any particular eye, the other three remaining open, or, indeed, as many as he chose, each several eye seeming to be controlled by his will and acting independently of the remainder. He could also revolve each eye separately in its orbit, looking backward with one and forward with another, upward with one and downward with another simultaneously.' He was of a savage, malignant disposition, delighting in ugly tricks, teasing children, torturing helpless animals, uttering profane and blasphemous words, and acting altogether like the monster, mental and physical, that he was. 'He could play the fiddle, though in a silly sort, having his notes on the left side, while closing the right pair of eyes. He also sang, but in a rough, screeching voice not to be listened to without disgust.'"

There is a recent report of a child born in Paris with its eyes in the top of its head. The infant seemed to be doing well and crowds of people have flocked to see it. Recent reports speak of a child born in Portland, Oregon, which had a median rudimentary eye between two normal eyes. Fournier describes an infant born with perfectly formed eyes, but with adherent eyelids and closed ocular aperture. Forlenze has seen the pupils adherent to the conjunctiva, and by dissection has given sight to the subject.

Dubois cites an instance of supernumerary eyelid. At the external angle of the eyelid was a fold of conjunctiva which extended 0.5 cm. in front of the conjunctiva, to which it did not adhere, therefore constituting a fourth eyelid. Fano presents a similar case in a child of four months, in whom no other anomaly, either of organs or of vision, was observed. On the right side, in front of the external half of the sclerotic, was observed a semilunar fold with the concavity inward, and which projected much more when the lower lid was depressed. When the eyelid rolled inward the fold rolled with the globe, but never reached so far as the circumference of the cornea and did not interfere with vision.

Total absence of both irides has been seen in a man of eighteen. Dixon reports a case of total aniridia with excellent sight in a woman of thirty-seven. In Guy's Hospital there was seen a case of complete congenital absence of the iris. Hentzschel speaks of a man with congenital absence of the iris who had five children, three of whom exhibited the same anomaly while the others were normal. Benson, Burnett, Demaux, Lawson, Morison, Reuling, Samelson, and others also report congenital deficiency of the irides in both eyes.

Jeaffreson describes a female of thirty, living in India, who was affected with complete ossification of the iris. It was immovable and quite beautiful when seen through the transparent cornea; the sight was only slightly impaired. No cause was traceable.

Multiple Pupils.—More than one pupil in the eye has often been noticed, and as many as six have been seen. They may be congenital or due to some pathologic disturbance after birth. Marcellus Donatus speaks of two pupils in one eye. Beer, Fritsche, and Heuermann are among the older writers who have noticed supernumerary pupils. Higgens in 1885 described a boy whose right iris was perforated by four pupils,—one above, one to the inner side, one below, and a fourth to the outer side. The first three were slit-shaped; the fourth was the largest and had the appearance as of the separation of the iris from its insertion. There were two pupils in the left eye, both to the outer side of the iris, one being slit-like and the other resembling the fourth pupil in the right eye. All six pupils commenced at the periphery, extended inward, and were of different sizes. The fundus could be clearly seen through all of the pupils, and there was no posterior staphyloma nor any choroidal changes. There was a rather high degree of myopia. This peculiarity was evidently congenital, and no traces of a central pupil nor marks of a past iritis could be found. Clinical Sketches a contains quite an extensive article on and several illustrations of congenital anomalies of the iris.

Double crystalline lenses are sometimes seen. Fritsch and Valisneri have seen this anomaly and there are modern references to it. Wordsworth presented to the Medical Society of London six members of one family, all of whom had congenital displacement of the crystalline lens outward and upward. The family consisted of a woman of fifty, two sons, thirty-five and thirty-seven, and three grandchildren—a girl of ten and boys of five and seven. The irides were tremulous.

Clark reports a case of congenital dislocation of both crystalline lenses. The lenses moved freely through the pupil into the anterior chambers. The condition remained unchanged for four years, when glaucoma supervened.

Differences in Color of the Two Eyes.—It is not uncommon to see people with different colored eyes. Anastasius I had one black eye and the other blue, from whence he derived his name "Dicore," by which this Emperor of the Orient was generally known. Two distinct colors have been seen in an iris. Berry gives a colored illustration of such a case.

The varieties of strabismus are so common that they will be passed without mention. Kuhn presents an exhaustive analysis of 73 cases of congenital defects of the movements of the eyes, considered clinically and didactically. Some or all of the muscles may be absent or two or more may be amalgamated, with anomalies of insertion, false, double, or degenerated, etc.

The influence of heredity in the causation of congenital defects of the eye is strikingly illustrated by De Beck. In three generations twelve members of one family had either coloboma iridis or irideremia. He performed two operations for the cure of cataract in two brothers. The operations were attended with difficulty in all four eyes and followed by cyclitis. The result was good in one eye of each patient, the eye most recently blind. Posey had a case of coloboma in the macular region in a patient who had a supernumerary tooth. He believes the defects were inherited, as the patient's mother also had a supernumerary tooth.

Nunnely reports cases of congenital malformation in three children of one family. The globes of two of them (a boy and a girl) were smaller than natural, and in the boy in addition were flattened by the action of the recti muscles and were soft; the sclera were very vascular and the cornea, conical, the irides dull, thin, and tremulous; the pupils were not in the axis of vision, but were to the nasal side. The elder sister had the same congenital condition, but to a lesser degree. The other boy in the family had a total absence of irides, but he could see fairly well with the left eye.

Anomalies of the Ears.—Bilateral absence of the external ears is quite rare, although there is a species of sheep, native of China, called the "Yungti," in which this anomaly is constant. Bartholinus, Lycosthenes, Pare, Schenck, and Oberteuffer have remarked on deficient external ears. Guys, the celebrated Marseilles litterateur of the eighteenth century, was born with only one ear. Chantreuil mentions obliteration of the external auditory canal in the new-born. Bannofont reports a case of congenital imperforation of the left auditory canal existing near the tympanic membrane with total deafness in that ear. Lloyd described a fetus showing absence of the external auditory meatus on both sides. Munro reports a case of congenital absence of the external auditory meatus of the right ear; and Richardson speaks of congenital malformation of the external auditory apparatus of the right side. There is an instance of absence of the auditory canal with but partial loss of hearing. Mussey reports several cases of congenitally deficient or absent aural appendages. One case was that in which there was congenital absence of the external auditory meatus of both ears without much impairment of hearing. In neither ear of N. W. Goddard, aged twenty-seven, of

Vermont, reported in 1834, was there a vestige of an opening or passage in the external ear, and not even an indentation. The Eustachian tube was closed. The integuments of the face and scalp were capable of receiving acoustic impressions and of transmitting them to the organs of hearing. The authors know of a student of a prominent New York University who is congenitally deficient in external ears, yet his hearing is acute. He hides his deformity by wearing his hair long and combed over his ears.

The knowledge of anomalous auricles is lost in antiquity. Figure 103 represents the head of an aegipan in the British Museum showing a supernumerary auricle. As a rule, supernumerary auricles are preauricular appendages. Warner, in a report of the examination of 50,000 children, quoted by Ballantyne, describes 33 with supernumerary auricles, represented by sessile or pedunculated outgrowths in front of the tragus. They are more commonly unilateral, always congenital, and can be easily removed, giving rise to no unpleasant symptoms. They have a soft and elastic consistency, and are usually composed of a hyaline or reticular cartilaginous axis covered with connective or adipose tissue and skin bearing fine hairs; sometimes both cartilage and fat are absent. They are often associated with some form of defective audition—harelip, ocular disturbance, club-feet, congenital hernia, etc. These supernumerary members vary from one to five in number and are sometimes hereditary. Reverdin describes a man having a supernumerary nipple on the right side of his chest, of whose five children three had preauricular appendages. Figure 104 represents a girl with a supernumerary auricle in the neck, described in the Lancet, 1888. A little girl under Birkett's care in Guy's Hospital more than answered to Macbeth's requisition, "Had I three ears I'd hear thee!" since she possessed two superfluous ones at the sides of the neck, somewhat lower than the angle of the jaw, which were well developed as to their external contour and made up of fibrocartilage. There is mentioned the case of a boy of six months on the left side of whose neck, over the middle anterior border of the sternocleidomastoid muscle, was a nipple-like projection 1/2 inch in length; a rod of cartilage was prolonged into it from a thin plate, which was freely movable in the subcutaneous tissue, forming a striking analogue to an auricle. Moxhay cites the instance of a mother who was frightened by the sight of a boy with hideous contractions in the neck, and who gave birth to a child with two perfect ears and three rudimentary auricles on the right side, and on the left side two rudimentary auricles.

In some people there is an excessive development of the auricular muscles, enabling them to move their ears in a manner similar to that of the lower animals. Of the celebrated instances the Abbe de Marolles, says Vigneul-Marville, bears witness in his "Memoires" that the Regent Crassot could easily move his ears. Saint Augustine mentions this anomaly.

Double tympanitic membrane is spoken of by Loeseke. There is sometimes natural perforation of the tympanum in an otherwise perfect ear, which explains how some people can blow tobacco-smoke from the ear. Fournier has seen several Spaniards and Germans who could perform this feat, and knew one man who could smoke a whole cigar without losing any smoke, since he made it leave either by his mouth, his ears, or in both ways. Fournier in the same article mentions that he has seen a woman with ears over four inches long.

Strange to say, there have been reports of cases in which the ossicles were deficient without causing any imperfection of hearing. Caldani mentions a case with the incus and malleus deficient, and Scarpa and Torreau quote instances of deficient ossicles. Thomka in 1895 reported a case of supernumerary tympanic ossicle, the nature of which was unknown, although it was neither an inflammatory product nor a remnant of Meckel's cartilage.

Absence of the Limbs.—Those persons born without limbs are either the subjects of intrauterine amputation or of embryonic malformation. Probably the most celebrated of this class was Marc Cazotte, otherwise known as "Pepin," who died in Paris in the last century at the age of sixty-two of a chronic intestinal disorder. He had no arms, legs, or scrotum, but from very jutting shoulders on each side were well-formed hands. His abdomen ended in a flattened buttock with badly-formed feet attached. He was exhibited before the public and was celebrated for his dexterity. He performed nearly all the necessary actions, exhibited skilfulness in all his movements, and was credited with the ability of coitus. He was quite intellectual, being able to write in several languages. His skeleton is preserved in the Musee Dupuytren. Flachsland speaks of a woman who three times had borne children without arms and legs. Hastings describes a living child born without any traces of arms or legs. Garlick has seen a child with neither upper nor lower extremities. In place of them were short stumps three or four inches long, closely resembling the ordinary stumps after amputation. The head, chest, body, and male genitals were well formed, and the child survived. Hutchinson reports the history of a child born without extremities, probably the result of intrauterine amputation. The flaps were healed at the deltoid insertion and just below the groin. Pare says he saw in Paris a man without arms, who by means of his head and neck could crack a whip or hold an axe. He ate by means of his feet, dealt and played cards, and threw dice with the same members, exhibiting such dexterity that finally his companions refused to play with him. He was proved to be a thief and a murderer and was finally hanged at Gueldres. Pare also relates having seen a woman in Paris who sewed, embroidered, and did other things with her feet. Jansen speaks of a man in Spain, born without arms, who could use his feet as well as most people use their arms. Schenck and Lotichius give descriptions of armless people.

Hulke describes a child of four whose upper limbs were absent, a small dimple only being in their place. He had free movement of the shoulders in every direction. and could grasp objects between his cheeks and his acromian process; the prehensile power of the toes was well developed, as he could pick up a coin thrown to him. A monster of the same conformation was the celebrated painter, Ducornet, who was born at Lille on the 10th of January, 1806. He was completely deprived of arms, but the rest of the body was well formed with the exception of the feet, of which the second toe was faulty. The deformity of the feet, however, had the happiest result, as the space between the great toe and its neighbor was much larger than ordinary and the toes much more mobile. He became so skilful in his adopted profession that he finally painted a picture eleven feet in height (representing Mary Magdalene at the feet of Christ after the resurrection), which was purchased by the Government and given to the city of Lille. Broca describes James Leedgwood, who was deprived of his arms and had only one leg. He exhibited great dexterity with his single foot, wrote, discharged a pistol, etc.; he was said to have been able to pick up a sewing-needle on a slippery surface with his eyes blindfolded. Capitan described to the Societe d'anthropologie de Paris a young man without arms, who was said to play a violin and cornet with his feet. He was able to take a kerchief from his pocket and to blow his nose; he could make a cigarette, light it, and put it in his mouth, play cards, drink from a glass, and eat with a fork by the aid of his dexterous toes. There was a creature exhibited some time since in the principal cities of France, who was called the "l'homme tronc." He was totally deprived of all his members. Curran describes a Hindoo, a prostitute of forty, with congenital absence of both upper extremities. A slight fleshy protuberance depended from the cicatrix of the humerus and shoulder-joint of the left side, and until the age of ten there was one on the right side. She performed many tricks with her toes. Caldani speaks of a monster without arms, Davis mentions one, and Smith describes a boy of four with his upper limbs entirely absent. Breschet has seen a child of nine with only portions of the upper arms and deformity of lower extremities and pelvis. Pare says that he saw in Paris in 1573, at the gate of St. Andrew des Arts, a boy of nine, a native of a small village near Guise, who had no legs and whose left foot was represented by a fleshy body hanging from the trunk; he had but two fingers hanging on his right hand, and had between his legs what resembled a virile penis. Pare attributes this anomaly to a default in the quantity of semen.

The figure and skeleton of Harvey Leach, called "Hervio Nono," is in the museum of the University College in London. The pelvis was comparatively weak, the femurs hardly to be recognized, and the right tibia and foot defective; the left foot was better developed, although far from being in due proportion to the trunk above. He was one of the most remarkable gymnasts of his day, and notwithstanding the distortion of his lower limbs had marvelous power and agility in them. As an arena-horseman, either standing or sitting, he was scarcely excelled. He walked and even ran quite well, and his power of leaping, partly with his feet and partly with his hands, was unusual. His lower limbs were so short that, erect, he touched the floor with his fingers, but he earned his livelihood as much with his lower as with his upper limbs. In his skeleton his left lower limb, between the hip and heel, measured 16 inches, while the right, between the same points, measured nine inches. Hare mentions a boy of five and a half whose head and trunk were the same as in any other child of like age. He was 22 1/2 inches high, had no spinal curvature, but was absolutely devoid of lower extremities. The right arm was two inches long and the left 2 1/4. Each contained the head and a small adjoining portion of the humerus. The legs were represented by masses of cellular tissue and fat covered by skin which projected about an inch. He was intelligent, had a good memory, and exhibited considerable activity. He seemed to have had more than usual mobility and power of flexion of the lower lumbar region. When on his back he was unable to rise up, but resting on the lower part of the pelvis he was able to maintain himself erect. He usually picked up objects with his teeth, and could hold a coin in the axilla as he rolled from place to place. His rolling was accomplished by a peculiar twisting of the thorax and bending of the pelvis. There was no history of maternal impression during pregnancy, no injury, and no hereditary disposition to anomalous members. Figure 112 represents a boy with congenital deficiency of the lower extremities. who was exhibited a few years ago in Philadelphia. In Figure 113, which represents a similar case in a girl whose photograph is deposited in the Mutter Museum of the College of Physicians, Philadelphia, we see how cleverly the congenital defect may be remedied by mechanical contrivance. With her crutches and artificial legs this girl was said to have moved about easily.

Parvin describes a "turtle-man" as an ectromelian, almost entering the class of phocomelians or seal-like monsters; the former term signifies abortive or imperfect formation of the members. The hands and feet were normally developed, but the arms, forearms, and legs are much shortened.

The "turtle-woman" of Demerara was so called because her mother when pregnant was frightened by a turtle, and also from the child's fancied resemblance to a turtle. The femur was six inches long, the woman had a foot of six bones, four being toes, viz., the first and second phalanges of the first and second toes. She had an acetabulum, capsule, and ligamentum teres, but no tibia or fibula; she also had a defective right forearm. She was never the victim of rachitis or like disease, but died of syphilis in the Colonial Hospital. In her twenty-second year she was delivered of a full-grown child free of deformity.

There was a woman living in Bavaria, under the observation of Buhl, who had congenital absence of both femurs and both fibulas. Almost all the muscles of the thigh existed, and the main attachment to the pelvis was by a large capsular articulation. Charpentier gives the portrait of a woman in whom there was a uniform diminution in the size of the limbs. Debout portrays a young man with almost complete absence of the thigh and leg, from whose right hip there depended a foot. Accrell describes a peasant of twenty-six, born without a hip, thigh, or leg on the right side. The external genital organs were in their usual place, but there was only one testicle in the scrotum. The man was virile. The rectum instead of opening outward and underneath was deflected to the right.

Supernumerary Limbs.—Haller reports several cases of supernumerary extremities. Plancus speaks of an infant with a complete third leg, and Dumeril cites a similar instance. Geoffroy-Saint-Hilaire presented to the Academie des Sciences in 1830 a child with four legs and feet who was in good health. Amman saw a girl with a large thigh attached to her nates. Below the thigh was a single leg made by the fusion of two legs. No patella was found and the knee was anchylosed. One of the feet of the supernumerary limb had six toes, while the other, which was merely an outgrowth, had two toes on it.

According to Jules Guerin, the child named Gustav Evrard was born with a thigh ending in two legs and two imperfect feet depending from the left nates.

Tucker describes a baby born in the Sloane Maternity in New York, October 1, 1894, who had a third leg hanging from a bony and fleshy union attached to the dorsal spine. The supernumerary leg was well formed and had a left foot attached to it. Larkin and Jones mention the removal of a meningocele and a supernumerary limb from an infant of four months. This limb contained three fingers only, one of which did not have a bony skeleton.

Pare says that on the day the Venetians and the Genevois made peace a monster was born in Italy which had four legs of equal proportions, and besides had two supernumerary arms from the elbows of the normal limbs. This creature lived and was baptized.

Anomalies of the Feet.—Hatte has seen a woman who bore a child that had three feet. Bull gives a description of a female infant with the left foot double or cloven.

There was only one heel, but the anterior portion consisted of an anterior and a posterior part. The anterior foot presented a great toe and four smaller ones, but deformed like an example of talipes equinovarus. Continuous with the outer edge of the anterior part and curving beneath it was a posterior part, looking not unlike a second foot, containing six well-formed toes situated directly beneath the other five. The eleven toes were all perfect and none of them were webbed.

There is a class of monsters called "Sirens" on account of their resemblance to the fabulous creatures of mythology of that name. Under the influence of compression exercised in the uterus during the early period of gestation fusion of the inferior extremities is effected. The accompanying illustration shows the appearance of these monsters, which are thought to resemble the enchantresses celebrated by Homer.

Anomalies of the Hand.—Blumenbach speaks of an officer who, having lost his right hand, was subsequently presented by his wife with infants of both sexes showing the same deformity. Murray cites the instance of a woman of thirty-eight, well developed, healthy, and the mother of normal children, who had a double hand. The left arm was abnormal, the flexion of the elbow imperfect, and the forearm terminated in a double hand with only rudimentary thumbs. In working as a charwoman she leaned on the back of the flexed carpus. The double hand could grasp firmly, though the maximum power was not so great as that of the right hand. Sensation was equally acute in all three of the hands. The middle and ring fingers of the supernumerary hand were webbed as far as the proximal joints, and the movements of this hand were stiff and imperfect. No single finger of the two hands could be extended while the other seven were flexed. Giraldes saw an infant in 1864 with somewhat the same deformity, but in which the disposition of the muscles and tendons permitted the ordinary movements.

Absence of Digits.—Maygrier describes a woman of twenty-four who instead of having a hand on each arm had only one finger, and each foot had but two toes. She was delivered of two female children in 1827 and one in 1829, each having exactly the same deformities. Her mother was perfectly formed, but the father had but one toe on his foot and one finger on his left hand.

Kohler gives photographs of quite a remarkable case of suppression and deformity of the digits of both the fingers and toes.

Figure 123 shows a man who was recently exhibited in Philadelphia. He had but two fingers on each hand and two toes on each foot, and resembles Kohler's case in the anomalous digital conformation.

Figure 124 represents an exhibitionist with congenital suppression of four digits on each hand.

Tubby has seen a boy of three in whom the first, second, and third toes of each foot were suppressed, the great toe and the little toe being so overgrown that they could be opposed. In this family for four generations 15 individuals out of 22 presented this defect of the lower extremity. The patient's brothers and a sister had exactly the same deformity, which has been called "lobster-claw foot."

Falla of Jedburgh speaks of an infant who was born without forearms or hands; at the elbow there was a single finger attached by a thin string of tissue. This was the sixth child, and it presented no other deformity. Falla also says that instances of intrauterine digital amputation are occasionally seen.

According to Annandale, supernumerary digits may be classified as follows:—

(1) A deficient organ, loosely attached by a narrow pedicle to the hand or foot (or to another digit).

(2) A more or less developed organ, free at its extremity, and articulating with the head or sides of a metacarpal, metatarsal, or phalangeal bone.

(3) A fully developed separate digit.

(4) A digit intimately united along its whole length with another digit, and having either an additional metacarpal or metatarsal bone of its own, or articulating with the head of one which is common to it and another digit.

Superstitions relative to supernumerary fingers have long been prevalent. In the days of the ancient Chaldeans it was for those of royal birth especially that divinations relative to extra digits were cast. Among the ancients we also occasionally see illustrations emblematic of wisdom in an individual with many fingers, or rather double hands, on each arm.

Hutchinson, in his comments on a short-limbed, polydactylous dwarf which was dissected by Ruysch, the celebrated Amsterdam anatomist, writes as follows.—

"This quaint figure is copied from Theodore Kerckring's 'Spicilegium Anatomicum,' published in Amsterdam in 1670. The description states that the body was that of an infant found drowned in the river on October 16, 1668. It was dissected by the renowned Ruysch. A detailed description of the skeleton is given. My reason for now reproducing the plate is that it offers an important item of evidence in reference to the development of short-limbed dwarfs. Although we must not place too much reliance on the accuracy of the draughtsman, since he has figured some superfluous lumbar vertebrae, yet there can be no doubt that the limbs are much too short for the trunk and head. This remark especially applies to the lower limbs and pelvis. These are exactly like those of the Norwich dwarf and of the skeleton in the Heidelberg Museum which I described in a recent number of the 'Archives.' The point of extreme interest in the present case is that this dwarfing of the limbs is associated with polydactylism. Both the hands have seven digits. The right foot has eight and the left nine. The conditions are not exactly symmetrical, since in some instances a metacarpal or metatarsal bone is wanting; or, to put it otherwise, two are welded together. It will be seen that the upper extremities are so short that the tips of the digits will only just touch the iliac crests.

"This occurrence of short limbs with polydactylism seems to prove conclusively that the condition may be due to a modification of development of a totally different nature from rickets. It is probable that the infant was not at full term. Among the points which the author has noticed in his description are that the fontanelle was double its usual size; that the orbits were somewhat deformed; that the two halves of the lower jaw were already united; and that the ribs were short and badly formed. He also, of course, draws attention to the shortness of the limbs, the stoutness of the long bones, and the supernumerary digits. I find no statement that the skeleton was deposited in any museum, but it is very possible that it is still in existence in Amsterdam, and if so it is very desirable that it should be more exactly described,"

In Figure 126, A represents division of thumb after Guyot-Daubes, shows a typical case of supernumerary fingers, and C pictures Morand's case of duplication of several toes.

Forster gives a sketch of a hand with nine fingers and a foot with nine toes. Voight records an instance of 13 fingers on each hand and 12 toes on each foot. Saviard saw an infant at the Hotel-Dieu in Paris in 1687 which had 40 digits, ten on each member. Annandale relates the history of a woman who had six fingers and two thumbs on each hand, and another who had eight toes on one foot.

Meckel tells of a case in which a man had 12 fingers and 12 toes, all well formed, and whose children and grandchildren inherited the deformity. Mason has seen nine toes on the left foot. There is recorded the account of a child who had 12 toes and six fingers on each hand, one fractured. Braid describes talipes varus in a child of a few months who had ten toes. There is also on record a collection of cases of from seven to ten fingers on each hand and from seven to ten toes on each foot. Scherer gives an illustration of a female infant, otherwise normally formed, with seven fingers on each hand, all united and bearing claw-like nails. On each foot there was a double halux and five other digits, some of which were webbed.

The influence of heredity on this anomaly is well demonstrated. Reaumur was one of the first to prove this, as shown by the Kelleia family of Malta, and there have been many corroboratory instances reported; it is shown to last for three, four, and even five generations; intermarriage with normal persons finally eradicates it.

It is particularly in places where consanguineous marriages are prevalent that supernumerary digits persist in a family. The family of Foldi in the tribe of Hyabites living in Arabia are very numerous and confine their marriages to their tribe. They all have 24 digits, and infants born with the normal number are sacrificed as being the offspring of adultery. The inhabitants of the village of Eycaux in France, at the end of the last century, had nearly all supernumerary digits either on the hands or feet. Being isolated in an inaccessible and mountainous region, they had for many years intermarried and thus perpetuated the anomaly. Communication being opened, they emigrated or married strangers and the sexdigitism vanished. Maupertuis recalls the history of a family living in Berlin whose members had 24 digits for many generations. One of them being presented with a normal infant refused to acknowledge it. There is an instance in the Western United States in which supernumerary digits have lasted through five generations. Cameron speaks of two children in the same family who were polydactylic, though not having the same number of supernumerary fingers.

Smith and Norwell report the case of a boy of fifteen both of whose hands showed webbing of the middle and ring fingers and accessory nodules of bone between the metacarpals, and six toes on each foot. The boy's father showed similar malformations, and in five generations 21 out of 28 individuals were thus malformed, ten females and 11 males. The deformity was especially transmitted in the female line.

Instances of supernumerary thumbs are cited by Panaroli, Ephemerides, Munconys, as well as in numerous journals since. This anomaly is not confined to man alone; apes, dogs, and other lower animals possess it. Bucephalus, the celebrated horse of Alexander, and the horse of Caesar were said to have been cloven-hoofed.

Hypertrophy of the digits is the result of many different processes, and true hypertrophy or gigantism must be differentiated from acromegaly, elephantiasis, leontiasis, and arthritis deformans, for which distinction the reader is referred to an article by Park. Park also calls attention to the difference between acquired gigantism, particularly of the finger and toes, and another condition of congenital gigantism, in which either after or before birth there is a relatively disproportionate, sometimes enormous, overgrowth of perhaps one finger or two, perhaps of a limited portion of a hand or foot, or possibly of a part of one of the limbs. The best collection of this kind of specimens is in the College of Surgeons in London.

Curling quotes a most peculiar instance of hypertrophy of the fingers in a sickly girl. The middle and ring fingers of the right hand were of unusual size, the middle finger measuring 5 1/2 inches in length four inches in circumference. On the left hand the thumb and middle fingers were hypertrophied and the index finger was as long as the middle one of the right hand. The middle finger had a lateral curvature outward, due to a displacement of the extensor tendon. This affection resembled acromegaly. Curling cites similar cases, one in a Spanish gentleman, Governor of Luzon, in the Philippine Islands, in 1850, who had an extraordinary middle finger, which he concealed by carrying it in the breast of his coat.

Hutchinson exhibited a photograph showing the absence of the radius and thumb, with shortening of the forearm. Conditions more or less approaching this had occurred in several members of the same family. In some they were associated with defects of development in the lower extremities also.

The varieties of club-foot—talipes varus, valgus, equinus, equino-varus, etc.—are so well known that they will be passed with mention only of a few persons who have been noted for their activity despite their deformity. Tyrtee, Parini, Byron, and Scott are among the poets who were club-footed; some writers say that Shakespeare suffered in a slight degree from this deformity. Agesilas, Genserie, Robert II, Duke of Normandy, Henry II, Emperor of the West, Otto II, Duke of Brunswick, Charles II, King of Naples, and Tamerlane were victims of deformed feet. Mlle. Valliere, the mistress of Louis XIV, was supposed to have both club-foot and hip-disease. Genu valgum and genu varum are ordinary deformities and quite common in all classes.

Transpositions of the character of the vertebrae are sometimes seen. In man the lumbar vertebrae have sometimes assumed the character of the sacral vertebrae, the sacral vertebrae presenting the aspect of lumbar vertebrae, etc. It is quite common to see the first lumbar vertebra presenting certain characteristics of the dorsal.

Numerical anomalies of the vertebrae are quite common, generally in the lumbar and dorsal regions, being quite rare in the cervical, although there have been instances of six or eight cervical vertebrae. In the lower animals the vertebrae are prolonged into a tail, which, however, is sometimes absent, particularly when hereditary influence exists. It has been noticed in the class of dogs whose tails are habitually amputated to improve their appearance that the tail gradually decreases in length. Some breeders deny this fact.

Human Tails.—The prolongation of the coccyx sometimes takes the shape of a caudal extremity in man. Broca and others claim that the sacrum and the coccyx represent the normal tail of man, but examples are not infrequent in which there has been a fleshy or bony tail appended to the coccygeal region. Traditions of tailed men are old and widespread, and tailed races were supposed to reside in almost every country. There was at one time an ancient belief that all Cornishmen had tails, and certain men of Kent were said to have been afflicted with tails in retribution for their insults to Thomas a Becket. Struys, a Dutch traveler in Formosa in the seventeenth century, describes a wild man caught and tied for execution who had a tail more than a foot long, which was covered with red hair like that of a cow.

The Niam Niams of Central Africa are reported to have tails smooth and hairy and from two to ten inches long. Hubsch of Constantinople remarks that both men and women of this tribe have tails. Carpus, or Berengarius Carpensis, as he is called, in one of his Commentaries said that there were some people in Hibernia with long tails, but whether they were fleshy or cartilaginous could not be known, as the people could not be approached. Certain supposed tailed races which have been described by sea-captains and voyagers are really only examples of people who wear artificial appendages about the waists, such as palm-leaves and hair. A certain Wesleyan missionary, George Brown, in 1876 spoke of a formal breeding of a tailed race in Kali, off the coast of New Britain. Tailless children were slain at once, as they would be exposed to public ridicule. The tailed men of Borneo are people afflicted with hereditary malformation analogous to sexdigitism. A tailed race of princes have ruled Rajoopootana, and are fond of their ancestral mark. There are fabulous stories told of canoes in the East Indies which have holes in their benches made for the tails of the rowers. At one time in the East the presence of tails was taken as a sign of brute force.

There was reported from Caracas the discovery of a tribe of Indians in Paraguay who were provided with tails. The narrative reads somewhat after this manner: One day a number of workmen belonging to Tacura Tuyn while engaged in cutting grass had their mules attacked by some Guayacuyan Indians. The workmen pursued the Indians but only succeeded in capturing a boy of eight. He was taken to the house of Senor Francisco Galeochoa at Posedas, and was there discovered to have a tail ten inches long. On interrogation the boy stated that he had a brother who had a tail as long as his own, and that all the tribe had tails.

Aetius, Bartholinus, Falk, Harvey, Kolping, Hesse, Paulinus, Strauss, and Wolff give descriptions of tails. Blanchard says he saw a tail fully a span in length: and there is a description in 1690 of a man by the name of Emanuel Konig, a son of a doctor of laws who had a tail half a span long, which grew directly downward from the coccyx and was coiled on the perineum, causing much discomfort. Jacob describes a pouch of skin resembling a tail which hung from the tip of the coccyx to the length of six inches. It was removed and was found to be thicker than the thumb, consisted of distinctly jointed portions with synovial capsules. Gosselin saw at his clinic a caudal appendix in an infant which measured about ten cm. Lissner says that in 1872 he assisted in the delivery of a young girl who had a tail consisting of a coccyx prolonged and covered with skin, and in 1884 he saw the same girl, at this time the tail measuring nearly 13 cm.

Virchow received for examination a tail three inches long amputated from a boy of eight weeks. Ornstein, chief physician of the Greek army, describes a Greek of twenty-six who had a hairless, conical tail, free only at the tip, two inches long and containing three vertebrae. He also remarks that other instances have been observed in recruits. Thirk of Broussa in 1820 described the tail of a Kurd of twenty-two which contained four vertebrae. Belinovski gives an account of a hip-joint amputation and extirpation of a fatty caudal extremity, the only one he had ever observed.

Before the Berlin Anthropological Society there were presented two adult male Papuans, in good health and spirits, who had been brought from New Guinea; their coccygeal bones projected 1 1/2 inches. Oliver Wendell Holmes in the Atlantic Monthly, June, 1890, says that he saw in London a photograph of a boy with a considerable tail. The "Moi Boy" was a lad of twelve, who was found in Cochin China, with a tail a foot long which was simply a mass of flesh. Miller tells of a West Point student who had an elongation of the coccyx, forming a protuberance which bulged very visibly under the skin. Exercise at the riding school always gave him great distress, and the protuberance would often chafe until the skin was broken, the blood trickling into his boots.

Bartels presents a very complete article in which he describes 21 persons born with tails, most of the tails being merely fleshy protuberances. Darwin speaks of a person with a fleshy tail and refers to a French article on human tails.

Science contains a description of a negro child born near Louisville, eight weeks old, with a pedunculated tail 2 1/2 inches long, with a base 1 1/4 inches in circumference. The tail resembled in shape a pig's tail and had grown 1/4 inch since birth. It showed no signs of cartilage or bone, and had its origin from a point slightly to the left of the median line and about an inch above the end of the spinal column.

Dickinson recently reported the birth of a child with a tail. It was a well-developed female between 5 1/2 and six pounds in weight. The coccyx was covered with the skin on both the anterior and posterior surfaces. It thus formed a tail of the size of the nail of the little finger, with a length of nearly 3/16 inch on the inner surface and 3/8 inch on the rear surface. This little tip could be raised from the body and it slowly sank back.

In addition to the familiar caudal projection of the human fetus, Dickinson mentions a group of other vestigial remains of a former state of things. Briefly these are:—

(1) The plica semilunaris as a vestige of the nictitating membrane of certain birds.

(2) The pointed ear, or the turned-down tip of the ears of many men.

(3) The atrophied muscles, such as those that move the ear, that are well developed in certain people, or that shift the scalp, resembling the action of a horse in ridding itself of flies.

(4) The supracondyloid foremen of the humerus.

(5) The vermiform appendix.

(6) The location and direction of the hair on the trunk and limbs.

(7) The dwindling wisdom-teeth.

(8) The feet of the fetus strongly deflected inward, as in the apes, and persisting in the early months of life, together with great mobility and a distinct projection of the great toe at an angle from the side of the foot.

(9) The remarkable grasping power of the hand at birth and for a few weeks thereafter, that permits young babies to suspend their whole weight on a cane for a period varying from half a minute to two minutes.

Horrocks ascribes to these anal tags a pathologic importance. He claims that they may be productive of fistula in ano, superficial ulcerations, fecal concretions, fissure in ano, and that they may hypertrophy and set up tenesmus and other troubles. The presence of human tails has given rise to discussion between friends and opponents of the Darwinian theory. By some it is considered a reversion to the lower species, while others deny this and claim it to be simply a pathologic appendix.

Anomalies of the Spinal Canal and Contents.—When there is a default in the spinal column, the vice of conformation is called spina bifida. This is of two classes: first, a simple opening in the vertebral canal, and, second, a large cleft sufficient to allow the egress of spinal membranes and substance. Figure 130 represents a large congenital sacral tumor.

Achard speaks of partial duplication of the central canal of the spinal cord. De Cecco reports a singular case of duplication of the lumbar segment of the spinal cord. Wagner speaks of duplication of a portion of the spinal cord.

Foot records a case of amyelia, or absence of the spinal cord, in a fetus with hernia cerebri and complete fissure of the spinal column. Nicoll and Arnold describe an anencephalous fetus with absence of spinal marrow; and Smith also records the birth of an amyelitic fetus.

In some persons there are exaggerated curvatures of the spine. The first of these curvatures is called kyphosis, in which the curvature is posterior; second, lordosis, in which the curvature is anterior; third, scoliosis, in which it is lateral, to the right or left.

Kyphosis is the most common of the deviations in man and is most often found in the dorsal region, although it may be in the lumbar region. Congenital kyphosis is very rare in man, is generally seen in monsters, and when it does exist is usually accompanied by lordosis or spine bifida. We sometimes observe a condition of anterior curvature of the lumbar and sacral regions, which might be taken for a congenital lordosis, but this is really a deformity produced after birth by the physiologic weight of the body. Figure 131 represents a case of lordosis caused by paralysis of the spinal muscles.

Analogous to this is what the accoucheurs call spondylolisthesis. Scoliosis may be a cervicodorsal, dorsolumbar, or lumbosacral curve, and the inclination of the vertebral column may be to the right or left. The pathologists divide scoliosis into a myopathic variety, in which the trouble is a physiologic antagonism of the muscles; or osteopathic, ordinarily associated with rachitis, which latter variety is generally accountable for congenital scoliosis. In some cases the diameter of the chest is shortened to an almost incredible degree, but may yet be compatible with life. Glover speaks of an extraordinary deformity of the chest with lateral curvature of the spine, in which the diameter from the pit of the stomach to the spinal integument was only 5 1/2 inches.

Supernumerary ribs are not at all uncommon in man, nearly every medical museum having some examples. Cervical ribs are not rare. Gordon describes a young man of seventeen in whom there was a pair of supernumerary ribs attached to the cervical vertebrae. Bernhardt mentions an instance in which cervical ribs caused motor and sensory disturbances. Dumerin of Lyons showed an infant of eight days which had an arrested development of the 2d, 3d, 4th, and 5th ribs. Cases of deficient ribs are occasionally met. Wistar in 1818 gives an account of a person in whom one side of the thorax was at rest while the other performed the movements of breathing in the usual manner.

In some cases we see fissure of the sternum, caused either by deficient union or absence of one of its constituent parts. In the most exaggerated cases these fissures permit the exit of the heart, and as a general rule ectopies of the heart are thus caused. Pavy has given a most remarkable case of sternal fissure in a young man of twenty-five, a native of Hamburg. He exhibited himself in one medical clinic after another all over Europe, and was always viewed with the greatest interest. In the median line, corresponding to the absence of sternum, was a longitudinal groove bounded on either side by a continuous hard ridge which articulated with the costal cartilages. The skin passed naturally over the chest from one side to another, but was raised at one part of the groove by a pulsatile swelling which occupied the position of the right auricle. The clavicle and the two margins of the sternum had no connections whatever, and below the groove was a hard substance corresponding to the ensiform cartilage, which, however, was very elastic, and allowed the patient, under the influence of the pectoral muscles, when the upper extremity was fixed, to open the groove to nearly the extent of three inches, which was more than twice its natural width. By approximating his arms he made the ends of his clavicles overlap. When he coughed, the right lung suddenly protruded from the chest through the groove and ascended a considerable distance above the clavicle into the neck. Between the clavicles another pulsatile swelling was easily felt but hardly seen, which was doubtless the arch of the aorta, as by putting the fingers on it one could feel a double shock, synchronous with distention and recoil of a vessel or opening and closing of the semilunar valves.

Madden pictures (Figs. 134 and 135) a Swede of forty with congenital absence of osseous structure in the middle line of the sternum, leaving a fissure 5 3/8 X 1 3/16 X 2 inches, the longest diameter being vertical. Madden also mentions several analogous instances on record. Groux's case was in a person of forty-five, and the fissure had the vertical length of four inches. Hodgen of St. Louis reports a case in which there was exstrophy of the heart through the fissure. Slocum reports the occurrence of a sternal fissure 3 X 1 1/2 inches in an Irishman of twenty-five. Madden also cites the case of Abbott in an adult negress and a mother. Obermeier mentions several cases. Gibson and Malet describe a presternal fissure uncovering the base of the heart. Ziemssen, Wrany, and Williams also record congenital fissures of the sternum.

Thomson has collected 86 cases of thoracic defects and summarizes his paper by saying that the structures deficient are generally the hair in the mammary and axillary regions, the subcutaneous fat over the muscles, nipples, and breasts, the pectorals and adjacent muscles, the costal cartilages and anterior ends of ribs, the hand and forearm; he also adds that there may be a hernia of the lung, not hereditary, but probably due to the pressure of the arm against the chest. De Marque gives a curious instance in which the chin and chest were congenitally fastened together. Muirhead cites an instance in which a firm, broad strip of cartilage resembling sternomastoid extended from below the left ear to the left upper corner of the sternum, being entirely separate from the jaw.

Some preliminary knowledge of embryology is essential to understand the formation of branchial fissures, and we refer the reader to any of the standard works on embryology for this information. Dzondi was one of the first to recognize and classify congenital fistulas of the neck. The proper classification is into lateral and median fissures. In a case studied by Fevrier the exploration of a lateral pharyngeal fistula produced by the introduction of the sound violent reflex phenomena, such as pallor of the face and irregular, violent beating of the heart. The rarest of the lateral class is the preauricular fissure, which has been observed by Fevrier, Le Dentu, Marchand, Peyrot, and Routier.

The median congenital fissures of the neck are probably caused by defective union of the branchial arches, although Arndt thinks that he sees in these median fistulas a persistence of the hypobranchial furrow which exists normally in the amphioxus. They are less frequent than the preceding variety.

The most typical form of malformation of the esophagus is imperforation or obliteration. Van Cuyck of Brussels in 1824 delivered a child which died on the third day from malnutrition. Postmortem it was found that the inferior extremity of the esophagus to the extent of about two inches was converted into a ligamentous cord. Porro describes a case of congenital obliteration of the esophagus which ended in a cecal pouch about one inch below the inferior portion of the glottidean aperture and from this point to the stomach only measured an inch; there was also tracheal communication. The child was noticed to take to the breast with avidity, but after a little suckling it would cough, become livid, and reject most of the milk through the nose, in this way almost suffocating at each paroxysm; it died on the third day.

In some cases the esophagus is divided, one portion opening into the bronchial or other thoracic organs. Brentano describes an infant dying ten days after birth whose esophagus was divided into two portions, one terminating in a culdesac, the other opening into the bronchi; the left kidney was also displaced downward. Blasius describes an anomalous case of duplication of the esophagus. Grashuys, and subsequently Vicq d'Azir, saw a dilatation of the esophagus resembling the crop of a bird.

Anomalies of the Lungs.—Carper describes a fetus of thirty-seven weeks in whose thorax he found a very voluminous thymus gland but no lungs. These organs were simply represented by two little oval bodies having no lobes, with the color of the tissue of the liver. The heart had only one cavity but all the other organs were perfectly formed. This case seems to be unique. Tichomiroff records the case of a woman of twenty-four who died of pneumonia in whom the left lung was entirely missing. No traces of a left bronchus existed. The subject was very poorly developed physically. Tichomiroff finds four other cases in literature, in all of which the left lung was absent. Theremin and Tyson record cases of the absence of the left lung.

Supplementary pulmonary lobes are occasionally seen in man and are taken by some authorities to be examples of retrogressive anomalies tending to prove that the derivation of the human race is from the quadrupeds which show analogous pulmonary malformation. Eckley reports an instance of supernumerary lobe of the right lung in close connection with the vena azygos major. Collins mentions a similar case. Bonnet and Edwards speak of instances of four lobes in the right lung. Testut and Marcondes report a description of a lung with six lobes.

Anomalies of the Diaphragm.—Diemerbroeck is said to have dissected a human subject in whom the diaphragm and mediastinum were apparently missing, but such cases must be very rare, although we frequently find marked deficiency of this organ. Bouchand reports an instance of absence of the right half of the diaphragm in an infant born at term. Lawrence mentions congenital deficiency of the muscular fibers of the left half of the diaphragm with displacement of the stomach. The patient died of double pneumonia. Carruthers, McClintock, Polaillon, and van Geison also record instances of congenital deficiency of part of the diaphragm. Recently Dittel reported unilateral defect in the diaphragm of an infant that died soon after birth. The stomach, small intestines, and part of the large omentum lay in the left pleural cavity; both the phrenic nerves were normal. Many similar cases of diaphragmatic hernia have been observed. In such cases the opening may be large enough to allow a great part of the visceral constituents to pass into the thorax, sometimes seriously interfering with respiration and circulation by the pressure which ensues. Alderson reports a fatal case of diaphragmatic hernia with symptoms of pneumothorax. The stomach, spleen, omentum, and transverse colon were found lying in the left pleura. Berchon mentions double perforation of the diaphragm with hernia of the epiploon. The most extensive paper on this subject was contributed by Bodwitch, who, besides reporting an instance in the Massachusetts General Hospital, gives a numerical analysis of all the cases of this affection found recorded in the writings of medical authors between the years 1610 and 1846. Hillier speaks of an instance of congenital diaphragmatic hernia in which nearly all the small intestines and two-thirds of the large passed into the right side of the thorax. Macnab reports an instance in which three years after the cure of empyema the whole stomach constituted the hernia. Recently Joly described congenital hernia of the stomach in a man of thirty-seven, who died from collapse following lymphangitis, persistent vomiting, and diarrhea. At the postmortem there was found a defect in the diaphragm on the left side, permitting herniation of the stomach and first part of the duodenum into the left pleural cavity. There was no history of traumatism to account for strangulation. Longworth cites an instance of inversion of the diaphragm in a human subject. Bartholinus mentions coalition of the diaphragm and liver; and similar cases are spoken of by Morgagni and the Ephemerides. Hoffman describes diaphragmatic junction with the lung.

Anomalies of the Stomach.—The Ephemerides contains the account of a dissection in which the stomach was found wanting, and also speaks of two instances of duplex stomach. Bartholinus, Heister, Hufeland, Morgagni, Riolan, and Sandifort cite examples of duplex stomach. Bonet speaks of a case of vomiting which was caused by a double stomach. Struthers reports two cases in which there were two cavities to the stomach. Struthers also mentions that Morgagni, Home, Monro, Palmer, Larry, Blasius, Hufeland, and Walther also record instances in which there was contraction in the middle of the stomach, accounting for their instances of duplex stomach. Musser reports an instance of hour-glass contraction of the stomach. Hart dissected the stomach of a woman of thirty which resembled the stomach of a predaceous bird, with patches of tendon on its surface. The right extremity instead of continuously contracting ended in a culdesac one-half as large as the greater end of the stomach. The duodenum proceeded from the depression marking the lesser arch of the organ midway between the cardiac orifice and the right extremity. Crooks speaks of a case in which the stomach of an infant terminated in a culdesac.

Hernia of the stomach is not uncommon, especially in diaphragmatic or umbilical deficiency. There are many cases on record, some terminating fatally from strangulation or exposure to traumatism. Paterson reports a case of congenital hernia of the stomach into the left portion of the thoracic cavity. It was covered with fat and occupied the whole left half of the thoracic cavity. The spleen, pancreas, and transverse colon were also superior to the diaphragm. Death was caused by a well-defined round perforation at the cardiac curvature the size of a sixpence.

Anomalies of the Intestines.—The Ephemerides contains the account of an example of double cecum, and Alexander speaks of a double colon, and there are other cases of duplication of the bowel recorded. There is an instance of coalition of the jejunum with the liver, and Treuner parallels this case. Aubery, Charrier Poelman, and others speak of congenital division of the intestinal canal. Congenital occlusion is quite frequently reported.

Dilatation of the colon frequently occurs as a transient affection, and by its action in pushing up the diaphragm may so seriously interfere with the action of the heart and lungs as to occasionally cause heart-failure. Fenwick has mentioned an instance of this nature. According to Osler there is a chronic form of dilatation of the colon in which the gut may reach an enormous size. The coats may be hypertrophied without evidence of any special organic change in the mucosa. The most remarkable instance has been reported by Formad. The patient, known as the "balloon-man," aged twenty-three at the time of his death, had had a distended abdomen from infancy. Postmortem the colon was found as large as that of an ox, the circumference ranging from 15 to 30 inches. The weight of the contents was 47 pounds. Cases are not uncommon in children. Osler reports three well-marked cases under his care. Chapman mentions a case in which the liver was displaced by dilatation of the sigmoid flexure. Mya reports two cases of congenital dilatation and hypertrophy of the colon (megacolon congenito). Hirsohsprung, Genersich, Faralli, Walker, and Griffiths all record similar instances, and in all these cases the clinical features were obstinate constipation and marked meteorismus.

Imperforate Anus.—Cases in which the anus is imperforate or the rectum ends in a blind pouch are occasionally seen. In some instances the rectum is entirely absent, the colon being the termination of the intestinal tract. There are cases on record in which the rectum communicated with the anus solely by a fibromuscular cord. Anorectal atresia is the ordinary imperforation of the anus, in which the rectum terminates in the middle of the sacral cavity. The rectum may be deficient from the superior third of the sacrum, and in this position is quite inaccessible for operation.

A compensatory coalition of the bowel with the bladder or urethra is sometimes present, and in these cases the feces are voided by the urinary passages. Huxham mentions the fusion of the rectum and colon with the bladder, and similar instances are reported by Dumas and Baillie. Zacutus Lusitanus describes an infant with an imperforate membrane over its anus who voided feces through the urethra for three months. After puncture of the membrane, the discharge came through the natural passage and the child lived; Morgagni mentions a somewhat similar case in a little girl living in Bologna, and other modern instances have been reported. The rectum may terminate in the vagina. Masters has seen a child who lived nine days in whom the sigmoid flexure of the colon terminated in the fundus of the bladder. Guinard pictures a case in which there was communication between the rectum and the bladder. In Figure 140 a represents the rectum; b the bladder; c the point of communication; g shows the cellular tissue of the scrotum.

There is a description of a girl of fourteen, otherwise well constituted and healthy, who had neither external genital organs nor anus. There was a plain dermal covering over the genital and anal region. She ate regularly, but every three days she experienced pain in the umbilicus and much intestinal irritation, followed by severe vomiting of stercoraceous matter; the pains then ceased and she cleansed her mouth with aromatic washes, remaining well until the following third day. Some of the urine was evacuated by the mammae. The examiners displayed much desire to see her after puberty to note the disposition of the menstrual flow, but no further observation of her case can be found.

Fournier narrates that he was called by three students, who had been trying to deliver a woman for five days. He found a well-constituted woman of twenty-two in horrible agony, who they said had not had a passage of the bowels for eight days, so he prescribed an enema. The student who was directed to give the enema found to his surprise that there was no anus, but by putting his finger in the vagina he could discern the floating end of the rectum, which was full of feces. There was an opening in this suspended rectum about the size of an undistended anus.

Lavage was practiced by a cannula introduced through the opening, and a great number of cherry stones agglutinated with feces followed the water, and labor was soon terminated. The woman afterward confessed that she was perfectly aware of her deformity, but was ashamed to disclose it before. There was an analogue of this case found by Mercurialis in a child of a Jew called Teutonicus.

Gerster reports a rare form of imperforate anus, with malposition of the left ureter, obliteration of the ostia of both ureters, with consequent hydronephrosis of a confluent kidney. There was a minute opening into the bladder, which allowed the passage of meconium through the urethra. Burge mentions the case of what he calls "sexless child," in which there was an imperforate anus and no pubic arch; the ureters discharged upon a tumor the size of a teacup extending from the umbilicus to the pubes. A postmortem examination confirmed the diagnosis of sexless child.

The Liver.—The Ephemerides, Frankenau, von Home, Molinetti, Schenok, and others speak of deficient or absent liver. Zacutus Lusitanus says that he once found a mass of flesh in place of the liver. Lieutaud is quoted as describing a postmortem examination of an adult who had died of hydropsy, in whom the liver and spleen were entirely missing. The portal vein discharged immediately into the vena cava; this case is probably unique, as no authentic parallel could be found.

Laget reports an instance of supernumerary lobe in the liver. Van Buren describes a supernumerary liver. Sometimes there is rotation, real or apparent, caused by transposition of the characteristics of the liver. Handy mentions such a case. Kirmisson reports a singular anomaly of the liver which he calls double displacement by interversion and rotation on the vertical axis. Actual displacements of the liver as well as what is known as wandering liver are not uncommon. The operation for floating liver will be spoken of later.

Hawkins reports a case of congenital obliteration of the ductus communis choledochus in a male infant which died at the age of four and a half months. Jaundice appeared on the eighth day and lasted through the short life. The hepatic and cystic ducts were pervious and the hepatic duct obliterated. There were signs of hepatic cirrhosis and in addition an inguinal hernia

The Gall-Bladder.—Harle mentions the case of a man of fifty, in whom he could find no gall-bladder; Patterson has seen a similar instance in a men of twenty-five. Purser describes a double gall-bladder.

The spleen has been found deficient or wanting by Lebby, Ramsay, and others, but more frequently it is seen doubled. Cabrolius, Morgagni, and others have found two spleens in one subject; Cheselden and Fallopius report three; Fantoni mentions four found in one subject; Guy-Patin has seen five, none as large as the ordinary organ; Hollerius, Kerckringius, and others have remarked on multiple spleens. There is a possibility that in some of the cases of multiple spleens reported the organ is really single but divided into several lobes. Albrecht mentions a case shown at a meeting of the Vienna Medical Society of a very large number of spleens found in the mesogastrium, peritoneum, on the mesentery and transverse mesocolon, in Douglas' pouch, etc. There was a spleen "the size of a walnut" in the usual position, with the splenic artery and vein in their normal position. Every one of these spleens had a capsule, was covered by peritoneum, and exhibited the histologic appearance of splenic tissue. According to the review of this article, Toldt explains the case by assuming that other parts of the celomic epithelium, besides that of the mesogastrium, are capable of forming splenic tissue. Jameson reports a case of double spleen and kidneys. Bainbrigge mentions a case of supernumerary spleen causing death from the patient being placed in the supine position in consequence of fracture of the thigh. Peevor mentions an instance of second spleen. Beclard and Guy-Patin have seen the spleen congenitally misplaced on the right side and the liver on the left; Borellus and Bartholinus with others have observed misplacement of the spleen.

The Pancreas.—Lieutaud has seen the pancreas missing and speaks of a double pancreatic duct that he found in a man who died from starvation; Bonet speaks of a case similar to this last.

There are several cases of complete transposition of the viscera on record. This bizarre anomaly was probably observed first in 1650 by Riolanus, but the most celebrated case was that of Morand in 1660, and Mery described the instance later which was the subject of the following quatrain:—

"La nature, peu sage et sans douse en debauche Placa le foie au cote gauche, Et de meme, vice versa Le coeur a le droite placa."

Young cites an example in a woman of eighty-five who died at Hammersmith, London. She was found dead in bed, and in a postmortem examination, ordered to discover if possible the cause of death, there was seen complete transposition of the viscera. The heart lay with its base toward the left, its apex toward the right, reaching the lower border of the 4th rib, under the right mamma. The vena cava was on the left side and passed into the pulmonary cavity of the heart, which was also on the left side, the aorta and systemic ventricle being on the right. The left splenic vein was lying on the superior vena cava, the liver under the left ribs, and the spleen on the right side underneath the heart. The esophagus was on the right of the aorta, and the location of the two ends of the stomach was reversed; the sigmoid flexure was on the right side. Davis describes a similar instance in a man.

Herrick mentions transposition of viscera in a man of twenty-five. Barbieux cites a case of transposition of viscera in a man who was wounded in a duel. The liver was to the left and the spleen and heart to the right etc. Albers, Baron, Beclard, Boyer, Bull, Mackensie, Hutchinson, Hunt, Murray, Dareste, Curran, Duchesne, Musser, Sabatier, Shrady, Vulpian, Wilson, and Wehn are among others reporting instances of transposition and inversion of the viscera.

Congenital extroversion or eventration is the result of some congenital deficiency in the abdominal wall; instances are not uncommon, and some patients live as long as do cases of umbilical hernia proper. Ramsey speaks of entire want of development of the abdominal parietes. Robertson, Rizzoli, Tait, Hamilton, Brodie, Denis, Dickie, Goyrand, and many others mention extroversion of viscera from parietal defects. The different forms of hernia will be considered in another chapter.

There seem to be no authentic cases of complete absence of the kidney except in the lowest grades of monstrosities. Becker, Blasius, Rhodius, Baillie, Portal, Sandifort, Meckel, Schenck, and Stoll are among the older writers who have observed the absence of one kidney. In a recent paper Ballowitz has collected 213 cases, from which the following extract has been made by the British Medical Journal:—

"Ballowitz (Virchow's Archiv, August 5, 1895) has collected as far as possible all the recorded cases of congenital absence of one kidney. Excluding cases of fused kidney and of partial atrophy of one kidney, he finds 213 cases of complete absence of one kidney, upon which he bases the following conclusions: Such deficiency occurs almost twice as often in males as in females, a fact, however, which may be partly accounted for by the greater frequency of necropsies on males. As to age, 23 occurred in the fetus or newly born, most having some other congenital deformity, especially imperforate anus; the rest were about evenly distributed up to seventy years of age, after which only seven cases occurred. Taking all cases together, the deficiency is more common on the left than on the right side; but while in males the left kidney is far more commonly absent than the right, in females the two sides show the defect equally. The renal vessels were generally absent, as also the ureter, on the abnormal side (the latter in all except 15 cases); the suprarenal was missing in 31 cases. The solitary kidney was almost always normal in shape and position, but much enlarged. Microscopically the enlargement would seem to be due rather to hyperplasia than to hypertrophy. The bladder, except for absence of the opening of one ureter, was generally normal. In a large number of cases there were associated deformities of the organs of generation, especially of the female organs, and these were almost invariably on the side of the renal defect; they affected the conducting portion much more than the glandular portion—that is, uterus, vagina, and Fallopian tubes in the female, and vas deferens or vesiculae seminales in the male, rather than the ovaries or testicles. Finally, he points out the practical bearing of the subject—for example, the probability of calculus causing sudden suppression of urine in such cases—and also the danger of surgical interference, and suggests the possibility of diagnosing the condition by ascertaining the absence of the opening of one ureter in the bladder by means of the cystoscope, and also the likelihood of its occurring where any abnormality of the genital organs is found, especially if this be unilateral."

Green reports the case of a female child in which the right kidney and right Fallopian tube and ovary were absent without any rudimentary structures in their place. Guiteras and Riesman have noted the absence of the right kidney, right ureter, and right adrenal in an old woman who had died of chronic nephritis. The left kidney although cirrhotic was very much enlarged.

Tompsett describes a necropsy made on a coolie child of nearly twelve months, in which it was seen that in the place of a kidney there were two left organs connected at the apices by a prolongation of the cortical substance of each; the child had died of neglected malarial fever. Sandifort speaks of a case of double kidneys and double ureters, and cases of supernumerary kidney are not uncommon, generally being segmentation of one of the normal kidneys. Rayer has seen three kidneys united and formed like a horseshoe. We are quite familiar with the ordinary "horseshoe kidney," in which two normal kidneys are connected.

There are several forms of displacement of the kidneys, the most common being the "floating kidney," which is sometimes successfully removed or fixed; Rayer has made an extensive study of this anomaly.

The kidney may be displaced to the pelvis, and Guinard quotes an instance in which the left kidney was situated in the pelvis, to the left of the rectum and back of the bladder. The ureter of the left side was very short. The left renal artery came from the bifurcation of the aorta and the primitive iliacs. The right kidney was situated normally, and received from the aorta two arteries, whose volume did not surpass the two arteries supplying the left suprarenal capsule, which was in its ordinary place. Displacements of the kidney anteriorly are very rare.

The ureters have been found multiple; Griffon reports the history of a male subject in whom the ureter on the left side was double throughout its whole length; there were two vesical orifices on the left side one above the other; and Morestin, in the same journal, mentions ureters double on both sides in a female subject. Molinetti speaks of six ureters in one person. Littre in 1705 described a case of coalition of the ureters. Allen describes an elongated kidney with two ureters. Coeyne mentions duplication of the ureters on both sides. Lediberder reports a case in which the ureter had double origin. Tyson cites an instance of four ureters in an infant. Penrose mentions the absence of the upper two-thirds of the left ureter, with a small cystic kidney, and there are parallel cases on record.

The ureters sometimes have anomalous terminations either in the rectum, vagina, or directly in the urethra. This latter disposition is realized normally in a number of animals and causes the incessant flow of urine, resulting in a serious inconvenience. Flajani speaks of the termination of the ureters in the pelvis; Nebel has seen them appear just beneath the umbilicus; and Lieutaud describes a man who died at thirty-five, from another cause, whose ureters, as large as intestines, terminated in the urethral canal, causing him to urinate frequently; the bladder was absent. In the early part of this century there was a young girl examined in New York whose ureters emptied into a reddish carnosity on the mons veneris. The urine dribbled continuously, and if the child cried or made any exertion it came in jets. The genital organs participated but little in the deformity, and with the exception that the umbilicus was low and the anus more anterior than natural, the child was well formed and its health good. Colzi reports a case in which the left ureter opened externally at the left side of the hymen a little below the normal meatus urinarius. There is a case described of a man who evidently suffered from a patent urachus, as the urine passed in jets as if controlled by a sphincter from his umbilicus. Littre mentions a patent urachus in a boy of eighteen. Congenital dilatation of the ureters is occasionally seen in the new-born. Shattuck describes a male fetus showing reptilian characters in the sexual ducts. There was ectopia vesicae and prolapse of the intestine at the umbilicus; the right kidney was elongated; the right vas deferens opened into the ureter. There was persistence in a separate condition of the two Mullerian ducts which opened externally inferiorly, and there were two ducts near the openings which represented anal pouches. Both testicles were in the abdomen. Ord describes a man in whom one of the Mullerian ducts was persistent.

Anomalies of the Bladder.—Blanchard, Blasius, Haller, Nebel, and Rhodius mention cases in which the bladder has been found absent and we have already mentioned some cases, but the instances in which the bladder has been duplex are much more frequent. Bourienne, Oberteuffer, Ruysch, Bartholinus, Morgagni, and Franck speak of vesical duplication. There is a description of a man who had two bladders, each receiving a ureter. Bussiere describes a triple bladder, and Scibelli of Naples mentions an instance in a subject who died at fifty-seven with symptoms of retention of urine. In the illustration, B represents the normal bladder, A and C the supplementary bladders, with D and E their respective points of entrance into B. As will be noticed, the ureters terminate in the supplementary bladders. Fantoni and Malgetti cite instances of quintuple bladders.

The Ephemerides speaks of a case of coalition of the bladder with the os pubis and another case of coalition with the omentum. Prochaska mentions vesical fusion with the uterus, and we have already described union with the rectum and intestine.

Exstrophy of the bladder is not rare, and is often associated with hypospadias, epispadias, and other malformations of the genitourinary tract. It consists of a deficiency of the abdominal wall in the hypogastric region, in which is seen the denuded bladder. It is remedied by many different and ingenious plastic operations.

In an occasional instance in which there is occlusion at the umbilicus and again at the neck of the bladder this organ becomes so distended as to produce a most curious deformity in the fetus. Figure 143 shows such a case.

The Heart.—Absence of the heart has never been recorded in human beings except in the case of monsters, as, for example, the omphalosites, although there was a case reported and firmly believed by the ancient authors,—a Roman soldier in whom Telasius said he could discover no vestige of a heart.

The absence of one ventricle has been recorded. Schenck has seen the left ventricle deficient, and the Ephemerides, Behr, and Kerckring speak of a single ventricle only in the heart. Riolan mentions a heart in which both ventricles were absent. Jurgens reported in Berlin, February 1, 1882, an autopsy on a child who had lived some days after birth, in which the left ventricle of the heart was found completely absent. Playfair showed the heart of a child which had lived nine months in which one ventricle was absent. In King's College Hospital in London there is a heart of a boy of thirteen in which the cavities consist of a single ventricle and a single auricle.

Duplication of the heart, notwithstanding the number of cases reported, has been admitted with the greatest reserve by Geoffroy-Saint-Hilaire and by a number of authors. Among the celebrated anatomists who describe duplex heart are Littre, Meckel, Collomb, Panum, Behr, Paullini, Rhodins, Winslow, and Zacutus Lusitanus.

The Ephemerides cites an instance of triple heart, and Johnston has seen a triple heart in a goose.

The phenomenon of "blue-disease," or congenital cyanosis, is due to the patency of the foremen ovale, which, instead of closing at birth, persists sometimes to adult life.

Perhaps the most unique collection of congenital malformations of the heart from persons who have reached the age of puberty was to be seen in London in 1895. In this collection there was an adult heart in which the foremen ovale remained open until the age of thirty-seven; there were but two pulmonary valves; there was another heart showing a large patent foramen ovale from a man of forty-six; and there was a septum ventriculorum of an adult heart from a woman of sixty-three, who died of carcinoma of the breast, in which the foremen ovale was still open and would admit the fore-finger. This woman had shown no symptoms of the malformation. There were also hearts in which the interventricular septum was deficient, the ductus arteriosus patent, or some valvular malformation present. All these persons had reached puberty.

Displacements of the heart are quite numerous. Deschamps of Laval made an autopsy on an old soldier which justified the expression, "He had a heart in his belly." This organ was found in the left lumbar region; it had, with its vessels, traversed an anomalous opening in the diaphragm. Franck observed in the Hospital of Colmar a woman with the heart in the epigastric region. Ramel and Vetter speak of the heart under the diaphragm.

Inversion of the heart is quite frequent, and we often find reports of cases of this anomaly. Fournier describes a soldier of thirty years, of middle height, well proportioned and healthy, who was killed in a duel by receiving a wound in the abdomen; postmortem, the heart was found in the position of the right lung; the two lungs were joined and occupied the left chest.

The anomalies of the vascular system are so numerous that we shall dismiss them with a slight mention. Malacarne in Torino in 1784 described a double aorta, and Hommelius mentions an analogous case. The following case is quite an interesting anatomic anomaly: A woman since infancy had difficulty in swallowing, which was augmented at the epoch of menstruation and after exercise; bleeding relieved her momentarily, but the difficulty always returned. At last deglutition became impossible and the patient died of malnutrition. A necropsy revealed the presence of the subclavicular artery passing between the tracheal artery and the esophagus, compressing this latter tube and opposing the passage of food.

Anomalies of the Breasts.—The first of the anomalies of the generative apparatus to be discussed, although not distinctly belonging under this head, will be those of the mammae.

Amazia, or complete absence of the breast, is seldom seen. Pilcher describes an individual who passed for a female, but who was really a male, in whom the breasts were absolutely wanting. Foerster, Froriep, and Ried cite instances associated with thoracic malformation. Greenhow reports a case in which the mammae were absent, although there were depressed rudimentary nipples and areolae. There were no ovaries and the uterus was congenitally imperfect.

There was a negress spoken of in 1842 in whom the right breast was missing, and there are cases of but one breast, mentioned by King, Paull, and others. Scanzoni has observed absence of the left mamma with absence of the left ovary.

Micromazia is not so rare, and is generally seen in females with associate genital troubles. Excessive development of the mammae, generally being a pathologic phenomenon, will be mentioned in another chapter. However, among some of the indigenous negroes the female breasts are naturally very large and pendulous. This is well shown in Figure 144, which represents a woman of the Bushman tribe nursing an infant. The breasts are sufficiently pendulous and loose to be easily thrown over the shoulder.

Polymazia is of much more frequent occurrence than is supposed. Julia, the mother of Alexander Severus, was surnamed "Mammea" because she had supernumerary breasts. Anne Boleyn, the unfortunate wife of Henry VIII of England, was reputed to have had six toes, six fingers, and three breasts. Lynceus says that in his time there existed a Roman woman with four mammae, very beautiful in contour, arranged in two lines, regularly, one above the other, and all giving milk in abundance. Rubens has pictured a woman with four breasts; the painting may be seen in the Louvre in Paris.

There was a young and wealthy heiress who addressed herself to the ancient faculty at Tubingen, asking, as she displayed four mammary, whether, should she marry, she would have three or four children at a birth. This was a belief with which some of her elder matron friends had inspired her, and which she held as a hindrance to marriage.

Leichtenstern, who has collected 70 cases of polymazia in females and 22 in males, thinks that accessory breasts or nipples are due to atavism, and that our most remote inferiorly organized ancestors had many breasts, but that by constantly bearing but one child, from being polymastic, females have gradually become bimastic. Some of the older philosophers contended that by the presence of two breasts woman was originally intended to bear two children.

Hirst says: "Supernumerary breasts and nipples are more common than is generally supposed. Bruce found 60 instances in 3956 persons examined (1.56 per cent). Leichtenstern places the frequency at one in 500. Both observers declare that men present the anomaly about twice as frequently as women. It is impossible to account for the accessory glands on the theory of reversion, as they occur with no regularity in situation, but may develop at odd places on the body. The most frequent position is on the pectoral surface below the true mammae and somewhat nearer the middle line, but an accessory gland has been observed on the left shoulder over the prominence of the deltoid, on the abdominal surface below the costal cartilages, above the umbilicus, in the axilla, in the groin, on the dorsal surface, on the labium majus, and on the outer aspect of the left thigh. Ahlfeld explains the presence of mammae on odd parts of the body by the theory that portions of the embryonal material entering into the composition of the mammary gland are carried to and implanted upon any portion of the exterior of the body by means of the amnion."

Possibly the greatest number of accessory mammae reported is that of Neugebauer in 1886, who found ten in one person. Peuch in 1876 collected 77 cases, and since then Hamy, Quinqusud, Whiteford, Engstrom, and Mitchell Bruce have collected cases. Polymazia must have been known in the olden times, and we still have before us the old images of Diana, in which this goddess is portrayed with numerous breasts, indicating her ability to look after the growing child. Figure 145 shows an ancient Oriental statue of Artemisia or Diana now at Naples.

Bartholinus has observed a Danish woman with three mammae, two ordinarily formed and a third forming a triangle with the others and resembling the breasts of a fat man. In the village of Phullendorf in Germany early in this century there was an old woman who sought alms from place to place, exhibiting to the curious four symmetrical breasts, arranged parallel. She was extremely ugly, and when on all fours, with her breasts pendulous, she resembled a beast. The authors have seen a man with six distinct nipples, arranged as regularly as those of a bitch or sow. The two lower were quite small. This man's body was covered with heavy, long hair, making him a very conspicuous object when seen naked during bathing. The hair was absent for a space of nearly an inch about the nipples. Borellus speaks of a woman with three mammae, two as ordinarily, the third to the left side, which gave milk, but not the same quantity as the others. Gardiner describes a mulatto woman who had four mammae, two of which were near the axillae, about four inches in circumference, with proportionate sized nipples. She became a mother at fourteen, and gave milk from all her breasts. In his "Dictionnaire Philosophique" Voltaire gives the history of a woman with four well-formed and symmetrically arranged breasts; she also exhibited an excrescence, covered with a nap-like hair, looking like a cow-tail. Percy thought the excrescence a prolongation of the coccyx, and said that similar instances were seen in savage men of Borneo.

Percy says that among some prisoners taken in Austria was found a woman of Valachia, near Roumania, exceedingly fatigued, and suffering intensely from the cold. It was January, and the ground was covered with three feet of snow. She had been exposed with her two infants, who had been born twenty days, to this freezing temperature, and died on the next day. An examination of her body revealed five mammae, of which four projected as ordinarily, while the fifth was about the size of that of a girl at puberty.

They all had an intense dark ring about them; the fifth was situated about five inches above the umbilicus. Percy injected the subject and dissected and described the mammary blood-supply. Hirst mentions a negress of nineteen who had nine mammae, all told, and as many nipples. The two normal glands were very large. Two accessory glands and nipples below them were small and did not excrete milk. All the other glands and nipples gave milk in large quantities. There were five nipples on the left and four on the right side. The patient's mother had an accessory mamma on the abdomen that secreted milk during the period of lactation.

Charpentier has observed in his clinic a woman with two supplementary axillary mammae with nipples. They gave milk as the ordinary mammae. Robert saw a woman who nourished an infant by a mamma on the thigh. Until the time of pregnancy this mamma was taken for an ordinary nevus, but with pregnancy it began to develop and acquired the size of a citron. Figure 147 is from an old wood-cut showing a child suckling at a supernumerary mamma on its mother's thigh while its brother is at the natural breast. Jenner speaks of a breast on the outer side of the thigh four inches below the great trochanter. Hare describes a woman of thirty-seven who secreted normal milk from her axillae. Lee mentions a woman of thirty-five with four mammae and four nipples; she suckled with the pectoral and not the axillary breasts. McGillicudy describes a pair of rudimentary abdominal mammae, and there is another similar case recorded. Hartung mentions a woman of thirty who while suckling had a mamma on the left labium majus. It was excised, and microscopic examination showed its structure to be that of a rudimentary nipple and mammary gland. Leichtenstern cites a case of a mamma on the left shoulder nearly under the insertion of the deltoid, and Klob speaks of an acromial accessory mamma situated on the shoulder over the greatest prominence of the deltoid. Hall reports the case of a functionally active supernumerary mamma over the costal cartilage of the 8th rib. Jussieu speaks of a woman who had three breasts, one of which was situated on the groin and with which she occasionally suckled; her mother had three breasts, but they were all situated on the chest. Saunois details an account of a female who had two supernumerary breasts on the back. Bartholinus (quoted by Meckel) and Manget also mention mammae on the back, but Geoffroy-Saint-Hilaire questions their existence. Martin gives a very clear illustration of a woman with a supernumerary breast below the natural organ. Sneddon, who has collected quite a number of cases of polymazia, quotes the case of a woman who had two swellings in each axilla in which gland-structure was made out, but with no external openings, and which had no anatomic connection with the mammary glands proper. Shortly after birth they varied in size and proportion, as the breasts were full or empty, and in five weeks all traces of them were lost. Her only married sister had similar enlargements at her third confinement.

Polymazia sometimes seems to be hereditary. Robert saw a daughter whose mother was polymastic, and Woodman saw a mother and eldest daughter who each had three nipples. Lousier mentions a woman wanting a mamma who transmitted this vice of conformation to her daughter. Handyside says he knew two brothers in both of whom breasts were wanting.

Supernumerary nipples alone are also seen, as many as five having been found on the same breast. Neugebauer reports eight supernumerary nipples in one case. Hollerus has seen a woman who had two nipples on the same breast which gave milk with the same regularity and the same abundance as the single nipple. The Ephemerides contains a description of a triple nipple. Barth describes "mamma erratica" on the face in front of the right ear which enlarged during menstruation.

Cases of deficiency of the nipples have been reported by the Ephemerides, Lentilius, Severinus, and Werckardus.

Cases of functional male mammae will be discussed in Chapter IX.

Complete absence of the hymen is very rare, if we may accept the statements of Devilliers, Tardieu, and Brouardel, as they have never seen an example in the numerous young girls they have examined from a medico-legal point of view.

Duplication or biperforation of the hymen is also a very rare anomaly of this membrane. In this instance the hymen generally presents two lateral orifices, more or less irregular and separated by a membranous band, which gives the appearance of duplicity. Roze reported from Strasburg in 1866 a case of this kind, and Delens has observed two examples of biperforate hymen, which show very well that this disposition of the membrane is due to a vice of conformation. The first was in a girl of eleven, in which the membrane was of the usual size and thickness, but was duplicated on either side. In her sister of nine the hymen was normally conformed. The second case was in a girl under treatment by Cornil in 1876 for vaginitis. Her brother had accused a young man of eighteen of having violated her, and on examination the hymen showed a biperforate conformation; there were two oval orifices, their greatest diameter being in the vertical plane; the openings were situated on each side of the median line, about five mm. apart; the dividing band did not appear to be cicatricial, but presented the same roseate coloration as the rest of the hymen. Since this report quite a number of cases have been recorded.

The different varieties of the hymen will be left to the works on obstetrics. As has already been observed, labor is frequently seriously complicated by a persistent and tough hymen.

Deficient vulva may be caused by the persistence of a thick hymen, by congenital occlusion, or by absolute absence in vulvar structure. Bartholinus, Borellus, Ephemerides, Julius, Vallisneri, and Baux are among the older writers who mention this anomaly, but as it is generally associated with congenital occlusion, or complete absence of the vagina, the two will be considered together.

Complete absence of the vagina is quite rare. Baux a reports a case of a girl of fourteen in whom "there was no trace of fundament or of genital organs." Oberteuffer speaks of a case of absent vagina. Vicq d'Azir is accredited with having seen two females who, not having a vagina, copulated all through life by the urethra, and Fournier sagely remarks that the extra large urethra may have been a special dispensation of nature. Bosquet describes a young girl of twenty with a triple vice of conformation—an obliterated vulva, closure of the vagina, and absence of the uterus. Menstrual hemorrhage took place from the gums. Clarke has studied a similar case which was authenticated by an autopsy.

O'Ferral of Dublin, Gooch, Davies, Boyd, Tyler Smith, Hancock, Coste, Klayskens, Debrou, Braid, Watson, and others are quoted by Churchill as having mentioned the absence of the vagina. Amussat observed a German girl who did not have a trace of a vagina and who menstruated regularly. Griffith describes a specimen in the Museum of St. Bartholomew's Hospital, London, in which the ovaries lay on the surface of the pelvic peritoneum and there was neither uterus nor vagina; the pelvis had some of the characteristics of the male type. Matthews Duncan has observed a somewhat similar case, the vagina not measuring more than an inch in length. Ferguson describes a prostitute of eighteen who had never menstruated. The labia were found well developed, but there was no vagina, uterus, or ovaries. Coitus had been through the urethra, which was considerably distended, though not causing incontinence of urine. Hulke reports a case of congenital atresia of the vagina in a brunette of twenty, menstruation occurring through the urethra. He also mentions the instance of congenital atresia of the vagina with hernia of both ovaries into the left groin in a servant of twenty, and the case of an imperforate vagina in a girl of nineteen with an undeveloped uterus.

Brodhurst reports an instance of absence of the vagina and uterus in a girl of sixteen who at four years of age showed signs of approaching puberty. At this early age the mons was covered with hair, and at ten the clitoris was three inches long and two inches in circumference. The mammae were well developed. The labia descended laterally and expanded into folds, resembling the scrotum.

Azema reports an instance of complete absence of the vagina and impermeability and probable absence of the col uterinus. The deficiencies were remedied by operation. Berard mentions a similar deformity and operation in a girl of eighteen. Gooding cites an instance of absent vagina in a married woman, the uterus discharging the functions. Gosselin reports a case in which a voluminous tumor was formed by the retained menstrual fluid in a woman without a vagina. An artificial vagina was created, but the patient died from extravasation of blood into the peritoneal cavity. Carter, Polaillon, Martin, Curtis, Worthington, Hall, Hicks, Moliere, Patry, Dolbeau, Desormeaux, and Gratigny also record instances of absence of the vagina.

There are some cases reported in extramedical literature which might be cited. Bussy Rabutin in his Memoires in 1639 speaks of an instance. The celebrated Madame Recamier was called by the younger Dumas an involuntary virgin; and in this connection could be cited the malicious and piquant sonnet—

Chateaubriand et Madame Recamier.

"Juliette et Rene s'aimaient d'amour si tendre Que Dien, sans les punir, a pu leur pardonner: Il n'avait pas voulu que l'une put donner Ce que l'autre ne pouvait prendre."

Duplex vagina has been observed by Bartholinus, Malacarne, Asch, Meckel, Osiander, Purcell, and other older writers. In more modern times reports of this anomaly are quite frequent. Hunter reports a case of labor at the seventh month in a woman with a double vagina, and delivery through the rectum. Atthill and Watts speak of double vagina with single uterus.

Robb of Johns Hopkins Hospital reports a case of double vagina in a patient of twenty suffering from dyspareunia. The vaginal orifice was contracted; the urethra was dilated and had evidently been used for coitus. A membrane divided the vagina into two canals, the cervix lying in the right half; the septum was also divided. Both the thumbs of the patient were so short that their tips could scarcely meet those of the little fingers. Double vagina is also reported by Anway, Moulton, Freeman, Frazer, Haynes, Lemaistre, Boardman, Dickson, Dunoyer, and Rossignol. This anomaly is usually associated with bipartite or double uterus. Wilcox mentions a primipara, three months pregnant, with a double vagina and a bicornate uterus, who was safely delivered of several children. Haller and Borellus have seen double vagina, double uterus, and double ovarian supply; in the latter case there was also a double vulva. Sanger speaks of a supernumerary vagina connecting with the other vagina by a fistulous opening, and remarks that this was not a case of patent Gartner's duct.

Cullingworth cites two cases in which there were transverse septa of the vagina. Stone reports five cases of transverse septa of the vagina. Three of the patients were young women who had never borne children or suffered injury. Pregnancy existed in each case. In the first the septum was about two inches from the introitus, and contained an opening about 1/2 inch in diameter which admitted the tip of the finger. The membrane was elastic and thin and showed no signs of inflammation. Menstruation had always been regular up to the time of pregnancy. The second was a duplicate of the first, excepting that a few bands extended from the cervix to the membranous septum. In the third the lumen of the vagina, about two inches from the introitus, was distinctly narrowed by a ridge of tissue. There was uterine displacement and some endocervicitis, but no history of injury or operation and no tendency to contraction. The two remaining cases occurred in patients seen by Dr. J. F. Scott. In one the septum was about 1 3/4 inches from the entrance to the vagina and contained an orifice large enough to admit a uterine probe. During labor the septum resisted the advance of the head for several hours, until it was slit in several directions. In the other, menstruation had always been irregular, intermissions being followed by a profuse flow of black and tarry blood, which lasted sometimes for fifteen days and was accompanied by severe pain. The septum was 1 1/2 inches from the vaginal orifice and contained an opening which admitted a uterine sound. It was very dense and tight and fully 1/8 inch in thickness.

Mordie reported a case of congenital deficiency of the rectovaginal septum which was successfully remedied by operation.

Anomalous Openings of the Vagina.—The vagina occasionally opens abnormally into the rectum, into the bladder, the urethra, or upon the abdominal parietes. Rossi reports from a hospital in Turin the case of a Piedmontese girl in whom there was an enormous tumor corresponding to the opening of the vaginal orifice; no traces of a vagina could be found. The tumor was incised and proved to be a living infant. The husband of the woman said that he had coitus without difficulty by the rectum, and examination showed that the vagina opened into the rectum, by which means impregnation had been accomplished. Bonnain and Payne have observed analogous cases of this abnormality of the vaginal opening and subsequent accouchement by the anus. Payne's case was of a woman of thirty-five, well formed, who had been in labor thirty-six hours, when the physician examined and looked in vain for a vaginal opening; the finger, gliding along the perineum, came in contact with the distended anus, in which was recognized the head of the fetus. The woman from prolongation of labor was in a complete state of prostration, which caused uterine inertia. Payne anesthetized the patient, applied the forceps, and extracted the fetus without further accident. The vulva of this woman five months afterward displayed all the characteristics of virginity, the vagina opened into the rectum, and menstruation had always been regular. This woman, as well as her husband, averred that they had no suspicion of the anomaly and that coitus (by the anus) had always been satisfactory.

Opening of the vagina upon the parietes, of which Le Fort has collected a number of cases, has never been observed in connection with a viable fetus.

Absence of the labia majora has been observed, especially by Pozzi, to the exclusion of all other anomalies. It is the rule in exstrophy of the bladder.

Absence of the nymphae has also been observed, particularly by Auvard and by Perchaux, and is generally associated with imperfect development of the clitoris. Constantinedes reports absence of the external organs of generation, probably also of the uterus and its appendages, in a young lady. Van Haartman, LeFort, Magee, and Ogle cite cases of absence of the external female organs. Riolan in the early part of the seventeenth century reported a case of defective nymphae; Neubauer in 1774 offers a contrast to this case in an instance of triple nymphae.

The nymphae are sometimes enormously enlarged by hypertrophy, by varicocele, or by elephantiasis, of which latter type Rigal de Gaillac has observed a most curious case. There is also a variety oœ enlargement of the clitoris which seems to be constant in some races; it may be a natural hypertrophy, or perhaps produced by artificial manipulation.

The peculiar conditions under which the Chinese women are obliged to live, particularly their mode of sitting, is said to have the effect of causing unusual development of the mons veneris and the labia majora. On the other hand, some of the lower African races have been distinguished by the deficiency in development of the labia majora, mons veneris, and genital hair. In this respect they present an approximation to the genitals of the anthropoid apes, among whom the orangoutang alone shows any tendency to formation of the labia majora.

The labial appendages of the Hottentot female have been celebrated for many years. Blumenbach and others of the earlier travelers found that the apron-like appearance of the genitals of the Hottentot women was due to abnormal hypertrophy of the labia and nymphae. According to John Knott, the French traveler, Le Vaillant, said that the more coquettish among the Hottentot girls are excited by extreme vanity to practice artificial elongation of the nympha and labia. They are said to pull and rub these parts, and even to stretch them by hanging weights to them. Some of them are said to spend several hours a day at this process, which is considered one of the important parts of the toilet of the Hottentot belle, this malformation being an attraction for the male members of the race. Merensky says that in Basutoland the elder women begin to practice labial manipulation on their female children shortly after infancy, and Adams has found this custom to prevail in Dahomey; he says that the King's seraglio includes 3000 members, the elect of his female subjects, all of whom have labia up to the standard of recognized length. Cameron found an analogous practice among the women of the shores of Lake Tanganyika. The females of this nation manipulated the skin of the lower part of the abdomens of the female children from infancy, and at puberty these women exhibit a cutaneous curtain over the genitals which reaches half-way down the thighs.

A corresponding development of the preputian clitorides, attaining the length of 18 mm. or even more, has been observed among the females of Bechuanaland. The greatest elongation measured by Barrow was five inches, but it is quite probable that it was not possible for him to examine the longest, as the females so gifted generally occupied very high social positions.

Morgagni describes a supernumerary left nympha, and Petit is accredited with seeing a case which exhibited neither nymphae, clitoris, nor urinary meatus. Mauriceau performed nymphotomy on a woman whose nymphae were so long as to render coitus difficult. Morand quotes a case of congenital malformation of the nymphae, to which he attributed impotency.

There is sometimes coalition of the labia and nymphae, which may be so firm and extensive as to obliterate the vulva. Debout has reported a case of absence of the vulva in a woman of twenty upon whom he operated, which was the result of the fusion of the labia minora, and this with an enlarged clitoris gave the external appearance of an hermaphrodite.

The absence of the clitoris coincides with epispadias in the male, and in atrophy of the vulva it is common to find the clitoris rudimentary; but a more frequent anomaly is hypertrophy of the clitoris.

Among the older authorities quoting instances of enlarged clitorides are Bartholinus, Schenck, Hellwig, Rhodius, Riolanus, and Zacchias. Albucasis describes an operation for enlarged clitoris, Chabert ligated one, and Riedlin gives an instance of an enlarged clitoris, in which there appeared a tumor synchronous with the menstrual epoch.

We learn from the classics that there were certain females inhabiting the borders of the Aegean Sea who had a sentimental attachment for one another which was called "Lesbian love," and which carried them to the highest degree of frenzy. The immortal effusions of Sappho contain references to this passion. The solution of this peculiar ardor is found in the fact that some of the females had enlarged clitorides, strong voices, robust figures, and imitated men. Their manner was imperative and authoritative to their sex, who worshiped them with perverted devotion. We find in Martial mention of this perverted love, and in the time of the dissolute Greeks and Romans ridiculous jealousies for unfaithfulness between these women prevailed. Aetius said that the Egyptians practiced amputation of the clitoris, so that enlargement of this organ must have been a common vice of conformation along the Nile. It was also said that the Egyptian women practiced circumcision on their females at the age of seven or eight, the time chosen being when the Nile was in flood. Bertherand cites examples of enlarged clitorides in Arab women; Bruce testifies to this circumstance in Abyssinia, and Mungo Park has observed it in the Mandingos and the Ibbos.

Sonnini says that the women of Egypt had a natural excrescence, fleshy in consistency, quite thick and pendulous, coming from the skin of the mons veneris.

Sonnini says that in a girl of eight he saw one of these caruncles which was 1/2 inch long, and another on a woman of twenty which was four inches long, and remarks that they seem peculiar only to women of distinct Egyptian origin.

Duhouset says that in circumcision the Egyptian women not only remove a great part of the body of the clitoris with the prepuce, but also adjacent portions of the nymphae; Gallieni found a similar operation customary on the upper banks of the Niger.

Otto at Breslau in 1824 reports seeing a negress with a clitoris 4 1/2 inches long and 1 1/2 inches in the transverse diameter; it projected from the vulva and when supine formed a complete covering for the vaginal orifice. The clitoris may at times become so large as to prevent coitus, and in France has constituted a legitimate cause for divorce. This organ is very sensitive, and it is said that in cases of supposed catalepsy a woman cannot bear titillation of the clitoris without some visible movement.

Columbus cites an example of a clitoris as long as a little finger; Haller mentions one which measured seven inches, and there is a record of an enlarged clitoris which resembled the neck of a goose and which was 12 inches long. Bainbridge reports a case of enlarged clitoris in a woman of thirty-two who was confined with her first child. This organ was five inches in length and of about the diameter of a quiescent penis. Figure 149 shows a well-marked case of hypertrophy of the clitoris. Rogers describes a woman of twenty-five in a reduced state of health with an enormous clitoris and warts about the anus; there were also manifestations of tuberculosis. On questioning her, it was found that she had formerly masturbated; later she had sexual intercourse several times with a young man, but after his death she commenced self-abuse again, which brought on the present enlargement. The clitoris was ligated and came away without leaving disfigurement. Cassano and Pedretti of Naples reported an instance of monstrous clitoris in 1860 before the Academy of Medicine.

In some cases ossification of the clitoris is observed Fournier speaks of a public woman in Venice who had an osseous clitoris; it was said that men having connection with her invariably suffered great pain, followed by inflammation of the penis.

There are a few instances recorded of bifid clitoris, and Arnaud cites the history of a woman who had a double clitoris. Secretain speaks of a clitoris which was in a permanent state of erection.

Complete absence of the ovaries is seldom seen, but there are instances in which one of the ovaries is missing. Hunter, Vidal, and Chaussier report in full cases of the absence of the ovaries, and Thudicum has collected 21 cases of this nature. Morgagni, Pears, and Cripps have published observations in which both ovaries were said to have been absent. Cripps speaks of a young girl of eighteen who had an infantile uterus and no ovaries; she neither menstruated nor had any signs of puberty. Lauth cites the case of a woman whose ovaries and uterus were rudimentary, and who exhibited none of the principal physiologic characteristics of her sex; on the other hand, Ruband describes a woman with only rudimentary ovaries who was very passionate and quite feminine in her aspect.

At one time the existence of genuine supernumerary ovaries was vigorously disputed, and the older records contain no instances, but since the researches of Beigel, Puech, Thudicum, Winckler, de Sinety, and Paladino the presence of multiple ovaries is an incontestable fact. It was originally thought that supernumerary ovaries as well as supernumerary kidneys were simply segmentations of the normal organs and connected to them by portions of the proper substance; now, however, by the recent reports we are warranted in admitting these anomalous structures as distinct organs. It has even been suggested that it is the persistence of these ovaries that causes the menstruation of which we sometimes hear as taking place after ovariotomy. Sippel records an instance of third ovary; Mangiagalli has found a supernumerary ovary in the body of a still-born child, situated to the inner side of the normal organ. Winckel discovered a large supernumerary ovary connected to the uterus by its own ovarian ligament. Klebs found two ovaries on one side, both consisting of true ovarian tissue, and connected by a band 3/5 inch long.

Doran divides supernumerary ovaries into three classes:—

(1) The ovarium succentauriatum of Beigel.

(2) Those cases in which two masses of ovarian tissue are separated by ligamentous bands.

(3) Entirely separate organs, as in Winckel's case.

Prolapsus or displacement of the ovaries into the culdesac of Douglas, the vaginal wall, or into the rectum can be readily ascertained by the resulting sense of nausea, particularly in defecation or in coitus. Munde, Barnes, Lentz, Madden, and Heywood Smith report instances, and Cloquet describes an instance of inguinal hernia of the ovary in which the uterus as well as the Fallopian tube were found in the inguinal canal. Debierre mentions that Puech has gathered 88 instances of inguinal hernia of the ovary and 14 of the crural type, and also adds that Otte cites the only instance in which crural ovarian hernia has been found on both sides. Such a condition with other associate malformations of the genitalia might easily be mistaken for an instance of hermaphroditic testicles.

The Fallopian tubes are rarely absent on either side, although Blasius reports an instance of deficient oviducts. Blot reports a case of atrophy, or rather rudimentary state of one of the ovaries, with absence of the tube on that side, in a woman of forty.

Doran has an instance of multiple Fallopian tubes, and Richard, in 1861, says several varieties are noticed. These tubes are often found fused or adherent to the ovary or to the uterus; but Fabricius describes the symphysis of the Fallopian tube with the rectum.

Absence of the uterus is frequently reported. Lieutaud and Richerand are each said to have dissected female subjects in whom neither the uterus nor its annexed organs were found. Many authors are accredited with mentioning instances of defective or deficient uteri, among them Bosquet, Boyer, Walther, Le Fort, Calori, Pozzi, Munde, and Strauch. Balade has reported a curious absence of the uterus and vagina in a girl of eighteen. Azem, Bastien, Bibb, Bovel, Warren, Ward, and many others report similar instances, and in several cases all the adnexa as well as the uterus and vagina were absent, and even the kidney and bladder malformed.

Phillips speaks of two sisters, both married, with congenital absence of the uterus. In his masterly article on "Heredity," Sedgwick quotes an instance of total absence of the uterus in three out of five daughters of the same family; two of the three were twice married.

Double uterus is so frequently reported that an enumeration of the cases would occupy several pages. Bicorn, bipartite, duplex, and double uteruses are so called according to the extent of the duplication. The varieties range all the way from slight increase to two distinct uteruses, with separate appendages and two vaginae. Meckel, Boehmer, and Callisen are among the older writers who have observed double uterus with associate double vagina. Figure 150 represents a transverse section of a bipartite uterus with a double vagina. The so-called uterus didelphus is really a duplex uterus, or a veritable double uterus, each segment having the appearance of a complete unicorn uterus more or less joined to its neighbor. Vallisneri relates the history of a woman who was poisoned by cantharides who had two uteruses, one opening into the vagina, the other into the rectum.

Morand, Bartholinus, Tiedemann, Ollivier, Blundell, and many others relate instances of double uterus in which impregnation had occurred, the fetus being retained until the full term.

Purcell of Dublin says that in the summer of 1773 he opened the body of a woman who died in the ninth month of pregnancy. He found a uterus of ordinary size and form as is usual at this period of gestation, which contained a full-grown fetus, but only one ovary attached to a single Fallopian tube. On the left side he found a second uterus, unimpregnated and of usual size, to which another ovary and tube were attached. Both of these uteruses were distinct and almost entirely separate.

Pregnancy with Double Uterus.—Hollander describes the following anomaly of the uterus which he encountered during the performance of a celiotomy:—

"There were found two uteruses, the posterior one being a normal organ with its adnexa; connected with this uterus was another one, anterior to it. The two uteruses had a common cervix; the anterior of the two organs had no adnexa, though there were lateral peritoneal ligaments; it had become pregnant." Hollander explains the anomaly by stating that probably the Mullerian ducts or one of them had grown excessively, leading to a folding off of a portion which developed into the anterior uterus.

Other cases of double uterus with pregnancy are mentioned on page 49.

When there is simultaneous pregnancy in each portion of a double uterus a complication of circumstances arises. Debierre quotes an instance of a woman who bore one child on July 16, 1870, and another on October 31st of the same year, and both at full term. She had only had three menstrual periods between the confinements. The question as to whether a case like this would be one of superfetation in a normal uterus, or whether the uterus was double, would immediately arise. There would also be the possibility that one of the children was of protracted gestation or that the other was of premature birth. Article 312 of the Civil Code of France accords a minimum of one hundred and eighty and a maximum of three hundred days for the gestation of a viable child. (See Protracted Gestation.)

Voight is accredited with having seen a triple uterus, and there are several older parallels on record. Thilow mentions a uterus which was divided into three small portions.

Of the different anomalous positions of the uterus, most of which are acquired, the only one that will be mentioned is that of complete prolapse of the uterus. In this instance the organ may hang entirely out of the body and even forbid locomotion.

Of 19 cases of hernia of the uterus quoted by Debierre 13 have been observed in the inguinal region, five on the right and seven on the left side. In the case of Roux in 1891 the hernia existed on both sides. The uterus has been found twice only in crural hernia and three times in umbilical hernia. There is one case recorded, according to Debierre, in which the uterus was one of the constituents of an obturator hernia. Sometimes its appendages are found with it. Doring, Ledesma, Rektorzick, and Scazoni have found the uterus in the sac of an inguinal hernia; Leotaud, Murray, and Hagner in an umbilical hernia. The accompanying illustration represents a hernia of the gravid womb through the linea alba.

Absence of the penis is an extremely rare anomaly, although it has been noted by Schenck, Borellus, Bouteiller, Nelaton, and others. Fortunatus Fidelis and Revolat describe a newly born child with absence of external genitals, with spina bifida and umbilical hernia. Nelaton describes a child of two entirely without a penis, but both testicles were found in the scrotum; the boy urinated by the rectum. Ashby and Wright mention complete absence of the penis, the urethra opening at the margin of the anus outside the external sphincter; the scrotum and testicles were well developed. Murphy gives the description of a well-formed infant apparently without a penis; the child passed urine through an opening in the lower part of the abdomen just above the ordinary location of the penis; the scrotum was present. Incisions were made into a small swelling just below the urinary opening in the abdomen which brought into view the penis, the glans being normal but the body very small. The treatment consisted of pressing out the glans daily until the wound healed; the penis receded spontaneously. It is stated that the organ would doubtless be equal to any requirements demanded of it. Demarquay quotes a somewhat similar case in an infant, but it had no urinary opening until after operation.

Among the older writers speaking of deficient or absent penis are Bartholinus, Bauhinus, Cattierus, the Ephemerides, Frank, Panaroli, van der Wiel, and others. Renauldin describes a man with a small penis and enormous mammae. Goschler, quoted by Jacobson, speaks of a well-developed man of twenty-two, with abundant hair on his chin and suprapubic region and the scrotum apparently perfect, with median rapine; a careful search failed to show any trace of a penis; on the anterior wall of the rectum four lines above the anus was an orifice which gave vent to urine; the right testicle and cord were normal, but there was an acute orchitis in the left. Starting from just in front of the anal orifice was a fold of skin 1 1/2 inches long and 3/4 inch high continuous with the rapine, which seemed to be formed of erectile tissue and which swelled under excitement, the enlargement lasting several minutes with usually an emission from the rectum. It was possible to pass a sound through the opening in the rectum to the bladder through a urethra 1 1/2 inches wide; the patient had control of the bladder and urinated from every three to five hours.

Many instances of rudimentary development of the penis have been recorded, most of them complicated with cryptorchism or other abnormality of the sexual organs. In other instances the organ is present, but the infantile type is present all through life; sometimes the subjects are weak in intellect and in a condition similar to cretinism. Kaufmann quotes a case in a weakly boy of twelve whose penis was but 3/4 inch long, about as thick as a goose-quill, and feeling as limp as a mere tube of skin; the corpora cavernosa were not entirely absent, but ran only from the ischium to the junction of the fixed portion of the penis, suddenly terminating at this point. Nothing indicative of a prostate could be found. The testicles were at the entrance of the inguinal canal and the glans was only slightly developed.

Binet speaks of a man of fifty-three whose external genitalia were of the size of those of a boy of nine. The penis was of about the size of the little finger, and contained on each side testicles not larger than a pea. There was no hair on the pubes or the face, giving the man the aspect of an old woman. The prostate was almost exterminated and the seminal vesicles were very primitive in conformation. Wilson was consulted by a gentleman of twenty-six as to his ability to perform the marital function. In size his penis and testicles hardly exceeded those of a boy of eight. He had never felt desire for sexual intercourse until he became acquainted with his intended wife, since when he had erections and nocturnal emissions. The patient married and became the father of a family; those parts which at twenty-six were so much smaller than usual had increased at twenty-eight to normal adult size. There are three cases on record in the older literature of penises extremely primitive in development. They are quoted by the Ephemerides, Plater, Schenck, and Zacchias. The result in these cases was impotency.

In the Army and Medical Museum at Washington are two injected specimens of the male organ divested of skin. From the meatus to the pubis they measure 6 1/2 and 5 1/2 inches; from the extremity to the termination of either crus 9 3/4 and 8 3/4 inches, and the circumferences are 4 3/4 and 4 1/4 inches. Between these two we can strike an average of the size of the normal penis.

In some instances the penis is so large as to forbid coitus and even inconvenience its possessor, measuring as much as ten or even more inches in length. Extraordinary cases of large penis are reported by Albinus (who mentions it as a cause for sterility), Bartholinus, Fabricius Hildanus, Paullini, Peyer, Plater, Schurig, Sinibaldus, and Zacchias. Several cases of enormous penises in the newborn have been observed by Wolff and others.

The penis palme, or suture de la verge of the French, is the name given to those examples of single cutaneous envelope for both the testicles and penis; the penis is adherent to the scrotum by its inferior face; the glans only is free and erection is impossible. Chretien cites an instance in a man of twenty-five, and Schrumpf of Wesserling describes an example of this rare anomaly. The penis and testes were inclosed in a common sac, a slight projection not over 1/4 inch long being seen from the upper part of this curious scrotum. When the child was a year old a plastic operation was performed on this anomalous member with a very satisfactory result. Petit describes an instance in which the penis was slightly fused with the scrotum.

There are many varieties of torsion of the penis. The glans itself may be inclined laterally, the curvature may be total, or there may be a veritable rotation, bringing the inferior face above and the superior face below. Gay describes a child with epispadias whose penis had undergone such torsion on its axis that its inferior surface looked upward to the left, and the child passed urine toward the left shoulder. Follin mentions a similar instance in a boy of twelve with complete epispadias, and Verneuil and Guerlin also record cases, both complicated with associate maldevelopment. Caddy mentions a youth of eighteen who had congenital torsion of the penis with out hypospadias or epispadias. There was a complete half-turn to the left, so that the slit-like urinary meatus was reversed and the frenum was above. Among the older writers who describe incurvation or torsion of the penis are Arantius, the Ephemerides, Haenel, Petit, Schurig, Tulpius, and Zacchias.

Zacutus Lusitans speaks of torsion of the penis from freezing. Paullini mentions a case the result of masturbation, and Hunter speaks of torsion of the penis associated with arthritis.

Ossification of the Penis.—MacClellann speaks of a man of fifty-two whose penis was curved and distorted in such a manner that urine could not be passed without pain and coitus was impossible. A bony mass was discovered in the septum between the corpora cavernosa; this was dissected out with much hemorrhage and the upward curvature was removed, but there resulted a slight inclination in the opposite direction. The formation of bone and cartilage in the penis is quite rare. Velpeau, Kauffmann, Lenhoseck, and Duploy are quoted by Jacobson as having seen this anomaly. There is an excellent preparation in Vienna figured by Demarquay, but no description is given. The Ephemerides and Paullini describe osseous penises.

The complete absence of the frenum and prepuce has been observed in animals but is very rare in man. The incomplete or irregular development is more frequent, but most common is excessive development of the prepuce, constituting phimosis, when there is abnormal adherence with the glans. Instances of phimosis, being quite common, will be passed without special mention. Deficient or absent prepuce has been observed by Blasius, Marcellus Donatus, and Gilibert. Partial deficiency is described by Petit Severinus, and others.

There may be imperforation or congenital occlusion of some portion of the urethra, causing enormous accumulation of urine in the bladder, but fortunately there is generally in such cases some anomalous opening of the urethra giving vent to the excretions. Tulpius mentions a case of deficient urethra. In the Ephemerides there is an account of a man who had a constant flow of semen from an abnormal opening in the abdomen. La Peyroma describes a case of impotence due to ejaculation of the spermatic ducts into the bladder instead of into the urethra, but remarks that there was a cicatrix of a wound of the neighboring parts. There are a number of instances in which the urethra has terminated in the rectum. Congenital dilatation of the urethral canal is very rare, and generally accompanied by other malformation.

Duplication of the urethra or the existence of two permeable canals is not accepted by all the authors, some of whom contend that one of the canals either terminates in a culdesac or is not separate in itself. Verneuil has published an article clearly exposing a number of cases, showing that it is possible for the urethra to have two or more canals which are distinct and have separate functions. Fabricius Hildanus speaks of a double aperture to the urethra; Marcellus Donatus describes duplicity of the urethra, one of the apertures being in the testicle; and there is another case on record in which there was a urethral aperture in the groin. A case of double urethra in a man of twenty-five living in Styria who was under treatment for gonorrhea is described, the supernumerary urethra opening above the natural one and receiving a sound to the depth of 17 cm. There was purulent gonorrhea in both urethrae. Vesalius has an account of a double urethral aperture, one of which was supposed to give spermatic fluid and the other urine. Borellus, Testa, and Cruveilhier have reported similar instances. Instances of double penis have been discussed under the head of diphallic terata, page 194.

Hypospadias and epispadias are names given to malformations of the urethra in which the wall of the canal is deficient either above or below. These anomalies are particularly interesting, as they are nearly always found in male hermaphrodites, the fissure giving the appearance of a vulva, as the scrotum is sometimes included, and even the perineum may be fissured in continuity with the other parts, thus exaggerating the deception. There seems to be an element of heredity in this malformation, and this allegation is exemplified by Sedgwick, who quotes a case from Heuremann in which a family of females had for generations given birth to males with hypospadias. Belloc mentions a man whose urethra terminated at the base of the frenum who had four sons with the same deformity. Picardat mentions a father and son, both of whom had double urethral orifices, one above the other, from one of which issued urine and from the other semen—a fact that shows the possibility of inheritance of this malformation. Patients in whom the urethra opens at the root of the penis, the meatus being imperforate, are not necessarily impotent; as, for instance, Fournier knew of a man whose urethra opened posteriorly who was the father of four children. Fournier supposed that the semen ejaculated vigorously and followed the fissure on the back of the penis to the uterus, the membrane of the vagina supplanting the deficient wall of the urethra. The penis was short, but about as thick as ordinary.

Gray mentions a curious case in a man afflicted with hypospadias who, suffering with delusions, was confined in the insane asylum at Utica. When he determined to get married, fully appreciating his physical defect, he resolved to imitate nature, and being of a very ingenious turn of mind, he busied himself with the construction of an artificial penis. While so engaged he had seized every opportunity to study the conformation of this organ, and finally prepared a body formed of cotton, six inches in length, and shaped like a penis, minus a prepuce. He sheathed it in pig's gut and gave it a slight vermilion hue. To the touch it felt elastic, and its shape was maintained by a piece of gutta-percha tubing, around which the cotton was firmly wound. It was fastened to the waist-band by means of straps, a central and an upper one being so arranged that the penis could be thrown into an erect position and so maintained. He had constructed a flesh-colored covering which completely concealed the straps. With this artificial member he was enabled to deceive his wife for fifteen months, and was only discovered when; she undressed him while he was in a state of intoxication. To further the deception he had told his wife immediately after their marriage that it was quite indecent for a husband to undress in the presence of his wife, and therefore she had always retired first and turned out the light. Partly from fear that his virile power would be questioned and partly from ignorance, the duration of actual coitus would approach an hour. When the discovery was made, his wife hid the instrument with which he had perpetrated a most successful fraud upon her, and the patient subsequently attempted coitus by contact with unsuccessful results, although both parties had incomplete orgasms. Shortly afterward evidences of mental derangement appeared and the man became the subject of exalted delusions. His wife, at the time of report, had filed application for divorce. Haslam reports a case in which loss of the penis was compensated for by the use of an ivory succedaneum. Parallel instances of this kind have been recorded by Ammann and Jonston.

Entire absence of the male sexual apparatus is extremely rare, but Blondin and Velpeau have reported cases.

Complete absence of the testicles, or anorchism, is a comparatively rare anomaly, and it is very difficult to distinguish between anorchism and arrest of development, or simple atrophy, which is much more common. Fisher of Boston describes the case of a man of forty-five, who died of pneumonia. From the age of puberty to twenty-five, and even to the day of death, his voice had never changed and his manners were decidedly effeminate. He always sang soprano in concert with females. After the age of twenty-five, however, his voice became more grave and he could not accompany females with such ease. He had no beard, had never shaved, and had never exhibited amorous propensities or desire for female society. When about twenty-one he became associated with a gay company of men and was addicted to the cup, but would never visit houses of ill-fame. On dissection no trace of testicles could be found; the scrotum was soft and flabby. The cerebellum was the exact size of that of a female child.

Individuals with one testicle are called monorchids, and may be divided into three varieties:—

(1) A solitary testicle divided in the middle by a deep fissure, the two lobes being each provided with a spermatic cord on the same side as the lobe.

(2) Testicles of the same origin, but with coalescence more general.

(3) A single testicle and two cords.

Gruber of St. Petersburg held a postmortem on a man in January, 1867, in whom the right half of the scrotum, the right testicle, epididymis, and the scrotal and inguinal parts of the right vas deferens were absent. Gruber examined the literature for thirty years up to the time of his report, and found 30 recorded postmortem examinations in which there was absence of the testicle, and in eight of these both testicles were missing. As a rule, natural eunuchs have feeble bodies, are mentally dull, and live only a short time. The penis is ordinarily defective and there is sometimes another associate malformation. They are not always disinclined toward the opposite sex.

Polyorchids are persons who have more than two testicles. For a long time the abnormality was not believed to exist, and some of the observers denied the proof by postmortem examination of any of the cases so diagnosed, but there is at present no doubt of the fact,—three, four, and five testicles having been found at autopsies. Russell, one of the older writers on the testicle, mentions a monk who was a triorchid, and was so salacious that his indomitable passion prevented him from keeping his vows of chastity. The amorous propensities and generative faculties of polyorchids have always been supposed greater than ordinary. Russell reports another case of a man with a similar peculiarity, who was prescribed a concubine as a reasonable allowance to a man thus endowed.

Morgagni and Meckel say that they never discovered a third testicle in dissections of reputed triorchids, and though Haller has collected records of a great number of triorchids, he has never been able to verify the presence of the third testicle on dissection. Some authors, including Haller, have demonstrated heredity in examples of polyorchism. There is an old instance in which two testicles, one above the other, were found on the right side and one on the left. Macann describes a recruit of twenty, whose scrotum seemed to be much larger on the right than on the left side, although it was not pendulous. On dissection a right and left testicle were found in their normal positions, but situated on the right side between the groin and the normal testicle was a supernumerary organ, not in contact, and having a separate and short cord. Prankard also describes a man with three testicles. Three cases of triorchidism were found in recruits in the British Army. Lane reports a supernumerary testis found in the right half of the scrotum of a boy of fifteen. In a necropsy held on a man killed in battle, Hohlberg discovered three fully developed testicles, two on the right side placed one above the other. The London Medical Record of 1884 quotes Jdanoff of St. Petersburg in mentioning a soldier of twenty-one who had a supernumerary testicle erroneously diagnosed as inguinal hernia. Quoted by the same reference, Bulatoff mentions a soldier who had a third testicle, which diagnosis was confirmed by several of his confreres. They recommended dismissal of the man from the service, as the third testicle, usually resting in some portion of the inguinal canal, caused extra exposure to traumatic influence.

Venette gives an instance of four testicles, and Scharff, in the Ephemerides, mentions five; Blasius mentions more than three testicles, and, without citing proof,

Buffon admits the possibility of such occurrence and adds that such men are generally more vigorous.

Russell mentions four, five, and even six testicles in one individual; all were not verified on dissection. He cites an instance of six testicles four of which were of usual size and two smaller than ordinary.

Baillie, the Ephemerides, and Schurig mention fusion of the testicles, or synorchidism, somewhat after the manner of the normal disposition of the batrachians and also the kangaroos, in the former of which the fusion is abdominal and in the latter scrotal. Kerckring has a description of an individual in whom the scrotum was absent.

In those cases in which the testicles are still in the abdominal cavity the individuals are termed cryptorchids. Johnson has collected the results of postmortem examinations of 89 supposed cryptorchids. In eight of this number no testicles were found postmortem, the number found in the abdomen was uncertain, but in 18 instances both testicles were found in the inguinal canal, and in eight only one was found in the inguinal canal, the other not appearing. The number in which the semen was examined microscopically was 16, and in three spermatozoa were found in the semen; one case was dubious, spermatozoa being found two weeks afterward on a boy's shirt. The number having children was ten. In one case a monorchid generated a cryptorchid child. Some of the cryptorchids were effeminate, although others were manly with good evidences of a beard. The morbid, hypochondriac, the voluptuous, and the imbecile all found a place in Johnson's statistics; and although there are evidences of the possession of the generative function, still, we are compelled to say that the chances are against fecundity of human cryptorchids. In this connection might be quoted the curious case mentioned by Geoffroy-Saint-Hilaire, of a soldier who was hung for rape. It was alleged that no traces of testicles were found externally or internally yet semen containing spermatozoa was found in the seminal vesicles. Spermatozoa have been found days and weeks after castration, and the individuals during this period were capable of impregnation, but in these cases the reservoirs were not empty, although the spring had ceased to flow. Beigel, in Virchow's Archives, mentions a cryptorchid of twenty-two who had nocturnal emissions containing spermatozoa and who indulged in sexual congress. Partridge describes a man of twenty-four who, notwithstanding his condition, gave evidences of virile seminal flow.

In some cases there is anomalous position of the testicle. Hough mentions an instance in which, from the great pain and sudden appearance, a small tumor lying against the right pubic bone was supposed to be a strangulated hernia. There were two well-developed testicles in the scrotum, and the hernia proved to be a third. McElmail describes a soldier of twenty-nine, who two or three months before examination felt a pricking and slight burning pain near the internal aperture of the internal inguinal canal, succeeded by a swelling until the tumor passed into the scrotum. It was found in the upper part of the scrotum above the original testicle, but not in contact, and was about half the size of the normal testicle; its cord and epididymis could be distinctly felt and caused the same sensation as pressure on the other testicle did.

Marshall mentions a boy of sixteen in whom the right half of the scrotum was empty, although the left was of normal size and contained a testicle. On close examination another testicle was found in the perineum; the boy said that while running he fell down, four years before, and on getting up suffered great pain in the groin. and this pain recurred after exertion. This testicle was removed successfully to the scrotum. Horsley collected 20 instances of operators who made a similar attempt, Annandale being the first one; his success was likely due to antisepsis, as previously the testicles had always sloughed. There is a record of a dog remarkable for its salacity who had two testicles in the scrotum and one in the abdomen; some of the older authors often indulged in playful humor on this subject.

Brown describes a child with a swelling in the perineum both painful and elastic to the touch. The child cried if pressure was applied to the tumor and there was every evidence that the tumor was a testicle. Hutcheson, quoted by Russell, has given a curious case in an English seaman who, as was the custom at that time, was impressed into service by H.M.S. Druid in 1807 from a trading ship off the coast of Africa. The man said he had been examined by dozens of ship-surgeons, but was invariably rejected on account of rupture in both groins. The scrotum was found to be an empty bag, and close examination showed that the testicles occupied the seats of the supposed rupture. As soon as the discovery was made the man became unnerved and agitated, and on re-examining the parts the testicles were found in the scrotum. When he found that there was no chance for escape he acknowledged that he was an impostor and gave an exhibition in which, with incredible facility, he pulled both testes up from the bottom of the scrotum to the external abdominal ring. At the word of command he could pull up one testicle, then another, and let them drop simultaneously; he performed other like feats so rapidly that the movements could not be distinguished.

In this connection Russell speaks of a man whose testicle was elevated every time the east wind blew, which caused him a sense of languor and relaxation; the same author describes a man whose testicles ascended into the inguinal canal every time he was in the company of women.

Inversion of the testicle is of several varieties and quite rare, it has been recognized by Sir Astley Cooper, Boyer, Maisonneuve, Royet, and other writers.

The anomalies of the vas deferens and seminal vesicles are of little interest and will be passed with mention of the case of Weber, who found the seminal vesicles double; a similar conformation has been seen in hermaphrodites.

CHAPTER VII

ANOMALIES OF STATURE, SIZE, AND DEVELOPMENT.

Giants.—The fables of mythology contain accounts of horrible monsters, terrible in ferocity, whose mission was the destruction of the life of the individuals unfortunate enough to come into their domains. The ogres known as the Cyclops, and the fierce anthropophages, called Lestrygons, of Sicily, who were neighbors of the Cyclops, are pictured in detail in the "Odyssey" of Homer. Nearly all the nations of the earth have their fairy tales or superstitions of monstrous beings inhabiting some forest, mountain, or cave; and pages have been written in the heroic poems of all languages describing battles between these monsters and men with superhuman courage, in which the giant finally succumbs.

The word giant is derived indirectly from the old English word "geant," which in its turn came from the French of the conquering Normans. It is of Greek derivation, "gigas", or the Latin, "gigas." The Hebrew parallel is "nophel," or plural, "nephilim."

Ancient Giants.—We are told in the Bible a that the bedstead of Og, King of Basham, was 9 cubits long, which in English measure is 16 1/2 feet. Goliath of Gath, who was slain by David, stood 6 cubits and a span tall—about 11 feet. The body of Orestes, according to the Greeks, was 11 1/2 feet long. The mythical Titans, 45 in number, were a race of Giants who warred against the Gods, and their descendants were the Gigantes. The height attributed to these creatures was fabulous, and they were supposed to heap up mountains to scale the sky and to help them to wage their battles. Hercules, a man of incredible strength, but who is said to have been not over 7 feet high, was dispatched against the Gigantes.

Pliny describes Gabbaras, who was brought to Rome by Claudius Caesar from Arabia and was between 9 and 10 feet in height, and adds that the remains of Posio and Secundilla, found in the reign of Augustus Caesar in the Sallustian Gardens, of which they were supposed to be the guardians, measured 10 feet 3 inches each. In common with Augustine, Pliny believed that the stature of man has degenerated, but from the remains of the ancients so far discovered it would appear that the modern stature is about the same as the ancient. The beautiful alabaster sarcophagus discovered near Thebes in 1817 and now in Sir John Soane's Museum in Lincoln's Inn Fields in London measures 9 feet 4 inches long. This unique example, the finest extant, is well worth inspection by visitors in London.

Herodotus says the shoes of Perseus measured an equivalent of about 3 feet, English standard. Josephus tells of Eleazar, a Jew, among the hostages sent by the King of Persia to Rome, who was nearly 11 feet high. Saxo, the grammarian, mentions a giant 13 1/2 feet high and says he had 12 companions who were double his height. Ferragus, the monster supposed to have been slain by Roland, the nephew of Charlemagne, was said to have been nearly 11 feet high. It was said that there was a giant living in the twelfth century under the rule of King Eugene II of Scotland who was 11 1/2 feet high.

There are fabulous stories told of the Emperor Maximilian. Some accounts say that he was between 8 1/2 and 9 feet high, and used his wife's bracelet for a finger-ring, and that he ate 40 pounds of flesh a day and drank six gallons of wine. He was also accredited with being a great runner, and in his earlier days was said to have conquered single-handed eight soldiers. The Emperors Charlemagne and Jovianus were also accredited with great height and strength.

In the olden times there were extraordinary stories of the giants who lived in Patagonia. Some say that Magellan gave the name to this country because its inhabitants measured 5 cubits. The naturalist Turner says that on the river Plata near the Brazilian coast he saw naked savages 12 feet high; and in his description of America, Thevenot confirms this by saying that on the coast of Africa he saw on a boat the skeleton of an American giant who had died in 1559, and who was 11 feet 5 inches in height. He claims to have measured the bones himself. He says that the bones of the leg measured 3 feet 4 inches, and the skull was 3 feet and 1 inch, just about the size of the skull of Borghini, who, however, was only of ordinary height. In his account of a voyage to the Straits of Magellan, Jacob Lemaire says that on December 17, 1615, he found at Port Desire several graves covered with stones, and beneath the stones were skeletons of men which measured between 10 and 11 feet. The ancient idea of the Spaniards was that the men of Patagonia were so tall that the Spanish soldiers could pass under their arms held out straight; yet we know that the Patagonians exhibit no exaggeration of height—in fact, some of the inhabitants about Terra del Fuego are rather diminutive. This superstition of the voyagers was not limited to America; there were accounts of men in the neighborhood of the Peak of Teneriffe who had 80 teeth in their head and bodies 15 feet in height.

Discoveries of "Giants' Bones."—Riolan, the celebrated anatomist, says that there was to be seen at one time in the suburbs of Saint Germain the tomb of the giant Isoret, who was reputed to be 20 feet tall; and that in 1509, in digging ditches at Rouen, near the Dominicans, they found a stone tomb containing a monstrous skeleton, the skull of which would hold a bushel of corn; the shin-bone measured about 4 feet, which, taken as a guide, would make his height over 17 feet. On the tomb was a copper plate which said that the tomb contained the remains of "the noble and puissant lord, the Chevalier Ricon de Vallemont." Plater, the famous physician, declares that he saw at Lucerne the true human bones of a subject that must have been at least 19 feet high.

Valence in Dauphine boasted of possessing the bones of the giant Bucart, the tyrant of the Vivarias, who was slain by his vassal, Count de Cabillon. The Dominicans had the shin-bone and part of the knee-articulation, which, substantiated by the frescoes and inscriptions in their possession, showed him to be 22 1/2 feet high. They claimed to have an os frontis in the medical school of Leyden measuring 9.1 X 12.2 X .5 inches, which they deduce must have belonged to a man 11 or 12 feet high.

It is said that while digging in France in 1613 there was disinterred the body of a giant bearing the title "Theutobochus Rex," and that the skeleton measured 25 feet long, 10 feet across the shoulders, and 5 feet from breast to back. The shin-bone was about 4 feet long, and the teeth as large as those of oxen. This is likely another version of the finding of the remains of Bucart.

Near Mezarino in Sicily in 1516 there was found the skeleton of a giant whose height was at least 30 feet; his head was the size of a hogshead, and each tooth weighed 5 ounces; and in 1548 and in 1550 there were others found of the height of 30 feet. The Athenians found near their city skeletons measuring 34 and 36 feet in height. In Bohemia in 758 it is recorded that there was found a human skeleton 26 feet tall, and the leg-bones are still kept in a medieval castle in that country. In September, 1691, there was the skull of a giant found in Macedonia which held 210 pounds of corn.

General Opinions.—All the accounts of giants originating in the finding of monstrous bones must of course be discredited, as the remains were likely those of some animal. Comparative anatomy has only lately obtained a hold in the public mind, and in the Middle Ages little was known of it. The pretended giants' remains have been those of mastodons, elephants, and other animals. From Suetonius we learn that Augustus Caesar pleased himself by adorning his palaces with so-called giants' bones of incredible size, preferring these to pictures or images. From their enormous size we must believe they were mastodon bones, as no contemporary animals show such measurements. Bartholinus describes a large tooth for many years exhibited as the canine of a giant which proved to be nothing but a tooth of a spermaceti whale (Cetus dentatus), quite a common fish. Hand described an alleged giant's skeleton shown in London early in the eighteenth century, and which was composed of the bones of the fore-fin of a small whale or of a porpoise.

The celebrated Sir Hans Sloane, who treated this subject very learnedly, arrived at the conclusion that while in most instances the bones found were those of mastodons, elephants, whales, etc., in some instances accounts were given by connoisseurs who could not readily be deceived. However, modern scientists will be loath to believe that any men ever existed who measured over 9 feet; in fact, such cases with authentic references are extremely rare Quetelet considers that the tallest man whose stature is authentically recorded was the "Scottish Giant" of Frederick the Great's regiment of giants. This person was not quite 8 feet 3 inches tall. Buffon, ordinarily a reliable authority, comes to a loose conclusion that there is no doubt that men have lived who were 10, 12, and even 15 feet tall; but modern statisticians cannot accept this deduction from the references offered.

From the original estimation of the height of Adam (Henrion once calculated that Adam's height was 123 feet and that of Eve 118) we gradually come to 10 feet, which seemed to be about the favorite height for giants in the Middle Ages. Approaching this century, we still have stories of men from 9 to 10 feet high, but no authentic cases. It was only in the latter part of the last century that we began to have absolutely authentic heights of giants, and to-day the men showing through the country as measuring 8 feet generally exaggerate their height several inches, and exact measurement would show that but few men commonly called giants are over 7 1/2 feet or weigh over 350 pounds. Dana says that the number of giants figuring as public characters since 1700 is not more than 100, and of these about 20 were advertised to be over 8 feet. If we confine ourselves to those accurately and scientifically measured the list is surprisingly small. Topinard measured the tallest man in the Austrian army and found that he was 8 feet 4 1/2 inches. The giant Winckelmeyer measured 8 feet 6 inches in height. Ranke measured

Marianne Wehde, who was born in Germany in the present century, and found that she measured 8 feet 4 1/4 inches when only sixteen and a half years old.

In giants, as a rule, the great stature is due to excessive growth of the lower extremities, the size of the head and that of the trunk being nearly the same as those of a man or boy of the same age. On the other hand, in a natural dwarf the proportions are fairly uniform, the head, however, being always larger in proportion to the body, just as we find in infants. Indeed, the proportions of "General Tom Thumb" were those of an ordinary infant of from thirteen to fifteen months old.

Figure 156 shows a portrait of two well-known exhibitionists of about the same age, and illustrates the possible extremes of anomalies in stature

Recently, the association of acromegaly with gigantism has been noticed, and in these instances there seems to be an acquired uniform enlargement of all the bones of the body. Brissaud and Meige describe the case of a male of forty-seven who presented nothing unusual before the age of sixteen, when he began to grow larger, until, having reached his majority, he measured 7 feet 2 inches in height and weighed about 340 pounds. He remained well and very strong until the age of thirty-seven, when he overlifted, and following this he developed an extreme deformity of the spine and trunk, the latter "telescoping into itself" until the nipples were on a level with the anterior superior spines of the ilium. For two years he suffered with debility, fatigue, bronchitis, night-sweats, headache, and great thirst. Mentally he was dull; the bones of the face and extremities showed the hypertrophies characteristic of acromegaly, the soft parts not being involved. The circumference of the trunk at the nipples was 62 inches, and over the most prominent portion of the kyphosis and pigeon-breast, 74 inches. The authors agree with Dana and others that there is an intimate relation between acromegaly and gigantism, but they go further and compare both to the growth of the body. They call attention to the striking resemblance to acromegaly of the disproportionate growth of the boy at adolescence, which corresponds so well to Marie's terse description of this disease: "The disease manifests itself by preference in the bones of the extremities and in the extremities of the bones," and conclude with this rather striking and aphoristic proposition: "Acromegaly is gigantism of the adult; gigantism is acromegaly of adolescence."

The many theories of the cause of gigantism will not be discussed here, the reader being referred to volumes exclusively devoted to this subject.

Celebrated Giants.—Mention of some of the most famous giants will be made, together with any associate points of interest.

Becanus, physician to Charles V, says that he saw a youth 9 feet high and a man and a woman almost 10 feet. Ainsworth says that in 1553 the Tower of London was guarded by three brothers claiming direct descent from Henry VIII, and surnamed Og, Gog, and Magog, all of whom were over 8 feet in height. In his "Chronicles of Holland" in 1557 Hadrianus Barlandus said that in the time of John, Earl of Holland, the giant Nicholas was so large that men could stand under his arms, and his shoe held 3 ordinary feet. Among the yeoman of the guard of John Frederick, Duke of Hanover, there was one Christopher Munster, 8 1/2 feet high, who died in 1676 in his forty-fifth year. The giant porter of the Duke of Wurtemberg was 7 1/2 feet high. "Big Sam," the porter at Carleton Palace, when George IV was Prince of Wales, was 8 feet high. The porter of Queen Elizabeth, of whom there is a picture in Hampton Court, painted by Zucchero, was 7 1/2 feet high; and Walter Parson, porter to James I, was about the same height. William Evans, who served Charles I, was nearly 8 feet; he carried a dwarf in his pocket.

In the seventeenth century, in order to gratify the Empress of Austria, Guy-Patin made a congress of all the giants and dwarfs in the Germanic Empire. A peculiarity of this congress was that the giants complained to the authorities that the dwarfs teased them in such a manner as to make their lives miserable.

Plater speaks of a girl in Basle, Switzerland, five years old, whose body was as large as that of a full-grown woman and who weighed when a year old as much as a bushel of wheat. He also mentions a man living in 1613, 9 feet high, whose hand was 1 foot 6 inches long. Peter van den Broecke speaks of a Congo negro in 1640 who was 8 feet high. Daniel, the porter of Cromwell, was 7 feet 6 inches high; he became a lunatic.

Frazier speaks of Chilian giants 9 feet tall. There is a chronicle which says one of the Kings of Norway was 8 feet high. Merula says that in 1538 he saw in France a Flemish man over 9 feet. Keysler mentions seeing Hans Brau in Tyrol in 1550, and says that he was nearly 12 feet high.

Jonston mentions a lad in Holland who was 8 feet tall. Pasumot mentions a giant of 8 feet.

Edmund Mallone was said to have measured 7 feet 7 inches. Wierski, a Polander, presented to Maximilian II, was 8 feet high. At the age of thirty-two there died in 1798 a clerk of the Bank of England who was said to have been nearly 7 1/2 feet high. The Daily Advertiser for February 23, 1745, says that there was a young colossus exhibited opposite the Mansion House in London who was 7 feet high, although but fifteen years old. In the same paper on January 31, 1753, is an account of MacGrath, whose skeleton is still preserved in Dublin. In the reign of George I, during the time of the Bartholomew Fair at Smithfield, there was exhibited an English man seventeen years old who was 8 feet tall.

Nicephorus tells of Antonius of Syria, in the reign of Theodosius, who died at the age of twenty-five with a height of 7 feet 7 inches. Artacaecas, in great favor with Xerxes, was the tallest Persian and measured 7 feet. John Middleton, born in 1752 at Hale, Lancashire, humorously called the "Child of Hale," and whose portrait is in Brasenose College, Oxford, measured 9 feet 3 inches tall. In his "History of Ripton," in Devonshire, 1854, Bigsby gives an account of a discovery in 1687 of a skeleton 9 feet long. In 1712 in a village in Holland there died a fisherman named Gerrit Bastiaansen who was 8 feet high and weighed 500 pounds. During Queen Anne's reign there was shown in London and other parts of England a most peculiar anomaly—a German giantess without hands or feet who threaded a needle, cut gloves, etc. About 1821 there was issued an engraving of Miss Angelina Melius, nineteen years of age and 7 feet high, attended by her page, Senor Don Santiago de los Santos, from the Island of Manilla, thirty-live years old and 2 feet 2 inches high. "The Annual Register" records the death of Peter Tuchan at Posen on June 18, 1825, of dropsy of the chest. He was twenty-nine years old and 8 feet 7 inches in height; he began to grow at the age of seven. This monster had no beard; his voice was soft; he was a moderate eater. There was a giant exhibited in St. Petersburg, June, 1829, 8 feet 8 inches in height, who was very thin and emaciated.

Dr. Adam Clarke, who died in 1832, measured a man 8 feet 6 inches tall. Frank Buckland, in his "Curiosities of Natural History," says that Brice, the French giant, was 7 feet 7 inches. Early in 1837 there was exhibited at Parma a young man formerly in the service of the King of the Netherlands who was 8 feet 10 inches high and weighed 401 pounds. Robert Hale, the "Norfolk Giant," who died in Yarmouth in 1843 at the age of forty-three, was 7 feet 6 inches high and weighed 452 pounds. The skeleton of Cornelius McGrath, now preserved in the Trinity College Museum, Dublin, is a striking example of gigantism. At sixteen years he measured 7 feet 10 inches.

O'Brien or Byrne, the Irish giant, was supposed to be 8 feet 4 inches in height at the time of his death in 1783 at the age of twenty-two. The story of his connection with the illustrious John Hunter is quite interesting. Hunter had vowed that he would have the skeleton of O'Brien, and O'Brien was equally averse to being boiled in the distinguished scientist's kettle. The giant was tormented all his life by the constant assertions of Hunter and by his persistence in locating him. Finally, when, following the usual early decline of his class of anomalies, O'Brien came to his death-bed, he bribed some fishermen to take his body after his death to the middle of the Irish Channel and sink it with leaden weights. Hunter, it is alleged, was informed of this and overbribed the prospective undertakers and thus secured the body. It has been estimated that it cost Hunter nearly 500 pounds sterling to gain possession of the skeleton of the "Irish Giant." The kettle in which the body was boiled, together with some interesting literature relative to the circumstances, are preserved in the Museum of the Royal College of Surgeons in London, and were exhibited at the meeting of the British Medical Association in 1895 with other Hunterian relics. The skeleton, which is now one of the features of the Museum, is reported to measure 92 3/4 inches in height, and is mounted alongside that of Caroline Crachami, the Sicilian dwarf, who was exhibited as an Italian princess in London in 1824. She did not grow after birth and died at the age of nine.

Patrick Cotter, the successor of O'Brien, and who for awhile exhibited under this name, claiming that he was a lineal descendant of the famous Irish King, Brian Boru, who he declared was 9 feet in height, was born in 1761, and died in 1806 at the age of forty-five. His shoe was 17 inches long, and he was 8 feet 4 inches tall at his death.

In the Museum of Madame Tussaud in London there is a wax figure of Loushkin, said to be the tallest man of his time. It measures 8 feet 5 inches, and is dressed in the military uniform of a drum-major of the Imperial Preobrajensky Regiment of Guards. To magnify his height there is a figure of the celebrated dwarf, "General Tom Thumb," in the palm of his hand. Figure 158 represents a well-known American giant, Ben Hicks who was called "the Denver Steeple."

Buffon refers to a Swedish giantess who he affirms was 8 feet 6 inches tall. Chang, the "Chinese Giant," whose smiling face is familiar to nearly all the modern world, was said to be 8 feet tall. In 1865, at the age of nineteen, he measured 7 feet 8 inches. At Hawick, Scotland, in 1870, there was an Irishman 7 feet 8 inches in height, 52 inches around the chest, and who weighed 22 stone. Figure 159 shows an American giantess known as "Leah, the Giantess." At the age of nineteen she was 7 feet 2 inches tall and weighed 165 pounds.

On June 17, 1871, there were married at Saint-Martins-in-the-Field in London Captain Martin Van Buren Bates of Kentucky and Miss Anna Swann of Nova Scotia, two celebrated exhibitionists, both of whom were over 7 feet. Captain Bates, familiarly known as the "Kentucky Giant," years ago was a familiar figure in many Northern cities, where he exhibited himself in company with his wife, the combined height of the two being greater than that of any couple known to history. Captain Bates was born in Whitesburg, Letcher County, Ky., on November 9, 1845. He enlisted in the Southern army in 1861, and though only sixteen years old was admitted to the service because of his size. At the close of the war Captain Bates had attained his great height of 7 feet 2 1/2 inches. His body was well proportioned and his weight increased until it reached 450 pounds. He traveled as a curiosity from 1866 to 1880, being connected with various amusement organizations. He visited nearly all the large cities and towns in the United States, Canada, Great Britain, France, Spain, Germany, Switzerland, Austria, and Russia. While in England in 1871 the Captain met Miss Anna H. Swann, known as the "Nova Scotia Giantess," who was two years the junior of her giant lover. Miss Swann was justly proud of her height, 7 feet 5 1/2 inches. The two were married soon afterward. Their combined height of 14 feet 8 inches marked them as the tallest married couple known to mankind.

Captain Bates' parents were of medium size. His father, a native of Virginia, was 5 feet 10 inches high and weighed 160 pounds. His mother was 5 feet 3 inches tall and weighed 125 pounds. The height of the father of Mrs. Anna Swann Bates was 6 feet and her mother was 5 feet and 2 inches high, weighing but 100 pounds.

A recent newspaper dispatch says: "Captain M. V. Bates, whose remarkable height at one time attracted the attention of the world, has recently retired from his conspicuous position and lives in comparative obscurity on his farm in Guilford, Medina County, O., half a mile east of Seville."

In 1845 there was shown in Paris Joachim Eleiceigui, the Spanish giant, who weighed 195 kilograms (429 pounds) and whose hands were 42 cm. (16 1/2 inches) long and of great beauty. In 1882 at the Alhambra in London there was a giantess by the name of Miss Marian, called the "Queen of the Amazons," aged eighteen years, who measured 2.45 meters (96 1/2 inches). William Campbell, a Scotchman, died at Newcastle in May 1878. He was so large that the window of the room in which the deceased lay and the brick-work to the level of the floor had to be taken out, in order that the coffin might be lowered with block and tackle three stories to the ground. On January 27, 1887, a Greek, although a Turkish subject, recently died of phthisis in Simferopol. He was 7 feet 8 inches in height and slept on three beds laid close together.

Giants of History.—A number of persons of great height, particularly sovereigns and warriors, are well-known characters of history, viz., William of Scotland, Edward III, Godefroy of Bouillon, Philip the Long, Fairfax, Moncey, Mortier,

Kleber; there are others celebrated in modern times. Rochester, the favorite of Charles II; Pothier, the jurist; Bank, the English naturalist; Gall, Billat-Savarin, Benjamin Constant, the painter David, Bellart, the geographer Delamarche, and Care, the founder of the Gentleman's Magazine, were all men of extraordinary stature.

Dwarfs.—The word "dwarf" is of Saxon origin (dwerg, dweorg) and corresponds to the "pumilio" or "nanus" of the Romans. The Greeks believed in the pygmy people of Thrace and Pliny speaks of the Spithamiens. In the "Iliad" Homer writes of the pygmies and Juvenal also describes them; but the fantasies of these poets have given these creatures such diminutive stature that they have deprived the traditions of credence. Herodotus relates that in the deserts of Lybia there were people of extreme shortness of stature. The Bible mentions that no dwarf can officiate at the altar. Aristotle and Philostratus speak of pygmy people descended from Pygmaeus, son of Dorus. In the seventeenth century van Helmont supposed that there were pygmies in the Canary Islands, and Abyssinia, Brazil, and Japan in the older times were repeatedly said to contain pygmy races. Relics of what must have been a pygmy race have been found in the Hebrides, and in this country in Kentucky and Tennessee.

Dr. Schweinfurth, the distinguished African traveler, confirms the statements of Homer, Herodotus, and Aristotle that there was a race of pygmies near the source of the Nile. Schweinfurth says that they live south of the country occupied by the Niam-Niam, and that their stature varies from 4 feet to 4 feet 10 inches. These people are called the Akkas, and wonderful tales are told of their agility and cunning, characteristics that seem to compensate for their small stature.

In 1860 Paul DuChaillu speaks of the existence of an African people called the Obongos, inhabiting the country of the Ashangos, a little to the south of the equator, who were about 1.4 meters in height. There have been people found in the Esquimaux region of very diminutive stature. Battel discovered another pygmy people near the Obongo who are called the Dongos. Kolle describes the Kenkobs, who are but 3 to 4 feet high, and another tribe called the Reebas, who vary from 3 to 5 feet in height. The Portuguese speak of a race of dwarfs whom they call the Bakka-bakka, and of the Yogas, who inhabit territory as far as the Loango. Nubia has a tribe of dwarfs called the Sukus, but little is known of them. Throughout India there are stories of dwarf tribes descended from the monkey-God, or Hoonuman of the mythologic poems.

In the works of Humboldt and Burgoa there is allusion to the tradition of a race of pygmies in the unexplored region of Chiapas near the Isthmus of Tehuantepec in Central America. There is an expedition of anthropologists now on the way to discover this people. Professor Starr of Chicago on his return from this region reported many colonies of undersized people, but did not discover any pygmy tribes answering to the older legendary descriptions. Figure 160 represents two dwarf Cottas measuring 3 feet 6 inches in height.

The African pygmies who were sent to the King of Italy and shown in Rome resembled the pygmy travelers of Akka that Schweinfurth saw at the court of King Munza at Monbuttu. These two pygmies at Rome were found in Central Africa and were respectively about ten and fifteen years old. They spoke a dialect of their own and different from any known African tongue; they were partly understood by an Egyptian sergeant, a native of Soudan, who accompanied them as the sole survivor of the escort with which their donor, Miani, penetrated Monbuttu. Miani, like Livingstone, lost his life in African travel. These dwarfs had grown rapidly in recent years and at the time of report. measured 1.15 and 1.02 meters. In 1874 they were under the care of the Royal Geographical Society of Italy. They were intelligent in their manner, but resented being lionized too much, and were prone to scratch ladies who attempted to kiss them.

The "Aztec Children" in 1851, at the ages of seven and six years, another pair of alleged indigenous pygmies, measured 33 3/4 and 29 1/2 inches in height and weighed 20 3/4 and 17 pounds respectively. The circumference of their heads did not equal that of an ordinary infant at birth.

It is known that at one time the ancients artificially produced dwarfs by giving them an insufficient alimentation when very young. They soon became rachitic from their deprivation of lime-salts and a great number perished, but those who survived were very highly prized by the Roman Emperors for their grotesque appearance. There were various recipes for dwarfing children. One of the most efficient in the olden times was said to have been anointing the backbone with the grease of bats, moles, dormice, and such animals; it was also said that puppies were dwarfed by frequently washing the feet and backbone, as the consequent drying and hardening of the parts were alleged to hinder their extension. To-day the growth of boys intended to be jockeys is kept down by excessive sweating.

Ancient Popularity of Dwarfs.—At one time a dwarf was a necessary appendage of every noble family. The Roman Emperors all had their dwarfs. Julia, the niece of Augustus, had a couple of dwarfs, Conopas and Andromeda, each of whom was 2 feet 4 inches in height. It was the fashion at one time to have dwarfs noted for their wit and wisdom. Philos of Cos, tutor of Ptolemy Philadelphus, was a dwarf, as were Carachus, the friend of Saladin; Alypius of Alexandria, who was only 2 feet high; Lucinus Calvus, who was only 3 feet high, and aesop, the famous Greek fabulist. Later in the Middle Ages and even to the last century dwarfs were seen at every Court. Lady Montagu describes the dwarfs at the Viennese Court as "devils bedaubed with diamonds." They had succeeded the Court Jester and exercised some parts of this ancient office. At this time the English ladies kept monkeys for their amusement. The Court dwarfs were allowed unlimited freedom of speech, and in order to get at truths other men were afraid to utter one of the Kings of Denmark made one of his dwarfs Prime Minister.

Charles IX in 1572 had nine dwarfs, of which four had been given to him by King Sigismund-Augustus of Poland and three by Maximilian II of Germany. Catherine de Medicis had three couples of dwarfs at one time, and in 1579 she had still five pygmies, named Merlin, Mandricart, Pelavine, Rodomont, and Majoski. Probably the last dwarf in the Court of France was Balthazar Simon, who died in 1662.

Sometimes many dwarfs were present at great and noble gatherings. In Rome in 1566 the Cardinal Vitelli gave a sumptuous banquet at which the table-attendants were 34 dwarfs. Peter the Great of Russia had a passion for dwarfs, and in 1710 gave a great celebration in honor of the marriage of his favorite, Valakoff, with the dwarf of the Princess Prescovie Theodorovna. There were 72 dwarfs of both sexes present to form the bridal party. Subsequently, on account of dangerous and difficult labor, such marriages were forbidden in Russia.

In England and in Spain the nobles had the portraits of their dwarfs painted by the celebrated artists of the day. Velasquez has represented Don Antonio el Ingles, a dwarf of fine appearance, with a large dog, probably to bring out the dwarf's inferior height. This artist also painted a great number of other dwarfs at the Court of Spain, and in one of his paintings he portrays the Infanta Marguerite accompanied by her male and female dwarfs. Reproductions of these portraits have been given by Garnier. In the pictures of Raphael, Paul Veronese, and Dominiquin, and in the "Triumph of Caesar" by Mantegna, representations of dwarfs are found, as well as in other earlier pictures representing Court events. At the present time only Russia and Turkey seem to have popular sympathy for dwarfs, and this in a limited degree.

Intellectual Dwarfs.—It must be remarked, however, that many of the dwarfs before the public have been men of extraordinary-intelligence, possibly augmented by comparison. In a postmortem discussed at a meeting of the Natural History Society at Bonn in 1868 it was demonstrated by Schaufhausen that in a dwarf subject the brain weighed 1/19 of the body, in contradistinction to the average proportion of adults, from 1 to 30 to 1 to 44. The subject was a dwarf of sixty-one who died in Coblentz, and was said to have grown after his thirtieth year. His height was 2 feet 10 inches and his weight 45 pounds. The circumference of the head was 520 mm. and the brain weighed 1183.33 am. and was well convoluted. This case was one of simple arrest of development, affecting all the organs of the body; he was not virile. He was a child of large parents; had two brothers and a sister of ordinary size and two brothers dwarfs, one 6 inches higher and the other his size.

Several personages famous in history have been dwarfs. Attila, the historian Procopius, Gregory of Tours, Pepin le Bref, Charles III, King of Naples, and Albert the Grand were dwarfs. About the middle of the seventeenth century the French episcopacy possessed among its members a dwarf renowned for his intelligence. This diminutive man, called Godeau, made such a success in literature that by the grace of Richelieu he was named the Archbishop of Grasse. He died in 1672. The Dutch painter Doos, the English painter Gibson (who was about 3 feet in height and the father of nine infants by a wife of about the same height), Prince Eugene, and the Spanish Admiral Gravina were dwarfs. Fleury and Garry, the actors

Hay, a member of Parliament from Sussex in the last century; Hussein-Pasha, celebrated for his reforms under Selim III; the Danish antiquarian and voyager, Arendt, and Baron Denon were men far below the average size Varro says that there were two gentlemen of Rome who from their decorations must have belonged to an Equestrian Order, and who were but 2 Roman cubits (about 3 feet) high. Pliny also speaks of them as preserved in their coffins.

It may be remarked that perhaps certain women are predisposed to give birth to dwarfs. Borwilaski had a brother and a sister who were dwarfs. In the middle of the seventeenth century a woman brought forth four dwarfs, and in the eighteenth century a dwarf named Hopkins had a sister as small as he was. Therese Souvray, the dwarf fiancee of Bebe, had a dwarf sister 41 inches high. Virey has examined a German dwarf of eight who was only 18 inches tall, i.e., about the length of a newly-born infant. The parents were of ordinary size, but had another child who was also a dwarf.

There are two species of dwarfs, the first coming into the world under normal conditions, but who in their infancy become afflicted with a sudden arrest of development provoked by some malady; the second are born very small, develop little, and are really dwarfs from their birth; as a rule they are well conformed, robust, and intelligent. These two species can be distinguished by an important characteristic. The rachitic dwarfs of the first class are incapable of perpetuating their species, while those of the second category have proved more than once their virility. A certain number of dwarfs have married with women of normal height and have had several children, though this is not, it is true, an indisputable proof of their generative faculties; but we have instances in which dwarfs have married dwarfs and had a family sometimes quite numerous. Robert Skinner (25 inches) and Judith (26 inches), his wife, had 14 infants, well formed, robust, and of normal height.

Celebrated Dwarfs.—Instances of some of the most celebrated dwarfs will be cited with a short descriptive mention of points of interest in their lives:—

Vladislas Cubitas, who was King of Poland in 1305, was a dwarf, and was noted for his intelligence, courage, and as a good soldier. Geoffrey Hudson, the most celebrated English dwarf, was born at Oakham in England in 1619. At the age of eight, when not much over a foot high, he was presented to Henriette Marie, wife of Charles I, in a pie; he afterward became her favorite. Until he was thirty he was said to be not more than 18 inches high, when he suddenly increased to about 45 inches. In his youth he fought several duels, one with a turkey cock, which is celebrated in the verse of Davenant. He became a popular and graceful courtier, and proved his bravery and allegiance to his sovereign by assuming command of a royalist company and doing good service therein. Both in moral and physical capacities he showed his superiority. At one time he was sent to France to secure a midwife for the Queen, who was a Frenchwoman. He afterward challenged a gentleman by the name of Croft to fight a duel, and would accept only deadly weapons; he shot his adversary in the chest; the quarrel grew out of his resentment of ridicule of his diminutive size. He was accused of participation in the Papist Plot and imprisoned by his political enemies in the Gate House at Westminster, where he died in 1682 at the advanced age of sixty-three. In Scott's "Peveril of the Peak" Hudson figures prominently. This author seemed fond of dwarfs.

About the same epoch Charles I had a page in his court named Richard Gibson, who was remarkable for his diminutive size and his ability as a miniature painter. This little artist espoused another of his class, Anne Shepherd, a dwarf of Queen Henriette Marie, about his size (45 inches). Mistress Gibson bore nine children, five of whom arrived at adult age and were of ordinary proportions. She died at the age of eighty; her husband afterward became the drawing master of Princesses Mary and Anne, daughters of James II; he died July 23, 1690, aged seventy-five years.

In 1730 there was born of poor fisher parents at Jelst a child named Wybrand Lokes. He became a very skilful jeweler, and though he was of diminutive stature he married a woman of medium height, by whom he had several children. He was one of the smallest men ever exhibited, measuring but 25 1/2 inches in height. To support his family better, he abandoned his trade and with great success exhibited himself throughout Holland and England. After having amassed a great fortune he returned to his country, where he died in 1800, aged seventy. He was very intelligent, and proved his power of paternity, especially by one son, who at twenty-three was 5 feet 3 inches tall, and robust.

Another celebrated dwarf was Nicolas Ferry, otherwise known as Bebe. He was born at Plaine in the Vosges in 1741; he was but 22 cm. (8 1/2 inches) long, weighed 14 ounces at birth, and was carried on a plate to the church for baptism. At five Bebe was presented to King Stanislas of Poland. At fifteen he measured 29 inches. He was of good constitution, but was almost an idiot; for example, he did not recognize his mother after fifteen days' separation. He was quite lax in his morals, and exhibited no evidences of good nature except his lively attachment for his royal master, who was himself a detestable character. He died at twenty-two in a very decrepit condition, and his skeleton is preserved in the Museum of Natural History in Paris. Shortly before his death Bebe became engaged to a female dwarf named Therese Souvray, who at one time was exhibited in Paris at the Theatre Conti, together with an older sister. Therese lived to be seventy-three, and both she and her sister measured only 30 inches in height. She died in 1819.

Aldrovandus gives a picture of a famous dwarf of the Duc de Crequi who was only 30 inches tall, though perfectly formed; he also speaks of some dwarfs who were not over 2 feet high.

There was a Polish gentleman named Joseph Borwilaski, born in 1739 who was famed all over Europe. He became quite a scholar, speaking French and German fairly well. In 1860, at the age of twenty-two, and 28 inches in height, he married a woman of ordinary stature, who bore him two infants well conformed. He was exhibited in many countries, and finally settled at Durham, England, where he died in 1837 at the almost incredible age of ninety-eight, and is buried by the side of the Falstaffian Stephen Kemble. Mary Jones of Shropshire, a dwarf 32 inches tall and much deformed, died in 1773 at the age of one hundred. These two instances are striking examples of great age in dwarfs and are therefore of much interest. Borwilaski's parents were tall in stature and three of his brothers were small; three of the other children measured 5 feet 6 inches. Diderot has written a history of this family.

Richeborg, a dwarf only 23 inches in height, died in Paris in 1858 aged ninety years. In childhood he had been a servant in the House of Orleans and afterward became their pensioner. During the Revolution he passed in and out of Paris as an infant in a nurse's arms, thus carrying dispatches memorized which might have proved dangerous to carry in any other manner.

At St. Philip's, Birmingham, there is the following inscription on a tomb: "In memory of Mannetta Stocker, who quitted this life on the 4th day of May, 1819, at the age of thirty-nine years, the smallest woman in the kingdom, and one of the most accomplished." She was born in Krauma, in the north of Austria, under normal conditions. Her growth stopped at the age of four, when she was 33 inches tall. She was shown in many villages and cities over Europe and Great Britain; she was very gay, played well on the piano, and had divers other accomplishments.

In 1742 there was shown in London a dwarf by the name of Robert Skinner, .63 meters in height, and his wife, Judith, who was a little larger. Their exhibition was a great success and they amassed a small fortune; during twenty-three years they had 14 robust and well-formed children. Judith died in 1763, and Robert grieved so much after her that he himself expired two years later.

Figure 161 shows a female dwarf with her husband and child, all of whom were exhibited some years since in the Eastern United States. The likeness of the child to the mother is already noticeable.

Buffon speaks of dwarfs 24, 21, and 18 inches high, and mentions one individual, aged thirty-seven, only 16 inches tall, whom he considers the smallest person on record. Virey in 1818 speaks of an English child of eight or nine who was but 18 inches tall. It had the intelligence of a child of three or four; its dentition was delayed until it was two years old and it did not walk until four. The parents of this child were of ordinary stature.

At the "Cosmorama" in Regent Street in 1848 there was a Dutch boy of ten exhibited. He was said to be the son of an apothecary and at the time of his birth weighed nine pounds. He continued to grow for six months and at the expiration of that time weighed 12 pounds; since then, however, he had only increased four pounds. The arrest of development seemed to be connected with hydrocephalus; although the head was no larger than that of a child of two, the anterior fontanelle was widely open, indicating that there was pressure within. He was strong and muscular; grave and sedate in his manner; cheerful and affectionate; his manners were polite and engaging; he was expert in many kinds of handicraft; he possessed an ardent desire for knowledge and aptitude for education.

Rawdon described a boy of five and a half, at the Liverpool Infirmary for Children, who weighed 10 1/2 pounds and whose height was 28 or 29 inches. He uttered no articulate sound, but evidently possessed the sense of hearing. His eyes were large and well formed, but he was apparently blind. He suckled, cut his teeth normally, but had tonic contractions of the spine and was an apparent idiot.

Hardie mentions a girl of sixteen and a half whose height was 40 inches and weight 35 1/2 pounds, including her clothes. During intrauterine life her mother had good health and both her parents had always been healthy. She seemed to stop growing at her fourth year. Her intellect was on a par with the rest of her body. Sometimes she would talk and again she would preserve rigid silence for a long time. She had a shuffling walk with a tendency to move on her toes. Her temporary teeth were shed in the usual manner and had been replaced by canines and right first molar and incisors on the right side. There was no indication of puberty except a slight development of the hips. She was almost totally imbecile, but could tell her letters and spell short words. The circumference of the head was 19 inches, and Ross pointed out that the tendon-reflexes were well marked, as well as the ankle-clonus; he diagnosed the case as one of parencephalus. Figure 162 represents a most curious case of a dwarf named Carrie Akers, who, though only 34 inches tall, weighed 309 pounds.

In recent years several dwarfs have commanded the popular attention, but none so much as "General Tom Thumb," the celebrated dwarf of Barnum's Circus. Charles Stratton, surnamed "Tom Thumb," was born at Bridgeport, Conn., on January 11, 1832; he was above the normal weight of the new-born. He ceased growing at about five months, when his height was less than 21 inches. Barnum, hearing of this phenomenon in his city, engaged him, and he was shown all over the world under his assumed name. He was presented to Queen Victoria in 1844, and in the following year he was received by the Royal Family in France. His success was wonderful, and even the most conservative journals described and commented on him. He gave concerts, in which he sang in a nasal voice; but his "drawing feat" was embracing the women who visited him. It is said that in England alone he kissed a million females; he prided himself on his success in this function, although his features were anything but inviting. After he had received numerous presents and had amassed a large fortune he returned to America in 1864, bringing with him three other dwarfs, the "Sisters Warren" and "Commodore Nutt." He married one of the Warrens, and by her had one child, Minnie, who died some months after birth of cerebral congestion. In 1883 Tom Thumb and his wife, Lavinia, were still living, but after that they dropped from public view and have since died.

In 1895 the wife of a dwarf named Morris gave birth to twins at Blaenavon, North Wales. Morris is only 35 inches in height and his wife is even smaller. They were married at Bartholmey Church and have since been traveling through England under the name of "General and Mrs. Small," being the smallest married couple in the world. At the latest reports the mother and her twins were doing well.

The Rossow Brothers have been recently exhibited to the public. These brothers, Franz and Carl, are twenty and eighteen years respectively. Franz is the eldest of 16 children and is said to weigh 24 pounds and measure 21 inches in height; Carl is said to weigh less than his brother but is 29 inches tall. They give a clever gymnastic exhibition and are apparently intelligent. They advertise that they were examined and still remain under the surveillance of the Faculty of Gottingen.

Next to the success of "Tom Thumb" probably no like attraction has been so celebrated as the "Lilliputians," whose antics and wit so many Americans have in late years enjoyed. They were a troupe of singers and comedians composed entirely of dwarfs; they exhibited much talent in all their performances, which were given for several years and quite recently in all the large cities of the United States. They showed themselves to be worthy rivals for honors in the class of entertainments known as burlesques. As near as could be ascertained, partly from the fact that they all spoke German fluently and originally gave their performance entirely in German, they were collected from the German and Austrian Empires.

The "Princess Topaze" was born near Paris in 1879. According to a recent report she is perfectly formed and is intelligent and vivacious. She is 23 1/2 inches tall and weighs 14 pounds. Her parents were of normal stature.

Not long since the papers recorded the death of Lucia Zarete, a Mexican girl, whose exact proportions were never definitely known; but there is no doubt that she was the smallest midget ever exhibited In this country. Her exhibitor made a fortune with her and her salary was among the highest paid to modern "freaks."

Miss H. Moritz, an American dwarf, at the age of twenty weighed 36 pounds and was only 22 inches tall.

Precocious development is characterized by a hasty growth of the subject, who at an early period of life attains the dimensions of an adult. In some of these instances the anomaly is associated with precocious puberty, and after acquiring the adult growth at an early age there is an apparent cessation of the development. In adult life the individual shows no distinguishing characters.

The first to be considered will be those cases, sometimes called "man-boys," characterized by early puberty and extraordinary development in infancy. Histories of remarkable children have been transmitted from the time of Vespasian. We read in the "Natural History" of Pliny that in Salamis, Euthimedes had a son who grew to 3 Roman cubits (4 1/2 feet) in three years; he was said to have little wit, a dull mind, and a slow and heavy gait; his voice was manly, and he died at three of general debility. Phlegon says that Craterus, the brother of King Antigonus, was an infant, a young man, a mature man, an old man, and married and begot children all in the space of seven years. It is said that King Louis II of Hungary was born so long before his time that he had no skin; in his second year he was crowned, in his tenth year he succeeded, in his fourteenth year he had a complete beard, in his fifteenth he was married, in his eighteenth he had gray hair, and in his twentieth he died. Rhodiginus speaks of a boy who when he was ten years impregnated a female. In 1741 there was a boy born at Willingham, near Cambridge, who had the external marks of puberty at twelve months, and at the time of his death at five years he had the appearance of an old man. He was called "prodigium Willinghamense." The Ephemerides and some of the older journals record instances of penile erection immediately after birth.

It was said that Philip Howarth, who was born at Quebec Mews, Portman Square, London, February 21, 1806, lost his infantile rotundity of form and feature after the completion of his first year and became pale and extremely ugly, appearing like a growing boy. His penis and testes increased in size, his voice altered, and hair grew on the pubes. At the age of three he was 3 feet 4 1/2 inches tall and weighed 51 1/4 pounds. The length of his penis when erect was 4 1/2 inches and the circumference 4 inches; his thigh-measure was 13 1/2 inches, his waist-measure 24 inches, and his biceps 7 inches. He was reported to be clever, very strong, and muscular. An old chronicle says that in Wisnang Parish, village of Tellurge, near Tygure, in Lordship Kiburge, there was born on the 26th of May, 1548, a boy called Henry Walker, who at five years was of the height of a boy of fourteen and possessed the genitals of a man. He carried burdens, did men's work, and in every way assisted his parents, who were of usual size.

There is a case cited by the older authors of a child born in the Jura region who at the age of four gave proof of his virility, at seven had a beard and the height of a man. The same journal also speaks of a boy of six, 1.62 meters tall, who was perfectly proportioned and had extraordinary strength. His beard and general appearance, together with the marks of puberty, gave him the appearance of a man of thirty.

In 1806 Dupuytren presented to the Medical Society in Paris a child 3 1/2 feet high, weighing 57 pounds, who had attained puberty.

There are on record six modern cases of early puberty in boys, one of whom died at five with the signs of premature senility; at one year he had shown signs of enlargement of the sexual organs. There was another who at three was 3 feet 6 3/4 inches high, weighed 50 pounds, and had seminal discharges. One of the cases was a child who at birth resembled an ordinary infant of five months. From four to fifteen months his penis enlarged, until at the age of three it measured when erect 3 inches. At this age he was 3 feet 7 inches high and weighed 64 pounds. The last case mentioned was an infant who experienced a change of voice at twelve months and showed hair on the pubes. At three years he was 3 feet 4 1/2 inches tall and weighed 51 1/4 pounds. Smith, in Brewster's Journal, 1829, records the case of a boy who at the age of four was well developed; at the age of six he was 4 feet 2 inches tall and weighed 74 pounds; his lower extremities were extremely short proportionally and his genitals were as well developed as those of an adult. He had a short, dark moustache but no hair on his chin, although his pubic hair was thick, black, and curly. Ruelle describes a child of three and a quarter years who was as strong and muscular as one at eight. He had full-sized male organs and long black hair on the pubes. Under excitement he discharged semen four or five times a day; he had a deep male voice, and dark, short hair on the cheek and upper lip.

Stone gives an account of a boy of four who looked like a child of ten and exhibited the sexual organs of a man with a luxuriant growth of hair on the pubes. This child was said to have been of great beauty and a miniature model of an athlete. His height was 4 feet 1/4 inch and weight 70 pounds; the penis when semiflaccid was 4 1/4 inches long; he was intelligent and lively, and his back was covered with the acne of puberty. A peculiar fact as regards this case was the statement of the father that he himself had had sexual indulgence at eight. Stone parallels this case by several others that he has collected from medical literature. Breschet in 1821 reported the case of a boy born October 20, 1817, who at three years and one month was 3 feet 6 3/4 inches tall; his penis when flaccid measured 4 inches and when erect 5 1/4 inches, but the testicles were not developed in proportion. Lopez describes a mulatto boy of three years ten and a half months whose height was 4 feet 1/2 inch and weight 82 pounds; he measured about the chest 27 1/2 inches and about the waist 27 inches; his penis at rest was 4 inches long and had a circumference of 3 1/2 inches, although the testes were not descended. He had evidences of a beard and his axillae were very hairy; it is said he could with ease lift a man weighing 140 pounds. His body was covered with acne simplex and had a strong spermatic odor, but it was not known whether he had any venereal appetite.

Johnson mentions a boy of seven with severe gonorrhea complicated with buboes which he had contracted from a servant girl with whom he slept. At the Hopital des Enfans Malades children at the breast have been observed to masturbate. Fournier and others assert having seen infantile masturbators, and cite a case of a girl of four who was habitually addicted to masturbation from her infancy but was not detected until her fourth year; she died shortly afterward in a frightful state of marasmus. Vogel alludes to a girl of three in whom repeated attacks of epilepsy occurred after six months' onanism. Van Bambeke mentions three children from ten to twenty months old, two of them females, who masturbated.

Bidwell describes a boy of five years and two months who during the year previous had erections and seminal emissions. His voice had changed and he had a downy moustache on his upper lip and hair on the pubes; his height was 4 feet 3 1/2 inches and his weight was 82 1/2 pounds. His penis and testicles were as well developed as those of a boy of seventeen or eighteen, but from his facial aspect one would take him to be thirteen. He avoided the company of women and would not let his sisters nurse him when he was sick.

Pryor speaks of a boy of three and a half who masturbated and who at five and a half had a penis of adult size, hair on the pubes, and was known to have had seminal emissions. Woods describes a boy of six years and seven months who had the appearance of a youth of eighteen. He was 4 feet 9 inches tall and was quite muscular. He first exhibited signs of precocious growth at the beginning of his second year and when three years old he had hair on the pubes. There is an instance in which a boy of thirteen had intercourse with a young woman at least a dozen times and succeeded in impregnating her. The same journal mentions an instance in which a boy of fourteen succeeded in impregnating a girl of the same age. Chevers speaks of a young boy in India who was sentenced to one year's imprisonment for raping a girl of three.

Douglass describes a boy of four years and three months who was 3 feet 10 1/2 inches tall and weighed 54 pounds; his features were large and coarse, and his penis and testes were of the size of those of an adult. He was unusually dull, mentally, quite obstinate, and self-willed. It is said that he masturbated on all opportunities and had vigorous erections, although no spermatozoa were found in the semen issued. He showed no fondness for the opposite sex. The history of this rapid growth says that he was not unlike other children until the third year, when after wading in a small stream several hours he was taken with a violent chill, after which his voice began to change and his sexual organs to develop.

Blanc quotes the case described by Cozanet in 1875 of Louis Beran, who was born on September 29, 1869, at Saint-Gervais, of normal size. At the age of six months his dimensions and weight increased in an extraordinary fashion. At the age of six years he was 1.28 meters high (4 feet 2 1/3 inches) and weighed 80 pounds. His puberty was completely manifested in every way; he eschewed the society of children and helped his parents in their labors. Campbell showed a lad of fourteen who had been under his observation for ten years. When fifteen months old this prodigy had hair on his pubes and his external genitals were abnormally larger end at the age of two years they were fully developed and had not materially changed in the following years. At times he manifested great sexual excitement. Between four and seven years he had seminal discharges, but it was not determined whether the semen contained spermatozoa. He had the muscular development of a man of twenty-five. He had shaved several years. The boy's education was defective from his failure to attend school.

The accompanying illustration represents a boy of five years and three months of age whose height at this time was 4 feet and his physical development far beyond that usual at this age, his external genitals resembling those of a man of twenty. His upper lip was covered by a mustache, and the hirsute growth elsewhere was similarly precocious.

The inscription on the tombstone of James Weir in the Parish of Carluke, Scotland, says that when only thirteen months old he measured 3 feet 4 inches in height and weighed 5 stone. He was pronounced by the faculty of Edinburgh and Glasgow to be the most extraordinary child of his age. Linnaeus saw a boy at the Amsterdam Fair who at the age of three weighed 98 pounds. In Paris, about 1822, there was shown an infant Hercules of seven who was more remarkable for obesity than general development. He was 3 feet 4 inches high, 4 feet 5 inches in circumference, and weighed 220 pounds. He had prominent eyebrows, black eyes, and his complexion resembled that of a fat cook in the heat. Borellus details a description of a giant child. There is quoted from Boston a the report of a boy of fifteen months weighing 92 pounds who died at Coney Island. He was said to have been of phenomenal size from infancy and was exhibited in several museums during his life.

Desbois of Paris mentions an extraordinary instance of rapid growth in a boy of eleven who grew 6 inches in fifteen days.

Large and Small New-born Infants.—There are many accounts of new-born infants who were characterized by their diminutive size. On page 66 we have mentioned Usher's instance of twins born at the one hundred and thirty-ninth day weighing each less than 11 ounces; Barker's case of a female child at the one hundred and fifty-eighth day weighing 1 pound; Newinton's case of twins at the fifth month, one weighing 1 pound and the other 1 pound 3 1/2 ounces; and on page 67 is an account of Eikam's five-months' child, weighing 8 ounces. Of full-term children Sir Everard Home, in his Croonian Oration in 1824, speaks of one borne by a woman who was traveling with the baggage of the Duke of Wellington's army. At her fourth month of pregnancy this woman was attacked and bitten by a monkey, but she went to term, and a living child was delivered which weighed but a pound and was between 7 and 8 inches long. It was brought to England and died at the age of nine, when 22 inches high. Baker mentions a child fifty days' old that weighed 1 pound 13 ounces and was 14 inches long. Mursick describes a living child who at birth weighed but 1 3/4 pounds. In June, 1896, a baby weighing 1 3/4 pounds was born at the Samaritan Hospital, Philadelphia.

Scott has recorded the birth of a child weighing 2 1/2 pounds, and another 3 1/4 pounds. In the Chicago Inter-Ocean there is a letter dated June 20, 1874, which says that Mrs. J. B. McCrum of Kalamazoo, Michigan, gave birth to a boy and girl that could be held in the palm of the hand of the nurse. Their aggregate weight was 3 pounds 4 ounces, one weighing 1 pound 8 ounces, the other 1 pound 12 ounces. They were less than 8 inches long and perfectly formed; they were not only alive but extremely vivacious.

There is an account of female twins born in 1858 before term. One weighed 22 1/2 ounces, and over its arm, forearm, and hand one could easily pass a wedding-ring. The other weighed 24 ounces. They both lived to adult life; the larger married and was the mother of two children, which she bore easily. The other did not marry, and although not a dwarf, was under-sized; she had her catamenia every third week. Post describes a 2-pound child.

On the other hand, there have been infants characterized by their enormous size at birth. Among the older writers, Cranz describes an infant which at birth weighed 23 pounds; Fern mentions a fetus of 18 pounds; and Mittehauser speaks of a new-born child weighing 24 pounds. Von Siebold in his "Lucina" has recorded a fetus which weighed 22 1/2 pounds. It is worthy of comment that so great is the rarity of these instances that in 3600 cases, in the Rotunda Hospital, Dublin, only one child reached 11 pounds.

There was a child born in Sussex in 1869 which weighed 13 1/2 pounds and measured 26 1/2 inches. Warren delivered a woman in Derbyshire of male twins, one weighing 17 pounds 8 ounces and the other 18 pounds. The placenta weighed 4 pounds, and there was an ordinary pailful of liquor amnii. Both the twins were muscular and well formed; the parents were of ordinary stature, and at last reports the mother was rapidly convalescing. Burgess mentions an 18-pound new-born child; end Meadows has seen a similar instance. Eddowes speaks of the birth of a child at Crewe, a male, which weighed 20 pounds 2 ounces and was 23 inches long. It was 14 1/2 inches about the chest, symmetrically developed, and likely to live. The mother, who was a schoolmistress of thirty-three, had borne two previous children, both of large size. In this instance the gestation had not been prolonged, the delivery was spontaneous, and there was no laceration of the parts.

Chubb says that on Christmas Day, 1852, there was a child delivered weighing 21 pounds. The labor was not severe and the other children of the family were exceptionally large. Dickinson describes a woman, a tertipara, who had a most difficult labor and bore an extremely large child. She had been thirty-six hours in parturition, and by evisceration and craniotomy was delivered of a child weighing 16 pounds. Her first child weighed 9 pounds, her second 20, and her third, the one described, cost her her life soon after delivery.

There is a history of a Swedish woman in Boston who was delivered by the forceps of her first child, which weighed 19 3/4 pounds and which was 25 3/4 inches long. The circumference of the head was 16 3/4 inches, of the neck 9 3/4, and of the thigh 10 3/4 inches.

Rice speaks of a child weighing 20 1/4 pounds at birth. Johnston describes a male infant who was born on November 26, 1848, weighing 20 pounds, and Smith another of the same weight. Baldwin quotes the case of a woman who after having three miscarriages at last had a child that weighed 23 pounds. In the delivery there was extensive laceration of the anterior wall of the vagina; the cervix and perineum, together with an inch of the rectum, were completely destroyed.

Beach describes a birth of a young giant weighing 23 3/4 pounds. Its mother was Mrs. Bates, formerly Anna Swann, the giantess who married Captain Bates. Labor was rather slow, but she was successfully delivered of a healthy child weighing 23 3/4 pounds and 30 inches long. The secundines weighed ten pounds and there were nine quarts of amniotic fluid.

There is a recent record of a Cesarian section performed on a woman of forty in her twelfth pregnancy and one month beyond term. The fetus, which was almost exsanguinated by amputation, weighed 22 1/2 pounds. Bumm speaks of the birth of a premature male infant weighing 4320 gm. (9 1/2 pounds) and measuring 54 cm. long. Artificial labor had been induced at the thirty-fifth week in the hope of delivering a living child, the three preceding infants having all been still-born on account of their large size. Although the mother's pelvis was wide, the disposition to bear huge infants was so great as to render the woman virtually barren.

Congenital asymmetry and hemihypertrophy of the body are most peculiar anomalies and must not be confounded with acromegaly or myxedema, in both of which there is similar lack of symmetric development. There seems to be no satisfactory clue to the causation of these abnormalisms. Most frequently the left side is the least developed, and there is a decided difference in the size of the extremities.

Finlayson reports a case of a child affected with congenital unilateral hypertrophy associated with patches of cutaneous congestion. Logan mentions hypertrophy in the right half of the body in a child of four, first noticed shortly after birth; Langlet also speaks of a case of congenital hypertrophy of the right side. Broca and Trelat were among the first observers to discuss this anomaly.

Tilanus of Munich in 1893 reported a case of hemihypertrophy in a girl of ten. The whole right half of the body was much smaller and better developed than the left, resulting in a limping gait. The electric reaction and the reflexes showed no abnormality. The asymmetry was first observed when the child was three. Mobius and Demme report similar cases.

Adams reports an unusual case of hemihypertrophy in a boy of ten. There was nothing noteworthy in the family history, and the patient had suffered from none of the diseases of childhood. Deformity was noticeable at birth, but not to such a degree relatively as at a later period. The increased growth affected the entire right half of the body, including the face, but was most noticeable in the leg, thigh, and buttock. Numerous telangiectatic spots were scattered irregularly over the body, but most thickly on the right side, especially on the outer surface of the leg. The accompanying illustration represents the child's appearance at the time of report.

Jacobson reports the history of a female child of three years with nearly universal giant growth (Riesenwuchs). At first this case was erroneously diagnosed as acromegaly. The hypertrophy affected the face, the genitals, the left side of the trunk, and all the limbs.

Milne records a case of hemihypertrophy in a female child of one year. The only deviation from uniform excess of size of the right side was shown in the forefinger and thumb, which were of the same size as on the other hand; and the left side showed no overgrowth in any of its members except a little enlargement of the second toe. While hypertrophy of one side is the usual description of such cases, the author suggests that there may be a condition of defect upon the other side, and he is inclined to think that in this case the limb, hand, and foot of the left side seemed rather below the average of the child's age. In this case, as in others previously reported, there were numerous telangiectatic spots of congestion scattered irregularly over the body. Milne also reported later to the Sheffield Medico-Chirurgical Society an instance of unilateral hypertrophy in a female child of nineteen months. The right side was involved and the anomaly was believed to be due to a deficiency of growth of the left side as well as over-development of the right. There were six teeth on the right side and one on the left.

Obesity.—The abnormality of the adipose system, causing in consequence an augmentation of the natural volume of the subject, should be described with other anomalies of size and stature. Obesity may be partial, as seen in the mammae or in the abdomen of both women and men, or it may be general; and it is of general obesity that we shall chiefly deal. Lipomata, being distinctly pathologic formations, will be left for another chapter.

The cases of obesity in infancy and childhood are of considerable interest, and we sometimes see cases that have been termed examples of "congenital corpulency." Figure 167 represents a baby of thirteen months that weighed 75 pounds. Figure 168 shows another example of infantile obesity, known as "Baby Chambers." Elliotson describes a female infant not a year old which weighed 60 pounds. There is an instance on record of a girl of four who weighed 256 pounds Tulpius mentions a girl of five who weighed 150 pounds and had the strength of a man. He says that the acquisition of fat did not commence until some time after birth. Ebstein reports an instance given to him by Fisher of Moscow of a child in Pomerania who at the age of six weighed 137 pounds and was 46 inches tall; her girth was 46 inches and the circumference of her head was 24 inches. She was the offspring of ordinary-sized parents, and lived in narrow and sometimes needy circumstances. The child was intelligent and had an animated expression of countenance.

Bartholinus mentions a girl of eleven who weighed over 200 pounds. There is an instance recorded of a young girl in Russia who weighed nearly 200 pounds when but twelve. Wulf, quoted by Ebstein, describes a child which died at birth weighing 295 ounces. It was well proportioned and looked like a child three months old, except that it had an enormous development of fatty tissue. The parents were not excessively large, and the mother stated that she had had children before of the same proportions. Grisolles mentions a child who was so fat at twelve months that there was constant danger of suffocation; but, marvelous to relate, it lost all its obesity when two and a half, and later was remarkable for its slender figure. Figure 169 shows a girl born in Carbon County, Pa., who weighed 201 pounds when nine years old. McNaughton describes Susanna Tripp, who at six years of age weighed 203 pounds and was 3 feet 6 inches tall and measured 4 feet 2 inches around the waist. Her younger sister, Deborah, weighed 119 pounds; neither of the two weighed over 7 pounds at birth and both began to grow at the fourth month. On October, 1788, there died at an inn in the city of York the surprising "Worcestershire Girl" at the age of five. She had an exceedingly beautiful face and was quite active. She was 4 feet in height and larger around the breast and waist; her thigh measured 18 inches and she weighed nearly 200 pounds. In February, 1814, Mr. S. Pauton was married to the only daughter of Thomas Allanty of Yorkshire; although she was but thirteen she was 13 stone weight (182 pounds). At seven years she had weighed 7 stone (98 pounds). Williams mentions several instances of fat children. The first was a German girl who at birth weighed 13 pounds; at six months, 42 pounds; at four years, 150 pounds; and at twenty years, 450 pounds. Isaac Butterfield, born near Leeds in 1781, weighed 100 pounds in 1782 and was 3 feet 13 inches tall. There was a child named Everitt, exhibited in London in 1780, who at eleven months was 3 feet 9 inches tall and measured around the loins over 3 feet. William Abernethy at the age of thirteen weighed 22 stone (308 pounds) and measured 57 inches around the waist. He was 5 feet 6 inches tall. There was a girl of ten who was 1.45 meters (4 feet 9 inches) high and weighed 175 pounds. Her manners were infantile and her intellectual development was much retarded. She spoke with difficulty in a deep voice; she had a most voracious appetite.

At a meeting of the Physical Society of Vienna on December 4, 1894, there was shown a girl of five and a half who weighed 250 pounds. She was just shedding her first teeth; owing to the excess of fat on her short limbs she toddled like an infant. There was no tendency to obesity in her family. Up to the eleventh month she was nursed by her mother, and subsequently fed on cabbage, milk, and vegetable soup. This child, who was of Russian descent, was said never to perspire.

Cameron describes a child who at birth weighed 14 pounds, at twelve months she weighed 69 pounds, and at seventeen months 98 pounds. She was not weaned until two years old and she then commenced to walk. The parents were not remarkably large. There is an instance of a boy of thirteen and a half who weighed 214 pounds. Kaestner speaks of a child of four who weighed 82 pounds, and Benzenberg noted a child of the same age who weighed 137. Hildman, quoted by Picat, speaks of an infant three years and ten months old who had a girth of 30 inches. Hillairet knew of a child of five which weighed 125 pounds. Botta cites several instances of preternaturally stout children. One child died at the age of three weighing 90 pounds, another at the age of five weighed 100 pounds, and a third at the age of two weighed 75 pounds.

Figure 170 represents Miss "Millie Josephine" of Chicago, a recent exhibitionist, who at the reputed age of thirteen was 5 feet 6 inches tall and weighed 422 pounds.

General Remarks.—It has been chiefly in Great Britain and in Holland that the most remarkable instances of obesity have been seen, especially in the former country colossal weights have been recorded. In some countries corpulency has been considered an adornment of the female sex. Hesse-Wartegg refers to the Jewesses of Tunis, who when scarcely ten years old are subjected to systematic treatment by confinement in narrow, dark rooms, where they are fed on farinaceous foods and the flesh of young puppies until they are almost a shapeless mass of fat. According to Ebstein, the Moorish women reach with astonishing rapidity the desired embonpoint on a diet of dates and a peculiar kind of meal.

In some nations and families obesity is hereditary, and generations come and go without a change in the ordinary conformation of the representatives. In other people slenderness is equally persistent, and efforts to overcome this peculiarity of nature are without avail.

Treatment of Obesity.—Many persons, the most famous of whom was Banting, have advanced theories to reduce corpulency and to improve slenderness; but they have been uniformly unreliable, and the whole subject of stature-development presents an almost unexplored field for investigation. Recently, Leichtenstein, observing in a case of myxedema treated with the thyroid gland that the subcutaneous fat disappeared with the continuance of the treatment, was led to adopt this treatment for obesity itself and reports striking results. The diet of the patient remained the same, and as the appetite was not diminished by the treatment the loss of weight was evidently due to other causes than altered alimentation. He holds that the observations in myxedema, in obesity, and psoriasis warrant the belief that the thyroid gland eliminates a material having a regulating influence upon the constitution of the panniculus adiposus and upon the nutrition of the skin in general. There were 25 patients in all; in 22 the effect was entirely satisfactory, the loss of weight amounting to as much as 9.5 kilos (21 pounds). Of the three cases in which the result was not satisfactory, one had nephritis with severe Graves' disease, and the third psoriasis. Charrin has used the injections of thyroid extract with decided benefit. So soon as the administration of the remedy was stopped the loss of weight ceased, but with the renewal of the remedy the loss of weight again ensued to a certain point, beyond which the extract seemed powerless to act. Ewald also reports good results from this treatment of obesity.

Remarkable Instances of Obesity.—From time immemorial fat men and women have been the object of curiosity and the number who have exhibited themselves is incalculable. Nearly every circus and dime museum has its example, and some of the most famous have in this way been able to accumulate fortunes.

Athenaeus has written quite a long discourse on persons of note who in the olden times were distinguished for their obesity. He quotes a description of Denys, the tyrant of Heraclea, who was so enormous that he was in constant danger of suffocation; most of the time he was in a stupor or asleep, a peculiarity of very fat people. His doctors had needles put in the back of his chairs to keep him from falling asleep when sitting up and thus incurring the danger of suffocation. In the same work Athenaeus speaks of several sovereigns noted for their obesity; among others he says that Ptolemy VII, son of Alexander, was so fat that, according to Posidonius, when he walked he had to be supported on both sides. Nevertheless, when he was excited at a repast, he would mount the highest couch and execute with agility his accustomed dance.

According to old chronicles the cavaliers at Rome who grew fat were condemned to lose their horses and were placed in retirement. During the Middle Ages, according to Guillaume in his "Vie de Suger," obesity was considered a grace of God.

Among the prominent people in the olden time noted for their embonpoint were Agesilas, the orator Licinius Calvus, who several times opposed Cicero, the actor Lucius, and others. Among men of more modern times we can mention William the Conqueror; Charles le Gros; Louis le Gros; Humbert II, Count of Maurienne; Henry I, King of Navarre; Henry III, Count of Champagne; Conan III, Duke of Brittany; Sancho I, King of Leon; Alphonse II, King of Portugal; the Italian poet Bruni, who died in 1635; Vivonne, a general under Louis XIV; the celebrated German botanist Dillenius; Haller; Frederick I, King of Wurtemberg, and Louis XVIII.

Probably the most famous of all the fat men was Daniel Lambert, born March 13, 1770, in the parish of Saint Margaret, Leicester. He did not differ from other youths until fourteen. He started to learn the trade of a die-sinker and engraver in Birmingham. At about nineteen he began to believe he would be very heavy and developed great strength. He could lift 500 pounds with ease and could kick seven feet high while standing on one leg. In 1793 he weighed 448 pounds; at this time he became sensitive as to his appearance. In June, 1809, he weighed 52 stone 11 pounds (739 pounds), and measured over 3 yards around the body and over 1 yard around the leg. He had many visitors, and it is said that once, when the dwarf Borwilaski came to see him, he asked the little man how much cloth he needed for a suit. When told about 3/4 of a yard, he replied that one of his sleeves would be ample. Another famous fat man was Edward Bright, sometimes called "the fat man of Essex." He weighed 616 pounds. In the same journal that records Bright's weight is an account of a man exhibited in Holland who weighed 503 pounds.

Wadd, a physician, himself an enormous man, wrote a treatise on obesity and used his own portrait for a frontispiece. He speaks of Doctor Beddoes, who was so uncomfortably fat that a lady of Clifton called him a "walking feather bed." He mentions Doctor Stafford, who was so enormous that this epitaph was ascribed to him:—

"Take heed, O good traveler! and do not tread hard, For here lies Dr. Stafford, in all this churchyard."

Wadd has gathered some instances, a few of which will be cited. At Staunton, January 2, 1816, there died Samuel Sugars, Gent., who weighed with a single wood coffin 50 stone (700 pounds). Jacob Powell died in 1764, weighing 660 pounds. It took 16 men to carry him to his grave. Mr. Baker of Worcester, supposed to be larger than Bright, was interred in a coffin that was larger than an ordinary hearse. In 1797 there was buried Philip Hayes, a professor of music, who was as heavy as Bright (616 pounds).

Mr. Spooner, an eminent farmer of Warwickshire, who died in 1775, aged fifty-seven, weighed 569 pounds and measured over 4 feet across the shoulders. The two brothers Stoneclift of Halifax, Yorkshire, together weighed 980 pounds.

Keysler in his travels speaks of a corpulent Englishman who in passing through Savoy had to use 12 chairmen; he says that the man weighed 550 pounds. It is recorded on the tombstone of James Parsons, a fat man of Teddington, who died March 7, 1743, that he had often eaten a whole shoulder of mutton and a peck of hasty pudding. Keysler mentions a young Englishman living in Lincoln who was accustomed to eat 18 pounds of meat daily. He died in 1724 at the age of twenty-eight, weighing 530 pounds. In 1815 there died in Trenaw, in Cornwall, a person known as "Giant Chillcot." He measured at the breast 6 feet 9 inches and weighed 460 pounds. One of his stockings held 6 gallons of wheat. In 1822 there was reported to be a Cambridge student who could not go out in the daytime without exciting astonishment. The fat of his legs overhung his shoes like the fat in the legs of Lambert and Bright. Dr. Short mentions a lady who died of corpulency in her twenty-fifth year weighing over 50 stone (700 pounds). Catesby speaks of a man who weighed 500 pounds, and Coe mentions another who weighed 584 pounds. Fabricius and Godart speak of obesity so excessive as to cause death. There is a case reported from the French of a person who weighed 800 pounds. Smetius speaks of George Fredericus, an office-holder in Brandenburgh, who weighed 427 pounds.

Dupuytren gives the history of Marie Francoise-Clay, who attained such celebrity for her obesity. She was born in poverty, reached puberty at thirteen, and married at twenty-five, at which age she was already the stoutest woman of her neighborhood notwithstanding her infirmity. She followed her husband, who was an old-clothes dealer, afoot from town to town. She bore six children, in whom nothing extraordinary was noticed. The last one was born when she was thirty-five years old. Neither the births, her travels, nor her poverty, which sometimes forced her to beg at church doors, arrested the progress of the obesity. At the age of forty she was 5 feet 1 inch high and one inch greater about the waist. Her head was small and her neck was entirely obliterated. Her breasts were over a yard in circumference and hung as low as the umbilicus. Her arms were elevated and kept from her body by the fat in her axillae. Her belly was enormous and was augmented by six pregnancies. Her thighs and haunches were in proportion to her general contour. At forty she ceased to menstruate and soon became afflicted with organic heart diseases

Fournier quotes an instance of a woman in Paris who at twenty-four, the time of her death, weighed 486 pounds. Not being able to mount any conveyance or carriage in the city, she walked from place to place, finding difficulty not in progression, but in keeping her equilibrium. Roger Byrne, who lived in Rosenalis, Queen's County, Ireland, died of excessive fatness at the age of fifty-four, weighing 52 stone. Percy and Laurent speak of a young German of twenty who weighed 450 pounds. At birth he weighed 13 pounds, at six months 42, and at four years 150 pounds. He was 5 feet 5 inches tall and the same in circumference. William Campbell, the landlord of the Duke of Wellington in Newcastle-on-Tyne, was 6 feet 4 inches tall and weighed 728 pounds. He measured 96 inches around the shoulders, 85 inches around the waist, and 35 inches around the calf. He was born at Glasgow in 1856, and was not quite twenty-two when last measured. To illustrate the rate of augmentation, he weighed 4 stone at nine months and at ten years 18 stone. He was one of a family of seven children. His appetite was not more than the average, and he was moderate as regards the use of liquors, but a great smoker Notwithstanding his corpulency, he was intelligent and affable.

Miss Conley, a member of an American traveling circus, who weighed 479 pounds, was smothered in bed by rolling over on her face; she was unable to turn on her back without assistance.

There was a girl who died at Plaisance near Paris in 1890 who weighed 470 pounds or more. In 1889 an impresario undertook to exhibit her; but eight men could not move her from her room, and as she could not pass through the door the idea was abandoned.

There was a colored woman who died near Baltimore who weighed 850 pounds, exceeding the great Daniel Lambert by 120 pounds. The journal reporting this case quotes the Medical Record as saying that there was a man in North Carolina, who was born in 1798, who was 7 feet 8 inches tall and weighed over 1000 pounds, probably the largest man that ever lived. Hutchison says that he Saw in the Infirmary at Kensington, under Porter's care, a remarkable example of obesity. The woman was only just able to walk about and presented a close resemblance to Daniel Lambert. Obesity forced her to leave her occupation. The accumulation of fat on the abdomen, back, and thighs was enormous.

According to a recent number of La Liberte, a young woman of Pennsylvania, although only sixteen years old, weighs 450 pounds. Her waist measures 61 inches in circumference and her neck 22 inches. The same paper says that on one of the quays of Paris may be seen a wine-shop keeper with whom this Pennsylvania girl could not compare. It is said that this curiosity of the Notre-Dame quarter uses three large chairs while sitting behind her specially constructed bar. There is another Paris report of a man living in Switzerland who weighs more than 40 stone (560 pounds) and eats five times as much as an ordinary person. When traveling he finds the greatest difficulty in entering an ordinary railway carriage, and as a rule contents himself in the luggage van. Figure 171 represents an extremely fat woman with a well-developed beard. To end this list of obese individuals, we mention an old gentleman living in San Francisco who, having previously been thin, gained 14 pounds in his seventieth year and 14 pounds each of seven succeeding years.

Simulation of Obesity.—General dropsy, elephantiasis, lipomata, myxedema, and various other affections in which there is a hypertrophic change of the connective tissues may be mistaken for general obesity; on the other hand, a fatty, pendulous abdomen may simulate the appearances of pregnancy or even of ovarian cyst.

Dercum of Philadelphia has described a variety of obesity which he has called "adiposis dolorosa," in which there is an enormous growth of fat, sometimes limited, sometimes spread all over the body, this condition differing from that of general lipomatosis in its rarity, in the mental symptoms, in the headache, and the generally painful condition complained of. In some of the cases examined by Dercum he found that the thyroid was indurated and infiltrated by calcareous deposits. The disease is not myxedema because there is no peculiar physiognomy, no spade-like hands nor infiltrated skin, no alteration of the speech, etc. Dercum considers it a connective- tissue dystrophy—a fatty metamorphosis of various stages, possibly a neuritis. The first of Dercum's cases was a widow of Irish birth, who died both alcoholic and syphilitic. When forty-eight or forty-nine her arms began to enlarge. In June, 1887, the enlargement affected the shoulders ,arms, back, and sides of the chest. The parts affected were elastic, and there was no pitting. In some places the fat was lobulated, in others it appeared as though filled with bundles of worms. The skin was not thickened and the muscles were not involved. In the right arm there was unendurable pain to the touch, and this was present in a lesser degree in the left arm. Cutaneous sensibility was lessened. On June 13th a chill was followed by herpes over the left arm and chest, and later on the back and on the front of the chest. The temperature was normal. The second case was a married Englishwoman of sixty-four. The enlarged tissue was very unevenly distributed, and sensibility was the same as in the previous case. At the woman's death she weighed 300 pounds, and the fat over the abdomen was three inches thick. The third case was a German woman in whom were seen soft, fat-like masses in various situations over either biceps, over the outer and posterior aspect of either arm, and two large masses over the belly; there was excessive prominence of the mons veneris. At the autopsy the heart weighed 8 1/2 ounces, and the fat below the umbilicus was seven inches thick.

Abnormal Leanness.—In contrast to the fat men are the so-called "living skeletons," or men who have attained notice by reason of absence of the normal adipose tissue. The semimythical poet Philotus was so thin that it was said that he fastened lead on his shoes to prevent his being blown away,—a condition the opposite of that of Dionysius of Heraclea, who, after choking to death from his fat, could hardly be moved to his grave.

In March, 1754, there died in Glamorganshire of mere old age and gradual decay a little Welshman, Hopkin Hopkins, aged seventeen years. He had been recently exhibited in London as a natural curiosity; he had never weighed over 17 pounds, and for the last three years of his life never more than 12 pounds. His parents still had six children left, all of whom were normal and healthy except a girl of twelve, who only weighed 18 pounds and bore marks of old age.

There was a "living skeleton" brought to England in 1825 by the name of Claude Seurat. He was born in 1798 and was in his twenty-seventh year. He usually ate in the course of a day a penny roll and drank a small quantity of wine. His skeleton was plainly visible, over which the skin was stretched tightly. The distance from the chest to the spine was less than 3 inches, and internally this distance was less. The pulsations of the heart were plainly visible. He was in good health and slept well. His voice was very weak and shrill. The circumference of this man's biceps was only 4 inches. The artist Cruikshank has made several drawings of Seurat.

Calvin Edson was another living skeleton. In 1813 he was in the army at the battle of Plattsburg, and had lain down in the cold and become benumbed. At this time he weighed 125 pounds and was twenty-five years old. In 1830 he weighed but 60 pounds, though 5 feet 4 inches tall. He was in perfect health and could chop a cord of wood without fatigue; he was the father of four children.

Salter speaks of a man in 1873 who was thirty-two years of age and only weighed 49 pounds. He was 4 feet 6 inches tall: his forehead measured in circumference 20 1/2 inches and his chest 27 inches. His genitals, both internal and external, were defectively developed. Figure 175 represents the well-known Ohio "living skeleton," J. W. Coffey, who has been exhibited all over the Continent. His good health and appetite were proverbial among his acquaintances.

In some instances the so-called "living skeletons" are merely cases of extreme muscular atrophy. As a prominent example of this class the exhibitionist, Rosa Lee Plemons at the age of eighteen weighed only 27 pounds. Figure 177 shows another case of extraordinary atrophic condition of all the tissues of the body associated with nondevelopment. These persons are always sickly and exhibit all the symptoms of progressive muscular atrophy, and cannot therefore be classed with the true examples of thinness, in which the health is but slightly affected or possibly perfect health is enjoyed.

CHAPTER VIII

LONGEVITY.

Scope of the Present Article.—The limits of space in this work render impossible a scientific discussion upon the most interesting subject of longevity, and the reader is referred to some of the modern works devoted exclusively to this subject. In reviewing the examples of extreme age found in the human race it will be our object to lay before the reader the most remarkable instances of longevity that have been authentically recorded, to cite the source of the information, when possible to give explanatory details, and to report any relative points of value and interest. Throughout the article occasional facts will be given to show in what degree character, habit, and temperament influence longevity, and in what state of mind and body and under what circumstances man has obtained the highest age.

General Opinions.—There have been many learned authorities who invariably discredit all accounts of extraordinary age, and contend that there has never been an instance of a man living beyond the century mark whose age has been substantiated by satisfactory proof. Such extremists as Sir G. Cornewall Lewis and Thoms contend that since the Christian era no person of royal or noble line mentioned in history whose birth was authentically recorded at its occurrence has reached one hundred years. They have taken the worst station in life in which to find longevity as their field of observation. Longevity is always most common in the middle and lower classes, in which we cannot expect to find the records preserved with historical correctness.

The Testimony of Statistics.—Walford in his wonderful "Encyclopedia of Insurance" says that in England the "Royal Exchange" for a period of one hundred and thirty-five years had insured no life which survived ninety-six. The "London Assurance" for the same period had no clients who lived over ninety, and the "Equitable" had only one at ninety-six. In an English Tontine there was in 1693 a person who died at one hundred; and in Perth there lived a nominee at one hundred and twenty-two and another at one hundred and seven. On the other hand, a writer in the Strand Magazine points out that an insurance investigator some years ago gathered a list of 225 centenarians of almost every social rank and many nationalities, but the majority of them Britons or Russians.

In reviewing Walford's statistics we must remember that it has only been in recent years that the middle and lower classes of people have taken insurance on their lives. Formerly only the wealthy and those exposed to early demise were in the habit of insuring.

Dr. Ogle of the English Registrar-General's Department gives tables of expectancy that show that 82 males and 225 females out of 1,000,000 are alive at one hundred years. The figures are based on the death-rates of the years 1871-80.

The researches of Hardy in the thirteenth, fourteenth, fifteenth, and sixteenth centuries are said to indicate that three-score-and-ten was considered old age; yet many old tombstones and monuments contain inscriptions recording age far beyond this, and even the pages of ordinary biographies disprove the alleged results of Hardy's research.

In all statistical work of an individual type the histories of the lower classes are almost excluded; in the olden times only the lives and movements of the most prominent are thought worthy of record. The reliable parish register is too often monopolized by the gentry, inferior births not being thought worth recording.

Many eminent scientists say that the natural term of the life of an animal is five times the period needed for its development. Taking twenty-one as the time of maturity in man, the natural term of human life would be one hundred and five. Sir Richard Owen fixes it at one hundred and three and a few months.

Censuses of Centenarians.—Dr. Farr, the celebrated English Registrar-General, is credited with saying that out of every 1,000,000 people in England only 223 live to be one hundred years old, making an average of one to 4484. French says that during a period of ten years, from 1881 to 1890, in Massachusetts, there were 203 deaths of persons past the age of one hundred, making an average, with a population of 394,484, of one in 1928. Of French's centenarians 165 were between one hundred and one hundred and five; 35 were between one hundred and five and one hundred and ten; five were between one hundred and ten and one hundred and fifteen; and one was one hundred and eighteen. Of the 203, 153 were females and 50 males. There are 508 people in Iowa who are more than ninety years of age. There are 21 who are more than one hundred years old. One person is one hundred and fifteen years old, two are one hundred and fourteen, and the remaining 18 are from one hundred to one hundred and seven.

In the British Medical Journal for 1886 there is an account of a report of centenarians. Fifty-two cases were analyzed. One who doubts the possibility of a man reaching one hundred would find this report of interest.

The Paris correspondent to the London Telegraph is accredited with the following:—

"A census of centenarians has been taken in France, and the results, which have been published, show that there are now alive in this country 213 persons who are over one hundred years old. Of these 147 are women, the alleged stronger sex being thus only able to show 66 specimens who are managing to still "husband out life's taper" after the lapse of a century. The preponderance of centenarians of the supposed weaker sex has led to the revival of some amusing theories tending to explain this phenomenon. One cause of the longevity of women is stated to be, for instance, their propensity to talk much and to gossip, perpetual prattle being highly conducive, it is said, to the active circulation of the blood, while the body remains unfatigued and undamaged. More serious theorists or statisticians, while commenting on the subject of the relative longevity of the sexes, attribute the supremacy of woman in the matter to the well-known cause, namely, that in general she leads a more calm and unimpassioned existence than a man, whose life is so often one of toil, trouble, and excitement. Setting aside these theories, however, the census of French centenarians is not devoid of interest in some of its details. At Rocroi an old soldier who fought under the First Napoleon in Russia passed the century limit last year. A wearer of the St. Helena medal—a distinction awarded to survivors of the Napoleonic campaigns, and who lives at Grand Fayt, also in the Nord—is one hundred and three years old, and has been for the last sixty-eight years a sort of rural policeman in his native commune. It is a rather remarkable fact in connection with the examples of longevity cited that in almost every instance the centenarian is a person in the humblest rank of life. According to the compilers of these records, France can claim the honor of having possessed the oldest woman of modern times. This venerable dame, having attained one hundred and fifty years, died peacefully in a hamlet in the Haute Garonne, where she had spent her prolonged existence, subsisting during the closing decade of her life on goat's milk and cheese. The woman preserved all her mental faculties to the last, but her body became attenuated to an extraordinary degree, and her skin was like parchment."

In the last ten years the St. James' Gazette has kept track of 378 centenarians, of whom 143 were men and 235 were women. A writer to the Strand Magazine tells of 14 centenarians living in Great Britain within the last half-dozen years.

It may be interesting to review the statistics of Haller, who has collected the greatest number of instances of extreme longevity. He found:—

```
1000 persons who lived from 100 to 110
  15 persons who lived from 130 to 140
  60    "      "      "       "   110 to 120
   6    "      "      "       "   140 to 150
  29    "      "      "       "   120 to 130
   1 person    "      "       "      to 169
```

Effect of Class-Influences, Occupation, etc.—Unfortunately for the sake of authenticity, all the instances of extreme age in this country have been from persons in the lower walks of life or from obscure parts of the country, where little else than hearsay could be procured to verify them. It must also be said that it is only among people of this class that we can expect to find parallels of the instances of extreme longevity of former times. The inhabitants of the higher stations of life, the population of thickly settled communities, are living in an age and under conditions almost incompatible with longevity. In fact, the strain of nervous energy made necessary by the changed conditions of business and mode of living really predisposes to premature decay.

Those who object to the reliability of reports of postcentenarianism seem to lose sight of these facts, and because absolute proof and parallel cannot be obtained they deny the possibility without giving the subject full thought and reason. As tending to substantiate the multitude of instances are the opinions of such authorities as Hufeland, Buffon, Haller, and Flourens. Walter Savage Landor on being told that a man in Russia was living at one hundred and thirty-two replied that he was possibly older, as people when they get on in years are prone to remain silent as to the number of their years—a statement that can hardly be denied. One of the strongest disbelievers in extreme age almost disproved in his own life the statement that there were no centenarians.

It is commonly believed that in the earliest periods of the world's history the lives of the inhabitants were more youthful and perfect; that these primitive men had gigantic size, incredible strength, and most astonishing duration of life. It is to this tendency that we are indebted for the origin of many romantic tales. Some have not hesitated to ascribe to our forefather Adam the height of 900 yards and the age of almost a thousand years; but according to Hufeland acute theologians have shown that the chronology of the early ages was not the same as that used in the present day. According to this same authority Hensler has proved that the year at the time of Abraham consisted of but three months, that it was afterward extended to eight, and finally in the time of Joseph to twelve. Certain Eastern nations, it is said, still reckon but three months to the year; this substantiates the opinion of Hensler, and, as Hufeland says, it would be inexplicable why the life of man should be shortened nearly one-half immediately after the flood.

Accepting these conclusions as correct, the highest recorded age, that of Methuselah, nine hundred years, will be reduced to about two hundred, an age that can hardly be called impossible in the face of such an abundance of reports, to which some men of comparatively modern times have approached, and which such substantial authorities as Buffon, Hufeland, and Flourens believed possible.

Alchemy and the "Elixir of Life."—The desire for long life and the acquisition of wealth have indirectly been the stimulus to medical and physical investigation, eventually evolving science as we have it now. The fundamental principles of nearly every branch of modern science were the gradual metamorphoses of the investigations of the old searchers after the "philosopher's stone" and "elixir of life." The long hours of study and experiment in the chase for this will-o'-the-wisp were of vast benefit to the coming generations; and to these deluded philosophers of the Middle Ages, and even of ancient times, we are doubtless indebted for much in this age of advancement.

With a credulous people to work upon, many of the claimants of the discovery of the coveted secret of eternal life must be held as rank impostors claiming ridiculous ages for themselves. In the twelfth century Artephius claimed that by the means of his discovery he had attained one thousand and twenty-five years. Shortly after him came Alan de Lisle of Flanders with a reputed fabulous age. In 1244 Albertus Magnus announced himself as the discoverer. In 1655 the celebrated Doctor Dee appeared on the scene and had victims by the score. Then came the Rosicrucians. Count Saint-Germain claimed the secret of the "philosopher's stone" and declared to the Court of Louis XV that he was two thousand years old, and a precursor of the mythical "Wandering Jew," who has been immortalized in prose and rhyme and in whose existence a great mass of the people recently believed. The last of the charlatans who claimed possession of the secret of perpetual life was Joseph Balsamo, who called himself "Count of

Cagliostro." He was born in Italy in 1743 and acquired a world-wide reputation for his alleged occult powers and acquisition of the "philosopher's stone." He died in 1795, and since then no one has generally inspired the superstitious with credence in this well-worn myth. The ill-fated Ponce de Leon when he discovered Florida, in spite of his superior education, announced his firm belief in the land of the "Fountain of Perpetual Youth," in the pursuit of which he had risked his fortune and life.

We wish to emphasize that we by no means assume the responsibility of the authenticity of the cases to be quoted, but expressing belief in their possibility, we shall mention some of the extraordinary instances of longevity derived from an exhaustive research of the literature of all times. This venerable gallery of Nestors will include those of all periods and nations, but as the modern references are more available greater attention will be given to them.

Turning first to the history of the earlier nations, we deduce from Jewish history that Abraham lived to one hundred and seventy-five; Isaac, likewise a tranquil, peaceful man, to one hundred and eighty; Jacob, who was crafty and cunning, to one hundred and forty-seven; Ishmael, a warrior, to one hundred and thirty-seven; and Joseph, to one hundred and ten. Moses, a man of extraordinary vigor, which, however, he exposed to great cares and fatigues, attained the advanced age of one hundred and twenty; and the warlike and ever-active Joshua lived to one hundred and ten. Lejoucourt gives the following striking parallels: John Glower lived to one hundred and seventy- two, and Abraham to one hundred and seventy-five; Susan, the wife of Gower, lived to one hundred and sixty-four, and Sarah, the wife of Abraham, to one hundred and twenty-seven. The eldest son of the Gower couple was one hundred and fifteen when last seen, and Isaac, the son of Abraham and Sarah, lived to one hundred and eighty.

However replete with fables may be the history of the Kings of Egypt, none attained a remarkable age, and the record of the common people is incomplete or unavailable.

If we judge from the accounts of Lucian we must form a high idea of the great age of the Seres, or ancient Chinese. Lucian ascribes this longevity to their habit of drinking excessive quantities of water.

Among the Greeks we find several instances of great age in men of prominence. Hippocrates divided life into seven periods, living himself beyond the century mark. Aristotle made three divisions,—the growing period, the stationary period, and the period of decline. Solon made ten divisions of life, and Varro made five.

Ovid ingeniously compares life to the four seasons. Epimenides of Crete is said to have lived one hundred and fifty-seven years, the last fifty-seven of which he slept in a cavern at night. Gorgias, a teacher, lived to one hundred and eight; Democritus, a naturalist, attained one hundred and nine; Zeno, the founder of the Stoics, lived to one hundred; and Diogenes, the frugal and slovenly, reached ninety years. Despite his life of exposure, Hippocrates lived to one hundred and nine; and Galen, the prince of physicians after him, who was naturally of a feeble constitution, lived past eighty, and few of the followers of his system of medicine, which stood for thirteen centuries, surpassed him in point of age.

Among the Romans, Orbilis, Corvinus, Fabius, and Cato, the enemy of the physicians, approximated the century mark.

A valuable collection relative to the duration of life in the time of the Emperor Vespasian has been preserved for us by Pliny from the records of a census, a perfectly reliable and creditable source. In 76 A. D. there were living in that part of Italy which lies between the Apennines and the Po 124 persons who had attained the age of one hundred and upward. There were 54 of one hundred; 57 of one hundred and ten; 2 of one hundred and twenty-five; 4 of one hundred and thirty; 4 of from one hundred and thirty-five to one hundred and thirty-seven, and 3 of one hundred and forty. In Placentia there was a man of one hundred and thirty and at Faventia a woman of one hundred and thirty-two. According to Hufeland, the bills of mortality of Ulpian agree in the most striking manner with those of our great modern cities.

Among hermits and ecclesiastics, as would be the natural inference from their regular lives, many instances of longevity are recorded. John was supposed to be ninety-three; Paul the hermit was one hundred and thirteen; Saint Anthony lived to one hundred and five; James the hermit to one hundred and four; Saint Epithanius lived to one hundred and fifteen; Simeon Stylites to one hundred and twelve; Saint Mungo was accredited with one hundred and eighty-five years (Spottiswood), and Saint David attained one hundred and forty-six. Saint Polycarpe suffered martyrdom at over one hundred, and Simon Cleophas was Bishop of Jerusalem at one hundred and twenty.

Brahmin priests of India are known to attain incredible age, and one of the secrets of the adepts of the Buddhist faith is doubtless the knowledge of the best means of attaining very old age. Unless cut off by violence or accident the priests invariably become venerable patriarchs.

Influence of Mental Culture.—Men of thought have at all times been distinguished for their age. Among the venerable sages are Appolonius of Tyana, a follower of Pythagoras, who lived to over one hundred; Xenophilus, also a Pythagorean, was one hundred and six; Demonax, a Stoic, lived past one hundred; Isocrates was ninety-eight, and Solon, Sophocles, Pindar, Anacreon, and Xenophon were octogenarians.

In more modern times we find men of science and literature who have attained advanced age. Kant, Buffon, Goethe, Fontenelle, and Newton were all over eighty. Michael Angelo and Titian lived to eighty-nine and ninety-nine respectively. Harvey, the discoverer of the circulation; Hans Sloane, the celebrated president of the Royal Society in London; Plater, the Swiss physician; Duverney, the anatomist, as well as his confrere, Tenon, lived to be octogenarians. Many men have displayed activity when past four score. Brougham at eighty-two and Lyndhurst at eighty-eight could pour forth words of eloquence and sagacity for hours at a time. Landor wrote his "Imaginary Conversations" when eighty-five, and Somerville his "Molecular Science" at eighty-eight; Isaac Walton was active with his pen at ninety; Hahnemann married at eighty and was working at ninety-one.

J. B. Bailey has published a biography of "Modern Methusalehs," which includes histories of the lives of Cornaro, Titian, Pletho, Herschell, Montefiore, Routh, and others. Chevreul, the centenarian chemist, has only lately died. Gladstone, Bismarck, and von Moltke exemplify vigor in age In the Senate of the United States, Senators Edmunds, Sherman, Hoar, Morrill, and other elderly statesmen display as much vigor as their youthful colleagues. Instances of vigor in age could be cited in every profession and these few examples are only mentioned as typical. At a recent meeting of the Society of English Naturalists, Lord Kelvin announced that during the last year 26 members had died at an average age of seventy-six and a half years; one reached the age of ninety-nine years, another ninety-seven, a third ninety-five, etc.

In commenting on the perfect compatibility of activity with longevity, the National Popular Review says:—

"Great men usually carry their full mental vigor and activity into old age. M. Chevreul, M. De Lesseps, Gladstone, and Bismarck are evidences of this anthropologic fact. Pius IX, although living in tempestuous times, reached a great age in full possession of all his faculties, and the dramatist Crebillon composed his last dramatic piece at ninety-four, while Michael Angelo was still painting his great canvases at ninety-eight, and Titian at ninety still worked with all the vigor of his earlier years. The Austrian General Melas was still in the saddle and active at eighty-nine, and would have probably won Marengo but for the inopportune arrival of Desaix. The Venetian Doge Henry Dandolo, born at the beginning of the eleventh century, who lost his eyesight when a young man, was nevertheless subsequently raised to the highest office in the republic, managed successfully to conduct various wars, and at the advanced age of eighty-three, in alliance with the French, besieged and captured Constantinople. Fontenelle was as gay-spirited at ninety-eight as in his fortieth year, and the philosopher Newton worked away at his tasks at the age of eighty-three with the same ardor that animated his middle age. Cornaro was as happy at ninety as at fifty, and in far better health at the age of ninety-five than he had enjoyed at thirty.

"These cases all tend to show the value and benefits to be derived from an actively cultivated brain in making a long life one of comfort and of usefulness to its owner. The brain and spirits need never grow old, even if our bodies will insist on getting rickety and in falling by the wayside. But an abstemious life will drag even the old body along to centenarian limits in a tolerable state of preservation and usefulness. The foregoing list can be lengthened out with an indefinite number of names, but it is sufficiently long to show what good spirits and an active brain will do to lighten up the weight of old age. When we contemplate the Doge Dandolo at eighty-three animating his troops from the deck of his galley, and the brave old blind King of Bohemia falling in the thickest of the fray at Crecy, it would seem as it there was no excuse for either physical, mental, or moral decrepitude short of the age of four score and ten."

Emperors and Kings, in short, the great ones of the earth, pay the penalty of their power by associate worriment and care. In ancient history we can only find a few rulers who attained four score, and this is equally the case in modern times. In the whole catalogue of the Roman and German Emperors, reckoning from Augustus to William I, only six have attained eighty years. Gordian, Valerian, Anastasius, and Justinian were octogenarians, Tiberius was eighty-eight at his death, and Augustus Caesar was eighty-six. Frederick the Great, in spite of his turbulent life, attained a rare age for a king, seventy-six. William I seems to be the only other exception.

Of 300 Popes who may be counted, no more than five attained the age of eighty. Their mode of life, though conducive to longevity in the minor offices of the Church, seems to be overbalanced by the cares of the Pontificate.

Personal Habits.—According to Hufeland and other authorities on longevity, sobriety, regular habits, labor in the open air, exercise short of fatigue, calmness of mind, moderate intellectual power, and a family life are among the chief aids to longevity. For this reason we find the extraordinary instances of longevity among those people who amidst bodily labor and in the open air lead a simple life, agreeable to nature. Such are farmers, gardeners, hunters, soldiers, and sailors. In these situations man may still maintain the age of one hundred and fifty or even one hundred and sixty.

Possibly the most celebrated case of longevity on record is that of Henry Jenkins. This remarkable old man was born in Yorkshire in 1501 and died in 1670, aged one hundred and sixty-nine. He remembered the battle of Flodden Field in 1513, at which time he was twelve years old. It was proved from the registers of the Chancery and other courts that he had appeared in evidence one hundred and forty years before his death and had had an oath administered to him. In the office of the King's Remembrancer is a record of a deposition in which he appears as a witness at one hundred and fifty-seven. When above one hundred he was able to swim a rapid stream.

Thomas Parr (or Parre), among Englishmen known as "old Parr," was a poor farmer's servant, born in 1483. He remained single until eighty. His first wife lived thirty-two years, and eight years after her death, at the age of one hundred and twenty, he married again. Until his one hundred and thirtieth year he performed his ordinary duties, and at this age was even accustomed to thresh. He was visited by Thomas, Earl of Arundel and Surrey, and was persuaded to visit the King in London. His intelligence and venerable demeanor impressed every one, and crowds thronged to see him and pay him homage. The journey to London, together with the excitement and change of mode of living, undoubtedly hastened his death, which occurred in less than a year. He was one hundred and fifty-two years and nine months old, and had lived under nine Kings of England. Harvey examined his body and at the necropsy his internal organs were found in a most perfect state. His cartilages were not even ossified, as is the case generally with the very aged. The slightest cause of death could not be discovered, and the general impression was that he died from being over-fed and too-well treated in London. His great-grandson was said to have died in this century in Cork at the age of one hundred and three. Parr is celebrated by a monument reared to his memory in Westminster Abbey.

The author of the Dutch dictionary entitled "Het algemen historish Vanderbok" says that there was a peasant in Hungary named Jean Korin who was one hundred and seventy-two and his wife was one hundred and sixty-four; they had lived together one hundred and forty-eight years, and had a son at the time of their death who was one hundred and sixteen.

Setrasch Czarten, or, as he is called by Baily, Petratsh Zartan, was also born in Hungary at a village four miles from Teneswaer in 1537. He lived for one hundred and eighty years in one village and died at the age of one hundred and eighty-seven, or, as another authority has it, one hundred and eighty-five. A few days before his death he had walked a mile to wait at the post-office for the arrival of travelers and to ask for succor, which, on account of his remarkable age, was rarely refused him. He had lost nearly all his teeth and his beard and hair were white. He was accustomed to eat a little cake the Hungarians call kalatschen, with which he drank milk. After each repast he took a glass of eau-de-vie. His son was living at ninety-seven and his descendants to the fifth generation embellished his old age. Shortly before his death Count Wallis had his portrait painted. Comparing his age with that of others, we find that he was five years older than the Patriarch Isaac, ten more than Abraham, thirty-seven more than Nahor, sixteen more than Henry Jenkins, and thirty-three more than "old Parr."

Sundry Instances of Great Age.—In a churchyard near Cardiff, Glamorganshire, is the following inscription: "Here lieth the body of William Edwards, of Cacreg, who departed this life 24th February, Anno Domini 1668, anno aetatis suae one hundred and sixty-eight."

Jonas Warren of Balydole died in 1787 aged one hundred and sixty-seven. He was called the "father of the fishermen" in his vicinity, as he had followed the trade for ninety-five years.

The Journal de Madrid, 1775, contains the account of a South American negress living in Spanish possessions who was one hundred and seventy-four years of age. The description is written by a witness, who declares that she told of events which confirmed her age. This is possibly the oft-quoted case that was described in the London Chronicle, October 5, 1780, Louisa Truxo, who died in South America at the age of one hundred and seventy-five.

Huteland speaks of Joseph Surrington, who died near Bergen, Norway, at the age of one hundred and sixty. Marvelous to relate, he had one living son of one hundred and three and another of nine. There has been recently reported from Vera Cruz, Mexico, in the town of Teluca, where the registers are carefully and efficiently kept, the death of a man one hundred and ninety-two years old—almost a modern version of Methuselah. Buffon describes a man who lived to be one hundred and sixty-five. Martin mentions a man of one hundred and eighty. There was a Polish peasant who reached one hundred and fifty-seven and had constantly labored up to his one hundred and forty-fifth year, always clad lightly, even in cold weather. Voigt admits the extreme age of one hundred and sixty.

There was a woman living in Moscow in 1848 who was said to be one hundred and sixty-eight; she had been married five times and was one hundred and twenty-one at her last wedding. D'Azara records the age of one hundred and eighty, and Roequefort speaks of two cases at one hundred and fifty.

There are stories of an Englishman who lived in the sixteenth century to be two hundred and seven, and there is a parallel case cited.

Van Owen tabulates 331 cases of deaths between 110 and 120, 91 between 120 and 130, 37 between 130 and 140, 11 at 150, and 17 beyond this age. While not vouching for the authenticity in each case, he has always given the sources of information.

Quite celebrated in English history by Raleigh and Bacon was the venerable Countess Desmond, who appeared at Court in 1614, being one hundred and forty years old and in full possession of all her powers, mental and physical. There are several portraits of her at this advanced age still to be seen. Lord Bacon also mentions a man named Marcus Appenius, living in Rimini, who was registered by a Vespasian tax-collector as being one hundred and fifty.

There are records of Russians who have lived to one hundred and twenty-five, one hundred and thirty, one hundred and thirty-five, one hundred and forty-five, and one hundred and fifty. Nemnich speaks of Thomas Newman living in Bridlington at one hundred and fifty-three years. Nemnich is confirmed in his account of Thomas Newman by his tombstone in Yorkshire, dated 1542.

In the chancel of the Honington Church, Wiltshire, is a black marble monument to the memory of G. Stanley, gent., who died in 1719, aged one hundred and fifty-one.

There was a Dane named Draakenburg, born in 1623, who until his ninety-first year served as a seaman in the royal navy, and had spent fifteen years of his life in Turkey as a slave in the greatest misery. He was married at one hundred and ten to a woman of sixty, but outlived her a long time, in his one hundred and thirtieth year he again fell in love with a young country girl, who, as may well be supposed, rejected him. He died in 1772 in his one hundred and forty-sixth year. Jean Effingham died in Cornwall in 1757 in his one hundred and forty-fourth year. He was born in the reign of James I and was a soldier at the battle of Hochstadt; he never drank strong liquors and rarely ate meat; eight days before his death he walked three miles.

Bridget Devine, the well-known inhabitant of Olean Street, Manchester died at the age of one hundred and forty-seven in 1845. On the register of the Cheshire Parish is a record of the death of Thomas Hough of Frodsam in 1591 at the age of one hundred and forty-one.

Peter Garden of Auchterless died in 1775 at the age of one hundred and thirty-one. He had seen and talked with Henry Jenkins about the battle of Flodden Field, at which the latter was present when a boy of twelve. It seems almost incredible that a man could say that he had heard the story of an event which had happened two hundred and sixty-three years before related by the lips of an eye-witness to that event; nevertheless, in this case it was true. A remarkable instance of longevity in one family has recently been published in the St. Thomas's Hospital Gazette. Mrs. B., born in 1630 (five years after the accession of Charles I), died March 13, 1732. She was tended in her last illness by her great-granddaughter, Miss Jane C., born 1718, died 1807, and Miss Sarah C., born 1725, died 1811. A great-niece of one of these two ladies, Mrs. W., who remembers one of them, was born in 1803, and is at the present time alive and well. It will be seen from the above facts that there are three lives only to bridge over the long period between 1630 and 1896, and that there is at present living a lady who personally knew Miss C., who had nursed a relative born in 1630. The last lady of this remarkable trio is hale and hearty, and has just successfully undergone an operation for cataract. Similar to the case of the centenarian who had seen Henry Jenkins was that of James Horrocks, who was born in 1744 and died in 1844. His father was born in 1657, one year before the death of the Protector, and had issue in early life. He married again at eighty-four to a woman of twenty-six, of which marriage James was the offspring in 1744. In 1844 this man could with verity say that he had a brother born during the reign of Charles II, and that his father was a citizen of the Commonwealth.

Among the Mission Indians of Southern California there are reported instances of longevity ranging from one hundred and twenty to one hundred and forty. Lieutenant Gibbons found in a village in Peru one hundred inhabitants who were past the century mark, and another credible explorer in the same territory records a case of longevity of one hundred and forty. This man was very temperate and always ate his food cold, partaking of meat only in the middle of the day. In the year of 1840 in the town of Banos, Ecuador, died "Old Morales," a carpenter, vigorous to his last days. He was an elderly man and steward of the Jesuits when they were expelled from their property near this location in 1767. In the year 1838 there was a witness in a judicial trial in South America who was born on the night of the great earthquake which destroyed the town of Ambato in 1698. How much longer this man who was cradled by an earthquake lived is not as yet reported. In the State of Vera Cruz, Mexico, as late as 1893 a man died at the age of one hundred and thirty-seven. The census of 1864 for the town of Pilaguin, Ecuador, lying 11,000 feet above the level of the sea and consisting of about 2000 inhabitants, gives 100 above seventy, 30 above ninety, five above one hundred, and one at one hundred and fifteen years.

Francis Auge died in Maryland in 1767 at the age of one hundred and thirty-four. He remembered the execution of Charles I and had a son born to him after he was one hundred.

There are several other instances in which men have displayed generative ability in old age. John Gilley, who died in Augusta, Maine, in 1813, was born in Ireland in 1690. He came to this country at the age of sixty, and continued in single blessedness until seventy-five, when he married a girl of eighteen, by whom he had eight children. His wife survived him and stated that he was virile until his one hundred and twentieth year. Baron Baravicino de Capelis died at Meran in 1770 at the age of one hundred and four, being the oldest man in Tyrol. His usual food was eggs, and he rarely tasted meat. He habitually drank tea and a well-sweetened cordial of his own recipe. He was married four times during his life, taking his fourth wife when he was eighty-four. By her he had seven children and at his death she was pregnant with the eighth child.

Pliny mentions cases of men begetting sons when past the age of eighty and Plot speaks of John Best of the parish of Horton, who when one hundred and four married a woman of fifty-six and begat a son. There are also records of a man in Stockholm of one hundred who had several children by a wife of thirty.

On August 7, 1776, Mary, the wife of Joseph Yates, at Lizard Common not far from London, was buried at the age of one hundred and twenty-seven. She had walked to London in 1666, and was hearty and strong at one hundred and twenty, and had married a third husband at ninety-two.

A case without parallel, of long survival of a deaf mute, is found in Mrs. Gray of Northfleet, Kent, who died in 1770, one hundred and twenty-one years old. She was noted for her cheerful disposition, and apparently enjoyed life in spite of her infirmity, which lasted one hundred and twenty-one years.

Macklin the actor was born in 1697 and died in 1797. Several years before his death he played "Shylock," displaying great vigor in the first act, but in the second his memory failed him, and with much grace and solemnity he advanced to the foot-lights and apologized for his inability to continue. It is worthy of remark that several instances of longevity in Roman actresses have been recorded. One Luceja, who came on the stage very young, performed a whole century, and even made her public appearance in her one hundred and twelfth year. Copiola was said to have danced before Augustus when past ninety.

Influence of Stimulants, etc.—There have been men who have attributed their long lives to their excesses in stimulants. Thomas Wishart of Annandale, Dumfries, died in 1760 at one hundred and twenty-four. He had chewed tobacco one hundred and seventeen years, contracting the habit when a child; his father gave it to him to allay hunger while shepherding in the mountains. John de la Somet of Virginia died in 1766 aged one hundred and thirty. He was a great smoker, and according to Eaton the habit agreed with his constitution, and was not improbably the cause of his long health and longevity. William Riddell, who died at one hundred and sixteen carefully avoided water all his life and had a love for brandy.

Possession of Faculties.—Eglebert Hoff was a lad driving a team in Norway when the news was brought that Charles I was beheaded. He died in Fishkill, N.Y., in 1764 at the age of one hundred and twenty-eight. He never used spectacles, read fluently, and his memory and senses were retained until his death, which was due to an accident. Nicolas Petours, curate of the parish of Baleene and afterward canon of the Cathedral of Constance, died at the age of one hundred and thirty-seven; he was always a healthy, vigorous man, and celebrated mass five days before his death. Mr. Evans of Spital Street, Spitalfields, London, died in 1780 aged one hundred and thirty-nine, having full possession of his mental faculties. Of interest to Americans is the case of David Kinnison, who, when one hundred and eleven, related to Lossing the historian the tale of the Boston Tea Party, of which he had been a member. He died in good mental condition at the age of one hundred and fifteen. Anthony Senish, a farmer of the village of Limoges, died in 1770 in his one hundred and eleventh year. He labored until two weeks before his death, had still his hair, and his sight had not failed him. His usual food was chestnuts and Turkish corn; he had never been bled or used any medicine. Not very long ago there was alive in Tacony, near Philadelphia, a shoemaker named R. Glen in his one hundred and fourteenth year. He had seen King William III, and all his faculties were perfectly retained; he enjoyed good health, walking weekly to Philadelphia to church. His third wife was but thirty years old.

Longevity in Ireland.—Lord Bacon said that at one time there was not a village in all Ireland in which there was not a man living upward of eighty. In Dunsford, a small village, there were living at one time 80 persons above the age of four score. Colonel Thomas Winslow was supposed to have died in Ireland on August 26, 1766, aged one hundred and forty-six. There was a man by the name of Butler who died at Kilkenny in 1769 aged one hundred and thirty-three. He rode after the hounds while yet a centenarian. Mrs. Eckelston, a widow in Phillipstown, Kings County, Ireland, died in 1690 at one hundred and forty-three.

There are a number of instances in which there is extraordinary renovation of the senses or even of the body in old age,—a new period of life, as it were, is begun. A remarkable instance is an old magistrate known to Hufeland, who lived at Rechingen and who died in 1791 aged one hundred and twenty. In 1787, long after he had lost all his teeth, eight new ones appeared, and at the end of six months they again dropped out, but their place was supplied by other new ones, and Nature, unwearied, continued this process until his death. All these teeth he had acquired and lost without pain, the whole number amounting to 150. Alice, a slave born in Philadelphia, and living in 1802 at the age of one hundred and sixteen, remembered William Penn and Thomas Story. Her faculties were well preserved, but she partially lost her eyesight at ninety-six, which, strange to say, returned in part at one hundred and two. There was a woman by the name of Helen Gray who died in her one hundred and fifth year, and who but a few years before her death had acquired a new set of teeth.

In Wilson's "Healthy Skin" are mentioned several instances of very old persons in whom the natural color of the hair returned after they had been gray for years. One of them was John Weeks, whose hair became brown again at one hundred and fourteen. Sir John Sinclair a mentions a similar case in a Scotchman who lived to one hundred and ten. Susan Edmonds when in her ninety-fifth year recovered her black hair, but previously to her death at one hundred and five again became gray. There was a Dr. Slave who at the age of eighty had a renewal of rich brown hair, which he maintained until his death at one hundred. There was a man in Vienna, aged one hundred and five, who had black hair long after his hair had first become white This man is mentioned as a parallel to Dr. Slave. Similar examples are mentioned in Chapter VI.

It is a remarkable fact that many persons who have reached an old age have lived on the smallest diet and the most frugal fare. Many of the instances of longevity were in people of Scotch origin who subsisted all their lives on porridges. Saint Anthony is said to have maintained life to one hundred and five on twelve ounces of bread daily. In 1792 in the Duchy of Holstein there was an industrious laborer named Stender who died at one hundred and three, his food for the most part of his life having been oatmeal and buttermilk. Throughout his life he had been particularly free from thirst, drinking little water and no spirits.

Heredity.—There are some very interesting instances of successive longevity. Lister speaks of a son and a father, from a village called Dent, who were witnesses before a jury at York in 1664. The son was above one hundred and the father above one hundred and forty. John Moore died in 1805 aged one hundred and seven. His father died at one hundred and five and his grandfather at one hundred and fifteen, making a total of three hundred and twenty-seven years for the three generations. Recently, Wynter mentions four sisters,—of one hundred, one hundred and three, one hundred and five, and one hundred and seven years respectively. On the register of Bremhill 1696, is the following remarkable entry: "Buried, September 29th, Edith Goldie, Grace Young, and Elizabeth Wiltshire, their united ages making three hundred." As late as 1886 in the district of Campinos there was a strong active man named Joseph Joachim de Prado, of good family, who was one hundred and seven years old. His mother died by accident at one hundred and twelve, and his maternal grandmother died at one hundred and twenty-two.

Longevity in Active Military Service.—One of the most remarkable proofs that under fickle fortune, constant danger, and the most destructive influences the life of man may be long preserved is exemplified in the case of an old soldier named Mittelstedt, who died in Prussia in 1792, aged one hundred and twelve. He was born at Fissalm in June, 1681. He entered the army, served under three Kings, Frederick I, Frederick William I, and Frederick II, and did active service in the Seven Years' War, in which his horse was shot under him and he was taken prisoner by the Russians. In his sixty-eight years of army service he participated in 17 general engagements, braved numerous dangers, and was wounded many times. After his turbulent life he married, and at last in 1790, in his one hundred and tenth year, he took a third wife. Until shortly before his death he walked every month to the pension office, a distance of two miles from his house.

Longevity in Physicians.—It may be of interest to the members of our profession to learn of some instances of longevity among confreres. Dr. R. Baynes of Rockland, Maine, has been mentioned in the list of "grand old men" in medicine; following in the footsteps of Hippocrates and Galen, he was practicing at ninety-nine. He lives on Graham's diet, which is a form of vegetarianism; he does not eat potatoes, but does eat fruit. His drink is almost entirely water, milk, and chocolate, and he condemns the use of tea, coffee, liquors, and tobacco. He has almost a perfect set of natural teeth and his sight is excellent. Like most men who live to a great age, Dr. Baynes has a "fad," to which he attributes a chief part in prolonging his life. This is the avoidance of beds, and except when away from home he has not slept on a bed or even on a mattress for over fifty years. He has an iron reclining chair, over which he spreads a few blankets and rugs.

The British Medical Journal speaks of Dr. Boisy of Havre, who is one hundred and three. It is said he goes his rounds every day, his practice being chiefly among the poor. At one time he practiced in India. He has taken alcoholic beverages and smoked tobacco since his youth, although in moderation. His father, it is added, died at the age of one hundred and eight. Mr. William R. Salmon, living near Cowbridge, Glamorganshire, recently celebrated his one hundred and sixth birthday. Mr. Salmon was born at Wickham Market in 1790, and became a member of the Royal College of Surgeons in 1809, the year in which Gladstone was born. He died April 11, 1896. In reference to this wonderful old physician the Journal of the American Medical Association, 1896, page 995, says—

"William Reynold Salmon, M.R.C.S., of Penllyn Court, Cowbridge, Glamorganshire, South Wales, completed his one hundred and sixth year on March 16th, and died on the 11th of the present month—at the time of his death the oldest known individual of indisputably authenticated age, the oldest physician, the oldest member of the Royal College of Surgeons, England, and the oldest Freemason in the world. His age does not rest upon tradition or repute. He was the son of a successful and esteemed practicing physician of Market Wickham, Suffolk, England, and there is in the possession of his two surviving relatives, who cared for his household for many years, his mother's diary, in which is inscribed in the handwriting of a lady of the eighteenth century, under the date, Tuesday, March 16, 1790, a prayer of thankfulness to God that she had passed her 'tryall,' and that a son was born, who she hoped 'would prosper, be a support to his parents, and make virtue his chief pursuit.' The Royal College of Surgeons verified this record many years ago, and it was subsequently again authenticated by the authorities of the Freemasons, who thereupon enshrined his portrait in their gallery as the oldest living Freemason. The Salmon family moved to Cowbridge in 1796, so that the doctor had lived exactly a century in the lovely and poetic Vale of Glamorgan, in the very heart of which Penllyn Court is situated. Here on his one hundred and sixth birthday—a man of over middle height, with still long, flowing hair, Druidical beard and mustache, and bushy eyebrows—Dr. Salmon was visited by one who writes:—

" 'Seen a few days ago, the Patriarch of Penllyn Court was hale and hearty. He eats well and sleeps well and was feeling better than he had felt for the last five years. On that day he rose at noon, dined at six, and retired at nine. Drank two glasses of port with his dinner, but did not smoke. He abandoned his favorite weed at the age of ninety, and had to discontinue his drives over his beautiful estate in his one hundredth year. One day is much the same as another, for he gives his two relatives little trouble in attending upon his wants. Dr. Salmon has not discovered the elixir of life, for the shadows of life's evening are stealing slowly over him. He cannot move about, his hearing is dulled, and the light is almost shut out from the "windows of his soul." Let us think of this remarkable man waiting for death uncomplainingly in his old-fashioned mansion, surrounded by the beautiful foliage and the broad expanse of green fields that he loved so much to roam when a younger man, in that sylvan Sleepy Hollow in the Vale of Glamorgan.'

"Eight weeks later he, who in youth had been 'the youngest surgeon in the army, died, the oldest physician in the world."

Dr. William Hotchkiss, said to have reached the age of one hundred and forty years, died in St. Louis April 1, 1895. He went to St. Louis forty years ago, and has always been known as the "color doctor." In his peculiar practice of medicine he termed his patients members of his "circles," and claimed to treat them by a magnetic process. Dr. A. J. Buck says that his Masonic record has been traced back one hundred years, showing conclusively that he was one hundred and twenty-one years old. A letter received from his old home in Virginia, over a year ago, says that he was born there in 1755.

It is comforting to the members of our profession, in which the average of life is usually so low, to be able to point out exceptions. It has been aptly said of physicians in general: "Aliis inserviendo consumuntur; aliis medendo moriuntur," or "In serving others they are consumed; in healing others they are destroyed."

Recent Instances of Longevity.—There was a man who died in Spain at the advanced age of one hundred and fifty-one, which is the most extraordinary instance from that country. It is reported that quite recently a Chinese centenarian passed the examination for the highest place in the Academy of Mandarins. Chevreul, born in 1786, at Angers, has only recently died after an active life in chemical investigation. Sir Moses Montefiore is a recent example of an active centenarian.

In the New York Herald of April 21, 1895, is a description and a portrait of Noah Raby of the Piscataway Poor Farm of New Jersey, to whom was ascribed one hundred and twenty-three years. He was discharged from active duty on the "Brandywine," U.S.N., eighty-three years ago. He relates having heard George Washington speak at Washington and at Portsmouth while his ship was in those places. The same journal also says that at Wichita, Kansas, there appeared at a municipal election an old negress named Mrs. Harriet McMurray, who gave her age as one hundred and fifteen. She had been a slave, and asserted that once on a visit to Alexandria with her master she had seen General Washington. From the

Indian Medical Record we learn that Lieutenant Nicholas Lavin of the Grand Armee died several years ago at the age of one hundred and twenty-five, leaving a daughter of seventy-eight. He was born in Paris in 1768, served as a hussar in several campaigns, and was taken a prisoner during the retreat from Moscow. After his liberation he married and made his residence in Saratoff.

CHAPTER IX

PHYSIOLOGIC AND FUNCTIONAL ANOMALIES.

In considering the anomalies of the secretions, it must be remembered that the ingestion of certain kinds of food and the administration of peculiar drugs in medicine have a marked influence in coloring secretions. Probably the most interesting of all these anomalies is the class in which, by a compensatory process, metastasis of the secretions is noticed.

Colored Saliva.—Among the older writers the Ephemerides contains an account of blue saliva; Huxham speaks of green saliva; Marcellus Donatus of yellow, and Peterman relates the history of a case of yellow saliva. Dickinson describes a woman of sixty whose saliva was blue; besides this nothing was definitely the matter with her. It seemed however, that the color was due to some chemic-pencil poisoning rather than to a pathologic process. A piece of this aniline pencil was caught in the false teeth. Paget cites an instance of blue saliva due to staining the tongue in the same manner. Most cases of anomalous coloring of this kind can be subsequently traced to artificial substances unconsciously introduced. Crocker mentions a woman who on washing her hands constantly found that the water was stained blue, but this was subsequently traced to the accidental introduction of an orchid leaf. In another instance there was a woman whose linen was at every change stained brown; this, however, was found to be due to a hair-wash that she was in the habit of using.

Among the older writers who have mentioned abnormal modes of exit of the urine is Baux, who mentions urine from the nipples; Paullini and the Ephemerides describe instances of urination from the eyes. Blancard, the Ephemerides, Sorbalt, and Vallisneri speak of urination by the mouth. Arnold relates the history of a case of dysuria in which urine was discharged from the nose, breasts, ears, and umbilicus; the woman was twenty-seven years old, and the dysuria was caused by a prolapsed uterus. There was an instance of anomalous discharge of urine from the body reported in Philadelphia many years ago which led to animated discussion. A case of dysuria in which the patient discharged urine from the stomach was reported early in this century from Germany. The patient could feel the accumulation of urine by burning pain in the epigastrium. Suddenly the pain would move to the soles of the feet, she would become nauseated, and large quantities of urine would soon be vomited. There was reported the case of an hysterical female who had convulsions and mania, alternating with anuria of a peculiar nature and lasting seven days. There was not a drop of urine passed during this time, but there were discharges through the mouth of alkaline waters with a strong ammoniacal odor.

Senter reports in a young woman a singular case of ischuria which continued for more than three years; during this time if her urine was not drawn off with the catheter she frequently voided it by vomiting; for the last twenty months she passed much gravel by the catheter; when the use of the instrument was omitted or unsuccessfully applied the vomitus contained gravel. Carlisle mentions a case in which there was vomiting of a fluid containing urea and having the sensible properties of urine. Curious to relate, a cure was effected after ligature of the superior thyroid arteries and sloughing of the thyroid gland. Vomiting of urine is also mentioned by Coley, Domine, Liron, Malago, Zeviani, and Yeats. Marsden reports a case in which, following secondary papular syphilis and profuse spontaneous ptyalism, there was vicarious secretion of the urinary constituents from the skin.

Instances of the anomalous exit of urine caused by congenital malformation or fistulous connections are mentioned in another chapter. Black urine is generally caused by the ingestion of pigmented food or drugs, such as carbolic acid and the anilines. Amatus Lusitanus, Bartholinus, and the Ephemerides speak of black urine after eating grapes or damson plums. The Ephemerides speaks of black urine being a precursor of death, but Piso, Rhodius, and Schenck say it is anomalous and seldom a sign of death. White urine, commonly known as chyluria, is frequently seen, and sometimes results from purulent cystitis. Though containing sediment, the urine looks as if full of milk. A case of this kind was seen in 1895 at the Jefferson Medical College Hospital, Philadelphia, in which the chyluria was due to a communication between the bladder and the thoracic duct.

Ackerman has spoken of metastasis of the tears, and Dixon gives an instance in which crying was not attended by the visible shedding of tears. Salomon reports a case of congenital deficiency of tears. Blood-stained tears were frequently mentioned by the older writers. Recently Cross has written an article on this subject, and its analogy is seen in the next chapter under hemorrhages from the eyes through the lacrimal duct.

The Semen.—The older writers spoke of metastasis of the seminal flow, the issue being by the skin (perspiration) and other routes. This was especially supposed to be the case in satyriasis, in which the preternatural exit was due to superabundance of semen, which could be recognized by its odor. There is no doubt that some people have a distinct seminal odor, a fact that will be considered in the section on "Human Odors."

The Ephemerides, Schurig, and Hoffman report instances of what they call fetid semen (possibly a complication of urethral disease). Paaw speaks of black semen in a negro, and the Ephemerides and Schurig mention instances of dark semen. Blancard records an instance of preternatural exit of semen by the bowel. Heers mentions a similar case caused by urethral fistula. Ingham mentions the escape of semen through the testicle by means of a fistula. Demarquay is the authority on bloody semen.

Andouard mentions an instance of blue bile in a woman, blue flakes being found in her vomit. There was no trace of copper to be found in this case. Andouard says that the older physicians frequently spoke of this occurrence.

Rhodius speaks of the sweat being sweet after eating honey; the Ephemerides and Paullini also mention it. Chromidrosis, or colored sweat, is an interesting anomaly exemplified in numerous reports. Black sweat has been mentioned by Bartholinus, who remarked that the secretion resembled ink; in other cases Galeazzi and Zacutus Lusitanus said the perspiration resembled sooty water. Phosphorescent sweat has been recorded. Paullini and the Ephemerides mention perspiration which was of a leek-green color, and Borellus has observed deep green perspiration. Marcard mentions green perspiration of the feet, possibly due to stains from colored foot-gear. The Ephemerides and Paullini speak of violet perspiration, and Bartholinus has described perspiration which in taste resembled wine.

Sir Benjamin Brodie has communicated the history of a case of a young girl of fifteen on whose face was a black secretion. On attempting to remove it by washing, much pain was caused. The quantity removed by soap and water at one time was sufficient to make four basins of water as black as if with India ink. It seemed to be physiologically analogous to melanosis. The cessation of the secretion on the forehead was followed by the ejection of a similar substance from the bowel, stomach, and kidney. The secretion was more abundant during the night, and at one time in its course an erysipelas-eruption made its appearance. A complete cure ultimately followed.

Purdon describes an Irish married woman of forty, the subject of rheumatic fever, who occasionally had a blue serous discharge or perspiration that literally flowed from her legs and body, and accompanied by a miliary eruption. It was on the posterior portions, and twelve hours previous was usually preceded by a moldy smell and a prickly sensation. On the abdomen and the back of the neck there was a yellowish secretion. In place of catamenia there was a discharge reddish-green in color. The patient denied having taken any coloring matter or chemicals to influence the color of her perspiration, and no remedy relieved her cardiac or rheumatic symptoms.

The first English case of chromidrosis, or colored sweat, was published by Yonge of Plymouth in 1709. In this affection the colored sweating appears symmetrically in various parts of the body, the parts commonly affected being the cheeks, forehead, side of the nose, whole face, chest, abdomen, backs of the hands, finger-tips, and the flexors, flexures at the axillae, groins, and popliteal spaces. Although the color is generally black, nearly every color has been recorded. Colcott Fox reported a genuine case, and Crocker speaks of a case at Shadwell in a woman of forty-seven of naturally dark complexion. The bowels were habitually sluggish, going three or four days at least without action, and latterly the woman had suffered from articular pains. The discolored sweat came out gradually, beginning at the sides of the face, then spreading to the cheeks and forehead. When seen, the upper half of the forehead, the temporal regions, and the skin between the ear and malar eminence were of a blackish-brown color, with slight hyperemia of the adjacent parts; the woman said the color had been almost black, but she had cleaned her face some. There was evidently much fat in the secretion; there was also seborrhea of the scalp. Washing with soap and water had very little effect upon it; but it was removed with ether, the skin still looking darker and redder than normal. After a week's treatment with saline purgatives the discoloration was much less, but the patient still had articular pains, for which alkalies were prescribed; she did not again attend. Crocker also quotes the case of a girl of twenty, originally under Mackay of Brighton. Her affection had lasted a year and was limited to the left cheek and eyebrow. Six months before the patch appeared she had a superficial burn which did not leave a distinct scar, but the surface was slightly granular. The deposit was distinctly fatty, evidently seborrheic and of a sepia-tint. The girl suffered from obstinate constipation, the bowels acting only once a week. The left side flushed more than the right In connection with this case may be mentioned one by White of Harvard, a case of unilateral yellow chromidrosis in a man. Demons gives the history of a case of yellow sweat in a patient with three intestinal calculi.

Wilson says that cases of green, yellow, and blue perspiration have been seen, and Hebra, Rayer, and Fuchs mention instances. Conradi records a case of blue perspiration on one-half the scrotum. Chojnowski records a case in which the perspiration resembled milk.

Hyperidrosis occurs as a symptom in many nervous diseases, organic and functional, and its presence is often difficult of explanation. The following are recent examples: Kustermann reports a case of acute myelitis in which there was profuse perspiration above the level of the girdle-sensation and none at all below. Sharkey reports a case of tumor of the pons varolii and left crus cerebri, in which for months there was excessive generalized perspiration; it finally disappeared without treatment. Hutchinson describes the case of a woman of sixty-four who for four years had been troubled by excessive sweating on the right side of the face and scalp. At times she was also troubled by an excessive flow of saliva, but she could not say if it was unilateral. There was great irritation of the right side of the tongue, and for two years taste was totally abolished. It was normal at the time of examination. The author offered no explanation of this case, but the patient gave a decidedly neurotic history, and the symptoms seem to point with some degree of probability to hysteria. Pope reports a peculiar case in which there were daily attacks of neuralgia preceded by sweating confined to a bald spot on the head. Rockwell reports a case of unilateral hyperidrosis in a feeble old man which he thought due to organic affection of the cervical sympathetic.

Dupont has published an account of a curious case of chronic general hyperidrosis or profuse sweating which lasted upward of six years. The woman thus affected became pregnant during this time and was happily delivered of an infant, which she nursed herself. According to Dupont, this hyperidrosis was independent of any other affection, and after having been combated fruitlessly by various remedies, yielded at last to fluid extract of aconitin.

Myrtle relates the case of a man of seventy-seven, who, after some flying pains and fever, began to sweat profusely and continued to do so until he died from exhaustion at the end of three months from the onset of the sweating. Richardson records another case of the same kind. Crocker quotes the case of a tailor of sixty-five in whom hyperidrosis had existed for thirty-five years. It was usually confined to the hands and feet, but when worst affected the whole body. It was absent as long as he preserved the horizontal posture, but came on directly when he rose; it was always increased in the summer months. At the height of the attack the man lost appetite and spirit, had a pricking sensation, and sometimes minute red papules appeared all over the hand. He had tried almost every variety of treatment, but sulphur did the most good, as it had kept the disease under for twelve months. Latterly, even that failed.

Bachman reports the history of a case of hyperidrosis cured by hypnotism.

Unilateral and localized sweating accompanies some forms of nervous disturbance. Mickle has discussed unilateral sweating in the general paralysis of the insane. Ramskill reports a case of sweating on one side of the face in a patient who was subject to epileptic convulsions. Takacs describes a case of unilateral sweating with proportionate nervous prostration. Bartholow and Bryan report unilateral sweating of the head. Cason speaks of unilateral sweating of the head, face, and neck. Elliotson mentions sweat from the left half of the body and the left extremities only. Lewis reports a case of unilateral perspiration with an excess of temperature of 3.5 degrees F. in the axilla of the perspiring side. Mills, White, Dow, and Duncan also cite instances of unilateral perspiration. Boquis describes a case of unilateral perspiration of the skin of the head and face, and instances of complete unilateral perspiration have been frequently recorded by the older writers,—Tebure, Marcellus Donatus, Paullini, and Hartmann discussing it. Hyperidrosis confined to the hands and feet is quite common.

Instances of bloody sweat and "stigmata" have been known through the ages and are most interesting anomalies. In the olden times there were people who represented that in their own persons they realized at certain periods the agonies of Gethsemane, as portrayed in medieval art, e.g., by pictures of Christ wearing the crown of thorns in Pilate's judgment hall. Some of these instances were, perhaps, of the nature of compensatory hemorrhage, substituting the menses or periodic hemorrhoids, hemoptysis, epistaxis, etc., or possibly purpura. Extreme religious frenzy or deep emotions might have been the indirect cause of a number of these bleeding zealots. There are instances on record in which fear and other similar emotions have caused a sweating of blood, the expression "sweating blood" being not uncommon.

Among the older writers, Ballonius, Marcolini, and Riedlin mention bloody sweat. The Ephemerides speaks of it in front of the hypochondrium. Paullini observed a sailor of thirty, who, falling speechless and faint during a storm on the deck of his ship, sweated a red perspiration from his entire body and which stained his clothes. He also mentions bloody sweat following coitus. Aristotle speaks of bloody sweat, and Pellison describes a scar which periodically opened and sweated blood. There were many cases like this, the scars being usually in the location of Christ's wounds.

De Thou mentions an Italian officer who in 1552, during the war between Henry II of France and Emperor Charles V, was threatened with public execution; he became so agitated that he sweated blood from every portion of the body. A young Florentine about to be put to death by an order of Pope Sixtus V was so overcome with grief that he shed bloody tears and sweated blood. The Ephemerides contains many instances of bloody tears and sweat occasioned by extreme fear, more especially fear of death. Mezeray mentions that the detestable Charles IX of France, being under constant agitation and emotion, sank under a disorder which was accompanied by an exudation of blood from every pore of his body. This was taken as an attempt of nature to cure by bleeding according to the theory of the venesectionists. Fabricius Hildanus mentions a child who, as a rule, never drank anything but water, but once, contrary to her habit, drank freely of white wine, and this was soon followed by hemorrhage from the gums, nose, and skin.

There is a case also related of a woman of forty-five who had lost her only son. One day she fancied she beheld him beseeching her to release his soul from purgatory by prayers and fasting every Friday. The following Friday, which was in the month of August, and for five succeeding Fridays she had a profuse bloody perspiration, the disorder disappearing on Friday, March 8th, of the following year. Pooley says that Maldonato, in his "Commentaries of Four Gospels," mentions a healthy and robust man who on hearing of his sentence of death sweated blood, and Zacchias noted a similar phenomenon in a young man condemned to the flames. Allusion may also be made to St. Luke, who said of Christ that in agony He prayed more earnestly, "and His sweat was, as it were, great drops of blood falling down to the ground."

Pooley quotes the case of a young woman of indolent habit who in a religious fanatical trance sweated blood. The stigmatists were often imposters who artificially opened their scars, and set the example for the really peculiar cases of bloody sweat, which among ignorant people was considered evidence of sympathy with the agony of the Cross.

Probably the best studied case on record is that of Louise Lateau of Bois d'Haine, which, according to Gray, occurred in 1869 in a village of Belgium when the girl was at the age of twenty-three; her previous life had offered nothing remarkable. The account is as follows: "One Friday Louise Lateau noticed that blood was flowing from one side of her chest, and this recurred every Friday. On each

Thursday morning an oval surface about one inch in length on the back of each hand became pink in color and smooth, whilst a similar oval surface on the palm of each hand became of the same hue, and on the upper surface of each foot a pinkish-white square appeared. Examined under a magnifying glass, the epidermis appeared at first without solution of continuity and delicate. About noon on Thursday a vesicle formed on the pink surfaces containing clear serum. In the night between Thursday and Friday, usually between midnight and one o'clock, the flow of blood began, the vesicle first rupturing. The amount of blood lost during the so called stigmata varied, and some observers estimated it at about one and three-quarter pints. The blood itself was of a reddish color, inclining to violet, about the hue therefore, of capillary blood, coagulating in the usual way, and the white and red corpuscles being normal in character and relative proportion. The flow ceased on Saturdays. During the flow of the blood the patient was in a rapt, ecstatic condition. The facial expression was one of absorption and far-off contemplation, changing often to melancholy, terror, to an attitude of prayer or contrition. The patient herself stated that at the beginning of the ecstasy she imagined herself surrounded by a brilliant light; figures then passed before her, and the successive scenes of the crucifixion were panoramically progressive. She saw Christ in person—His clothing, His wounds, His crown of thorns, His cross—as well as the Apostles, the holy women, and the assembled Jews. During the ecstasy the circulation of the skin and heart was regular, although at times a sudden flash or pallor overspread the face, according with the play of the expression. From midday of Thursdays, when she took a frugal meal, until eight o'clock on Saturday mornings the girl took no nourishment, not even water, because it was said that she did not feel the want of it and could not retain anything upon her stomach. During this time the ordinary secretions were suspended."

Fournier mentions a statesman of forty-five who, following great Cabinet labors during several years and after some worriment, found that the day after indulging in sexual indiscretions he would be in a febrile condition, with pains in the thighs, groins, legs, and penis. The veins of these parts became engorged, and subsequently blood oozed from them, the flow lasting several days. The penis was the part most affected. He was under observation for twenty months and presented the same phenomena periodically, except that during the last few months they were diminished in every respect. Fournier also mentions a curious case of diapedesis in a woman injured by a cow. The animal struck her in the epigastric region, she fell unconscious, and soon after vomited great quantities of blood, and continued with convulsive efforts of expulsion to eject blood periodically from every eight to fifteen days, losing possibly a pound at each paroxysm. There was no alteration of her menses. A physician gave her astringents, which partly suppressed the vomiting, but the hemorrhage changed to the skin, and every day she sweated blood from the chest, back of the thighs, feet, and the extremities of the fingers. When the blood ceased to flow from her skin she lost her appetite, became oppressed, and was confined to her bed for some days. Itching always preceded the appearance of a new flow. There was no dermal change that could be noticed.

Fullerton mentions a girl of thirteen who had occasional oozing of blood from her brow, face, and the skin under the eyes. Sometimes a pound of clots was found about her face and pillow. The blood first appeared in a single clot, and, strange to say, lumps of fleshy substance and minute pieces of bone were discharged all day. This latter discharge became more infrequent, the bone being replaced by cartilaginous substance. There was no pain, discoloration, swelling, or soreness, and after this strange anomaly disappeared menstruation regularly commenced. Van Swieten mentions a young lady who from her twelfth year at her menstrual periods had hemorrhages from pustules in the skin, the pustules disappearing in the interval.

Schmidt's Jahrbucher for 1836 gives an account of a woman who had diseased ovaries and a rectovesicovaginal fistula, and though sometimes catamenia appeared at the proper place it was generally arrested and hemorrhage appeared on the face. Chambers mentions a woman of twenty-seven who suffered from bloody sweat after the manner of the stigmatists, and Petrone mentions a young man of healthy antecedents, the sweat from whose axillae and pubes was red and very pungent. Petrone believes it was due to a chromogenic micrococcus, and relieved the patient by the use of a five per cent solution of caustic potash. Chloroform, ether, and phenol had been tried without success. Hebra mentions a young man in whom the blood spurted from the hand in a spiral jet corresponding to the direction of the duct of the sweat-gland. Wilson refers to five cases of bloody sweat.

There is a record of a patient who once or twice a day was attacked with swelling of the scrotum, which at length acquired a deep red color and a stony hardness, at which time the blood would spring from a hundred points and flow in the finest streams until the scrotum was again empty.

Hill describes a boy of four who during the sweating stage of malaria sweated blood from the head and neck. Two months later the skin-hemorrhages ceased and the boy died, vomiting blood and with bloody stools.

Postmortem sweating is described in the Ephemerides and reported by Hasenest and Schneider. Bartholinus speaks of bloody sweat in a cadaver

In considering the anomalies of lactation we shall first discuss those of color and then the extraordinary places of secretion. Black milk is spoken of by the Ephemerides and Paullini. Red milk has been observed by Cramer and Viger. Green milk has been observed by Lanzonius, Riverius, and Paullini. The Ephemerides also contains an account of green milk. Yellow milk has been mentioned in the Ephemerides and its cause ascribed to eating rhubarb.

It is a well-known fact that some cathartics administered to nursing mothers are taken from the breast by their infants, who, notwithstanding its indirect mode of administration, exhibit the effects of the original drug. The same is the case with some poisons, and instances of lead-poisoning and arsenic-poisoning have been seen in children who have obtained the toxic substance in the mother's milk. There is one singular case on record in which a child has been poisoned from the milk of its mother after she had been bitten by a serpent.

Paullini and the Ephemerides give instances of milk appearing in the perspiration, and there are numerous varieties of milk-metastasis recorded Dolaeus and Nuck mention the appearance of milk in the saliva. Autenreith mentions metastasis of milk through an abdominal abscess to the thigh, and Balthazaar also mentions excretion of milk from the thigh. Bourdon mentions milk from the thigh, labia, and vulva. Klein speaks of the metastasis of the milk to the lochia. Gardane speaks of metastasis to the lungs, and there is another case on record in which this phenomenon caused asphyxia. Schenck describes excretion of milk from the bladder and uterus. Jaeger in 1770 at Tubingen describes the metastasis of milk to the umbilicus, Haen to the back, and Schurig to a wound in the foot. Knackstedt has seen an abscess of the thigh which contained eight pounds of milk. Hauser gives the history of a case in which the kidneys secreted milk vicariously.

There is the history of a woman who suffered from metastasis of milk to the stomach, and who, with convulsive action of the chest and abdomen, vomited it daily. A peculiar instance of milk in a tumor is that of a Mrs. Reed, who, when pregnant with twins, developed an abdominal tumor from which 25 pounds of milk was drawn off.

There is a French report of secretion of milk in the scrotum of a man of twenty-one. The scrotum was tumefied, and to the touch gave the sensation of a human breast, and the parts were pigmented similar to an engorged breast. Analysis showed the secretion to have been true human milk.

Cases of lactation in the new-born are not infrequent. Bartholinus, Baricelli, Muraltus, Deusingius, Rhodius, Schenck, and Schurig mention instances of it.

Cardanus describes an infant of one month whose breasts were swollen and gave milk copiously. Battersby cites a description of a male child three weeks old whose breasts were full of a fluid, analysis proving it to have been human milk; Darby, in the same journal, mentions a child of eight days whose breasts were so engorged that the nurse had to milk it. Faye gives an interesting paper in which he has collected many instances of milk in the breasts of the new-born. Jonston details a description of lactation in an infant. Variot mentions milk-secretion in the new-born and says that it generally takes place from the eighth to the fifteenth day and not in the first week. He also adds that probably mammary abscesses in the new-born could be avoided if the milk were squeezed out of the breasts in the first days. Variot says that out of 32 children of both sexes, aged from six to nine months, all but six showed the presence of milk in the breasts. Gibb mentions copious milk-secretion in an infant, and Sworder and Menard have seen young babes with abundant milk-secretion.

Precocious Lactation.—Bochut says that he saw a child whose breasts were large and completely developed, offering a striking contrast to the slight development of the thorax. They were as large as a stout man's fist, pear-shaped, with a rosy areola, in the center of which was a nipple. These precocious breasts increased in size at the beginning of the menstrual epoch (which was also present) and remained enlarged while the menses lasted. The vulva was covered with thick hair and the external genitalia were well developed. The child was reticent, and with a doll was inclined to play the role of mother.

Baudelocque mentions a girl of eight who suckled her brother with her extraordinarily developed breasts. In 1783 this child milked her breasts in the presence of the Royal Academy at Paris. Belloc spoke of a similar case. There is another of a young negress who was able to nourish an infant; and among the older writers we read accounts of young virgins who induced lactation by applying infants to their breasts. Bartholinus, Benedictus, Hippocrates, Lentilius, Salmuth, and Schenck mention lactation in virgins.

De la Coide describes a case in which lactation was present, though menstruation had always been deficient. Dix, at the Derby Infirmary, has observed two females in whom there was continued lactation, although they had never been pregnant. The first was a chaste female of twenty-five, who for two years had abundant and spontaneous discharge of milk that wetted the linen; and the other was in a prostitute of twenty, who had never been pregnant, but who had, nevertheless, for several months an abundant secretion of healthy milk. Zoologists know that a nonpregnant bitch may secrete milk in abundance. Delafond and de Sinnety have cited instances.

Lactation in the aged has been frequently noticed. Amatus Lusitanus and Schenck have observed lactation in old women; in recent years Dunglison has collected some instances. Semple relates the history of an elderly woman who took charge of an infant the mother of which had died of puerperal infection. As a means of soothing the child she allowed it to take the nipple, and, strange to say, in thirty-six hours milk appeared in her breasts, and soon she had a flow as copious as she had ever had in her early married life. The child thrived on this production of a sympathetic and spontaneous lactation. Sir Hans Sloane mentions a lady of sixty-eight who though not having borne a child for twenty years, nursed her grandchildren one after another.

Montegre describes a woman in the Department of Charente who bore two male children in 1810. Not having enough milk for both, and being too poor to secure the assistance of a midwife, in her desperation she sought an old woman named Laverge, a widow of sixty-five, whose husband had been dead twenty-nine years. This old woman gave the breast to one of the children, and in a few days an abundant flow of milk was present. For twenty-two months she nursed the infant, and it thrived as well as its brother, who was nursed by their common mother—in fact, it was even the stronger of the two.

Dargan tells of a case of remarkable rejuvenated lactation in a woman of sixty, who, in play, placed the child to her breast, and to her surprise after three weeks' nursing of this kind there appeared an abundant supply of milk, even exceeding in amount that of the young mother.

Blanchard mentions milk in the breasts of a woman of sixty, and Krane cites a similar instance. In the Philosophical Transactions there is an instance of a woman of sixty-eight having abundant lactation.

Warren, Boring, Buzzi, Stack, Durston, Egan, Scalzi, Fitzpatrick, and Gillespie mention rejuvenation and renewed lactation in aged women. Ford has collected several cases in which lactation was artificially induced by women who, though for some time not having been pregnant themselves, nursed for others.

Prolonged lactation and galactorrhea may extend through several pregnancies. Green reports the case of a woman of forty-seven, the mother of four children, who after each weaning had so much milk constantly in her breasts that it had to be drawn until the next birth. At the time of report the milk was still secreting in abundance. A similar and oft-quoted case was that of Gomez Pamo, who described a woman in whom lactation seemed indefinitely prolonged; she married at sixteen, two years after the establishment of menstruation. She became pregnant shortly after marriage, and after delivery had continued lactation for a year without any sign of returning menstruation. Again becoming pregnant, she weaned her first child and nursed the other without delay or complication. This occurrence took place fourteen times. She nursed all 14 of her children up to the time that she found herself pregnant again, and during the pregnancies after the first the flow of milk never entirely ceased; always after the birth of an infant she was able to nurse it. The milk was of good quality and always abundant, and during the period between her first pregnancy to seven years after the birth of her last child the menses had never reappeared. She weaned her last child five years before the time of report, and since then the milk had still persisted in spite of all treatment. It was sometimes so abundant as to necessitate drawing it from the breast to relieve painful tension.

Kennedy describes a woman of eighty-one who persistently menstruated through lactation, and for forty-seven years had uninterruptedly nursed many children, some of which were not her own. Three years of this time she was a widow. At the last reports she had a moderate but regular secretion of milk in her eighty-first year.

In regard to profuse lacteal flow, Remy is quoted as having seen a young woman in Japan from whom was taken 12 1/2 pints of milk each day, which is possibly one of the most extreme instance of continued galactorrhea on record.

Galen refers to gynecomastia or gynecomazia; Aristotle says he has seen men with mammae a which were as well developed as those of a woman, and Paulus aegineta recognized the fact in the ancient Greeks. Subsequently Albucasis discusses it in his writings. Bartholinus, Behr, Benedictus, Borellus, Bonet, the Ephemerides, Marcellus Donatus, Schenck, Vesalius, Schacher, Martineau, and Buffon all discuss the anomalous presence of milk in the male breast. Puech says that this condition is found in one out of 13,000 conscripts.

To Bedor, a marine surgeon, we owe the first scientific exposition of this subject, and a little later Villeneuve published his article in the French dictionary. Since then many observations have been made on this subject, and quite recently Laurent has published a most exhaustive treatise upon it.

Robert describes an old man who suckled a child, and Meyer discusses the case of a castrated man who was said to suckle children. It is said that a Bishop of Cork, who gave one-half crown to an old Frenchman of seventy, was rewarded by an exhibition of his breasts, which were larger than the Bishop had ever seen in a woman. Petrequin speaks of a male breast 18 inches long which he amputated, and Laurent gives the photograph of a man whose breasts measured 30 cm. in circumference at the base, and hung like those of a nursing woman.

In some instances whole families with supernumerary breasts are seen. Handyside gives two instances of quadruple breasts in brothers. Blanchard speaks of a father who had a supernumerary nipple on each breast and his seven sons had the same deformities; it was not noticed in the daughters. The youngest son transmitted this anomaly to his four sons. Petrequin describes a man with three mammae, two on the left side, the third being beneath the others. He had three sons with accessory mammae on the right side and two daughters with the same anomaly on the left side. Savitzky reports a case of gynecomazia in a peasant of twenty-one whose father, elder brother, and a cousin were similarly endowed. The patient's breasts were 33 cm. in circumference and 15 cm. from the nipple to the base of the gland; they resembled normal female mammae in all respects. The penis and the other genitalia were normal, but the man had a female voice and absence of facial hair. There was an abundance of subcutaneous fat and a rather broad pelvis.

Wiltshire said that he knew a gynecomast in the person of a distinguished naturalist who since the age of puberty observed activity in his breasts, accompanied with secretion of milky fluid which lasted for a period of six weeks and occurred every spring. This authority also mentions that the French call husbands who have well-developed mammae "la couvade;" the Germans call male supernumerary breasts "bauchwarze," or ventral nipples. Hutchinson describes several cases of gynecomazia, in which the external genital organs decreased in proportion to the size of the breast and the manners became effeminate. Cameron, quoted by Snedden, speaks of a fellow-student who had a supernumerary nipple, and also says he saw a case in a little boy who had an extra pair of nipples much wider than the ordinary ones. Ansiaux, surgeon of Liege, saw a conscript of thirteen whose left mamma was well developed like that of a woman, and whose nipple was surrounded by a large areola. He said that this breast had always been larger than the other, but since puberty had grown greatly; the genital organs were well formed. Morgan examined a seaman of twenty-one, admitted to the Royal Naval Hospital at Hong Kong, whose right mamma, in size and conformation, had the appearance of the well developed breast of a full-grown woman. It was lobulated and had a large, brown-colored areola; the nipple, however, was of the same size as that on the left breast. The man stated that he first observed the breast to enlarge at sixteen and a half years; since that time it had steadily increased, but there was no milk at any time from the nipple; the external genital organs were well and fully developed. He complained of no pain or uneasiness except when in drilling aloft his breast came in contact with the ropes.

Gruger of St. Petersburg divides gynecomazia into three classes:—

(1) That in which the male generative organs are normal;

(2) In which they are deformed;

(3) In which the anomaly is spurious, the breast being a mass of fat or a new growth.

The same journal quotes an instance (possibly Morgan's case) in a young man of twenty-one with a deep voice, excellent health, and genitals well developed, and who cohabited with his wife regularly. When sixteen his right breast began to enlarge, a fact that he attributed to the pressure of a rope. Glandular substance could be distinctly felt, but there was no milk-secretion. The left breast was normal. Schuchardt has collected 272 cases of gynecomazia.

Instances of Men Suckling Infants.—These instances of gynecomazia are particularly interesting when the individuals display ability to suckle infants. Hunter refers to a man of fifty who shared equally with his wife the suckling of their children. There is an instance of a sailor who, having lost his wife, took his son to his own breast to quiet him, and after three or four days was able to nourish him. Humboldt describes a South American peasant of thirty-two who, when his wife fell sick immediately after delivery, sustained the child with his own milk, which came soon after the application to the breast; for five months the child took no other nourishment. In Franklin's "Voyages to the Polar Seas" he quotes the instance of an old Chippewa who, on losing his wife in childbirth, had put his infant to his breast and earnestly prayed that milk might flow; he was fortunate enough to eventually produce enough milk to rear the child. The left breast, with which he nursed, afterward retained its unusual size. According to Mehliss some missionaries in Brazil in the sixteenth century asserted that there was a whole Indian nation whose women had small and withered breasts, and whose children owed their nourishment entirely to the males. Hall exhibited to his class in Baltimore a negro of fifty-five who had suckled all his mistress' family. Dunglison reports this case in 1837, and says that the mammae projected seven inches from the chest, and that the external genital organs were well developed. Paullini and Schenck cite cases of men suckling infants, and Blumenbach has described a male-goat which, on account of the engorgement of the mammae, it was necessary to milk every other day of the year.

Ford mentions the case of a captain who in order to soothe a child's cries put it to his breast, and who subsequently developed a full supply of milk. He also quotes an instance of a man suckling his own children, and mentions a negro boy of fourteen who secreted milk in one breast. Hornor and Pulido y Fernandez also mention similar instances of gynecomazia.

Human Odors.—Curious as it may seem, each individual as well as each species is in life enveloped with an odor peculiarly its own, due to its exhaled breath, its excretions, and principally to its insensible perspiration. The faculty of recognizing an odor in different individuals, although more developed in savage tribes, is by no means unknown in civilized society. Fournier quotes the instance of a young man who, like a dog, could smell the enemy by scent, and who by smell alone recognized his own wife from other persons.

Fournier also mentions a French woman, an inhabitant of Naples, who had an extreme supersensitiveness of smell. The slightest odor was to her intolerable; sometimes she could not tolerate the presence of certain individuals. She could tell in a numerous circle which women were menstruating. This woman could not sleep in a bed which any one else had made, and for this reason discharged her maid, preparing her own toilet and her sleeping apartments. Cadet de Gassieourt witnessed this peculiar instance, and in consultation with several of the physicians of Paris attributed this excessive sensitiveness to the climate. There is a tale told of a Hungarian monk who affirmed that he was able to decide the chastity of females by the sense of smell alone. It is well known that some savage tribes with their large, open nostrils not only recognize their enemies but also track game the same as hounds.

Individual Odors.—Many individuals are said to have exhaled particularly strong odors, and history is full of such instances. We are told by Plutarch that Alexander the Great exhaled an odor similar to that of violet flowers, and his undergarments always smelled of this natural perfume. It is said that Cujas offered a particular analogy to this. On the contrary, there are certain persons spoken of who exhaled a sulphurous odor. Martial said that Thais was an example of the class of people whose odor was insupportable. Schmidt has inserted in the Ephemerides an account of a journeyman saddler, twenty-three years of age, of rather robust constitution, whose hands exhaled a smell of sulphur so powerful and penetrating as to rapidly fill any room in which he happened to be. Rayer was once consulted by a valet-de-chambre who could never keep a place in consequence of the odor he left behind him in the rooms in which he worked.

Hammond is quoted with saying that when the blessed Venturni of Bergamons officiated at the altar people struggled to come near him in order to enjoy the odor he exhaled. It was said that St. Francis de Paul, after he had subjected himself to frequent disciplinary inflictions, including a fast of thirty-eight to forty days, exhaled a most sensible and delicious odor. Hammond attributes the peculiar odors of the saints of earlier days to neglect of washing and, in a measure, to affections of the nervous system. It may be added that these odors were augmented by aromatics, incense, etc., artificially applied. In more modern times Malherbe and Haller were said to diffuse from their bodies the agreeable odor of musk. These "human flowers," to use Goethe's expression, are more highly perfumed in Southern latitudes.

Modifying Causes.—According to Brieude, sex, age, climate, habits, ailments, the passions, the emotions, and the occupations modify the difference in the humors exhaled, resulting in necessarily different odors. Nursing infants have a peculiar sourish smell, caused by the butyric acid of the milk, while bottle-fed children smell like strong butter. After being weaned the odors of the babies become less decided. Boys when they reach puberty exhibit peculiar odors which are similar to those of animals when in heat. These odors are leading symptoms of what Borden calls "seminal fever" and are more strongly marked in those of a voluptuous nature. They are said to be caused by the absorption of spermatic fluid into the circulation and its subsequent elimination by the skin. This peculiar circumstance, however, is not seen in girls, in whom menstruation is sometimes to be distinguished by an odor somewhat similar to that of leather. Old age produces an odor similar to that of dry leaves, and there have been persons who declared that they could tell approximately the age of individuals by the sense of smell.

Certain tribes and races of people have characteristic odors. Negroes have a rank ammoniacal odor, unmitigated by cleanliness; according to Pruner-Bey it is due to a volatile oil set free by the sebaceous follicles. The Esquimaux and Greenlanders have the odors of their greasy and oily foods, and it is said that the Cossacks, who live much with their horses, and who are principally vegetarians, will leave the atmosphere charged with odors several hours after their passage in numbers through a neighborhood. The lower race of Chinamen are distinguished by a peculiar musty odor, which may be noticed in the laundry shops of this country. Some people, such as the low grade of Indians, have odors, not distinctive, and solely due to the filth of their persons. Food and drink, as have been mentioned, markedly influence the odor of an individual, and those perpetually addicted to a special diet or drink have a particular odor.

Odor after Coitus.—Preismann in 1877 makes the statement that for six hours after coitus there is a peculiar odor noticeable in the breath, owing to a peculiar secretion of the buccal glands. He says that this odor is most perceptible in men of about thirty-five, and can be discerned at a distance of from four to six feet. He also adds that this fact would be of great medicolegal value in the early arrest of those charged with rape. In this connection the analogy of the breath immediately after coitus to the odor of chloroform has been mentioned. The same article states that after coitus naturally foul breath becomes sweet.

The emotions are said to have a decided influence on the odor of an individual. Gambrini, quoted by Monin, mentions a young man, unfortunate in love and violently jealous, whose whole body exhaled a sickening, pernicious, and fetid odor. Orteschi met a young lady who, without any possibility of fraud, exhaled the strong odor of vanilla from the commissures of her fingers.

Rayer speaks of a woman under his care at the Hopital de la Charite affected with chronic peritonitis, who some time before her death exhaled a very decided odor of musk. The smell had been noticed several days, but was thought to be due to a bag of musk put purposely into the bed to overpower other bad smells. The woman, however, gave full assurance that she had no kind of perfume about her and that her clothes had been frequently changed. The odor of musk in this case was very perceptible on the arms and other portions of the body, but did not become more powerful by friction. After continuing for about eight days it grew fainter and nearly vanished before the patient's death. Speranza relates a similar case.

Complexion.—Pare states that persons of red hair and freckled complexion have a noxious exhalation; the odor of prussic acid is said to come from dark individuals, while blondes exhale a secretion resembling musk. Fat persons frequently have an oleaginous smell.

The disorders of the nervous system are said to be associated with peculiar odors. Fevre says the odor of the sweat of lunatics resembles that of yellow deer or mice, and Knight remarks that the absence of this symptom would enable him to tell whether insanity was feigned or not. Burrows declares that in the absence of further evidence he would not hesitate to pronounce a person insane if he could perceive certain associate odors. Sir William Gull and others are credited with asserting that they could detect syphilis by smell. Weir Mitchell has observed that in lesions of nerves the corresponding cutaneous area exhaled the odor of stagnant water. Hammond refers to three cases under his notice in which specific odors were the results of affections of the nervous system. One of these cases was a young woman of hysterical tendencies who exhaled the odor of violets, which pervaded her apartments. This odor was given off the left half of the chest only and could be obtained concentrated by collecting the perspiration on a handkerchief, heating it with four ounces of spirit, and distilling the remaining mixture. The administration of the salicylate of soda modified in degree this violaceous odor. Hammond also speaks of a young lady subject to chorea whose insensible perspiration had an odor of pineapples; a hypochondriac gentleman under his care smelled of violets. In this connection he mentions a young woman who, when suffering from intense sick headache, exhaled an odor resembling that of Limburger cheese.

Barbier met a case of disordered innervation in a captain of infantry, the upper half of whose body was subject to such offensive perspiration that despite all treatment he had to finally resign his commission.

In lethargy and catalepsy the perspiration very often has a cadaverous odor, which has probably occasionally led to a mistaken diagnosis of death. Schaper and de Meara speak of persons having a cadaveric odor during their entire life.

Various ingesta readily give evidence of themselves by their influence upon the breath. It has been remarked that the breath of individuals who have recently performed a prolonged necropsy smells for some hours of the odor of the cadaver. Such things as copaiba, cubebs, sandalwood, alcohol, coffee, etc., have their recognizable fragrance. There is an instance of a young woman taking Fowler's solution who had periodic offensive axillary sweats that ceased when the medicine was discontinued.

Henry of Navarre was a victim of bromidrosis; proximity to him was insufferable to his courtiers and mistresses, who said that his odor was like that of carrion. Tallemant says that when his wife, Marie de Medicis, approached the bridal night with him she perfumed her apartments and her person with the essences of the flowers of her country in order that she might be spared the disgusting odor of her spouse. Some persons are afflicted with an excessive perspiration of the feet which often takes a disgusting odor. The inguinoscrotal and inguinovulvar perspirations have an aromatic odor like that of the genitals of either sex.

During menstruation, hyperidrosis of the axillae diffuses an aromatic odor similar to that of acids or chloroform, and in suppression of menses, according to the Ephemerides, the odor is as of hops.

Odors of Disease.—The various diseases have their own peculiar odors. The "hospital odor," so well known, is essentially variable in character and chiefly due to an aggregation of cutaneous exhalations. The wards containing women and children are perfumed with butyric acid, while those containing men are influenced by the presence of alkalies like ammonia.

Gout, icterus, and even cholera (Drasch and Porker) have their own odors. Older observers, confirmed by Doppner, say that all the plague-patients at Vetlianka diffused an odor of honey. In diabetes there is a marked odor of apples. The sweat in dysentery unmistakably bears the odor of the dejecta. Behier calls the odor of typhoid that of the blood, and Berard says that it attracts flies even before death. Typhus has a mouse-like odor, and the following diseases have at different times been described as having peculiar odors,—measles, the smell of freshly plucked feathers; scarlatina, of bread hot from the oven; eczema and impetigo, the smell of mold; and rupia, a decidedly offensive odor.

The hair has peculiar odors, differing in individuals. The hair of the Chinese is known to have the odor of musk, which cannot be washed away by the strongest of chemicals. Often the distinctive odor of a female is really due to the odor of great masses of hair. It is said that wig-makers simply by the sense of smell can tell whether hair has been cut from the living head or from combings, as hair loses its odor when it falls out. In the paroxysms of hysteroepilepsy the hair sometimes has a specific odor of ozone. Taenia favosa gives to the scalp an odor resembling that of cat's urine.

Sexual Influence of Odors.—In this connection it may be mentioned that there is a peculiar form of sexual perversion, called by Binet "fetichism," in which the subject displays a perverted taste for the odors of handkerchiefs, shoes, underclothing, and other articles of raiment worn by the opposite sex. Binet maintains that these articles play the part of the "fetich" in early theology. It is said that the favors given by the ladies to the knights in the Middle Ages were not only tokens of remembrance and appreciation, but sexual excitants as well. In his remarkable "Osphresiologie," Cloquet calls attention to the sexual pleasure excited by the odors of flowers, and tells how Richelieu excited his sexual functions by living in an atmosphere loaded with these perfumes. In the Orient the harems are perfumed with intense extracts and flowers, in accordance with the strong belief in the aphrodisiac effect of odors.

Krafft-Ebing quotes several interesting cases in which the connection between the olfactory and sexual functions is strikingly verified.

"The case of Henry III shows that contact with a person's perspiration may be the exciting cause of passionate love. At the betrothal feast of the King of Navarre and Margaret of Valois he accidentally dried his face with a garment of Maria of Cleves which was moist with her perspiration. Although she was the bride of the Prince of Conde, Henry immediately conceived such a passion for her that he could not resist it, and, as history shows, made her very unhappy. An analogous instance is related of Henry IV, whose passion for the beautiful Gabrielle is said to have originated at the instant when, at a ball, he wiped his brow with her handkerchief."

Krafft-Ebing also says that "one learns from reading the work of Ploss ('Das Weib') that attempts to attract a person of the opposite sex by means of the perspiration may be discerned in many forms in popular psychology. In reference to this a custom is remarkable which holds among the natives of the Philippine Islands when they become engaged. When it becomes necessary for the engaged pair to separate they exchange articles of wearing apparel, by means of which each becomes assured of faithfulness. These objects are carefully preserved, covered with kisses, and smelled."

The love of perfumes by libertines and prostitutes, as well as sensual women of the higher classes, is quite marked. Heschl reported a case of a man of forty-five in whom absence of the olfactory sense was associated with imperfect development of the genitals; it is also well known that olfactory hallucinations are frequently associated with psychoses of an erotic type.

Garnier has recently collected a number of observations of fetichism, in which he mentions individuals who have taken sexual satisfaction from the odors of shoes, night-dresses, bonnets, drawers, menstrual napkins, and other objects of the female toilet. He also mentions creatures who have gloated over the odors of the blood and excretions from the bodies of women, and gives instances of fetichism of persons who have been arrested in the streets of Paris for clipping the long hair from young girls. There are also on record instances of homosexual fetichism, a type of disgusting inversion of the sexual instinct, which, however, it is not in the province of this work to discuss.

Among animals the influence of the olfactory perceptions on the sexual sense is unmistakable. According to Krafft Ebing, Althaus shows that animals of opposite sexes are drawn to each other by means of olfactory perceptions, and that almost all animals at the time of rutting emit a very strong odor from their genitals. It is said that the dog is attracted in this way to the bitch several miles away. An experiment by Schiff is confirmatory. He extirpated the olfactory nerves of puppies, and found that as they grew the male was unable to distinguish the female. Certain animals, such as the musk-ox, civet-cat, and beaver, possess glands on their sexual organs that secrete materials having a very strong odor. Musk, a substance possessing the most penetrating odor and used in therapeutics, is obtained from the preputial follicles of the musk-deer of Thibet; and castor, a substance less penetrating, is obtained from the preputial sacs of the beaver. Virgin moths (Bombyx) carried in boxes in the pockets of entomologists will on wide commons cause the appearance of males of the same species.

Bulimia is excessive morbid hunger, also called canine appetite. While sometimes present in healthy people, it is most often seen in idiots and the insane, and is a symptom of diabetes mellitus. Mortimer mentions a boy of twelve who, while laboring under this affliction, in six days devoured food to the extent of 384 pounds and two ounces. He constantly vomited, but his craving for food was so insatiable that if not satisfied he would devour the flesh off his own bones. Martyn, Professor of Botany at Cambridge in the early part of the last century, tells of a boy ten years old whose appetite was enormous. He consumed in one week 373 pounds of food and drink. His urine and stools were voided in normal quantities, the excess being vomited. A pig was fed on what he vomited, and was sold in the market. The boy continued in this condition for a year, and at last reports was fast failing. Burroughs mentions a laborer at Stanton, near Bury, who ate an ordinary leg of veal at a meal, and fed at this extravagant rate for many days together. He would eat thistles and other similar herbs greedily. At times he would void worms as large as the shank of a clay-pipe, and then for a short period the bulimia would disappear.

Johnston mentions a case of bulimia in a man who devoured large quantities of raw flesh. There is an instance on record of a case of canine appetite in which nearly 400 pounds of solid and fluid elements were taken into the body in six days and again ejected. A recovery was effected by giving very concentrated food, frequently repeated in small quantities. Mason mentions a woman in St. Bartholomew's Hospital in London in the early part of this century who was wretched unless she was always eating. Each day she consumed three quartern-loaves, three pounds of beef-steak, in addition to large quantities of vegetables, meal, etc., and water. Smith describes a boy of fourteen who ate continuously fifteen hours out of the twenty-four, and who had eight bowel movements each day. One year previous his weight was 105 pounds, but when last seen he weighed 284 pounds and was increasing a half pound daily. Despite his continuous eating, this boy constantly complained of hunger.

Polydipsia is an abnormal thirst; it may be seen in persons otherwise normal, or it may be associated with diseases—such as diabetes mellitus or diabetes insipidus. Mackenzie quotes a case from Trousseau, in which an individual afflicted with diabetes insipidus passed 32 liters of urine daily and drank enormous quantities of water. This patient subjected himself to severe regimen for eight months,—although one day, in his agonies, he seized the chamber-pot and drank its contents at once. Mackenzie also mentions an infant of three who had polydipsia from birth and drank daily nearly two pailfuls of water. At the age of twenty-two she married a cobbler, unaware of her propensity, who found that his earnings did not suffice to keep her in water alone, and he was compelled to melt ice and snow for her. She drank four pailfuls a day, the price being 12 sous; water in the community was scarce and had to be bought. This woman bore 11 children. At the age of forty she appeared before a scientific commission and drank in their presence 14 quarts of water in ten hours and passed ten quarts of almost colorless urine. Dickinson mentions that he has had patients in his own practice who drank their own urine. Mackenzie also quotes Trousseau's history of a man who drank a liter of strong French brandy in two hours, and habitually drank the same quantity daily. He stated that he was free from the effects of alcohol; on several occasions on a wager he took 20 liters of wine, gaining his wager without visibly affecting his nervous system.

There is an instance of a man of fifty-eight who could not live through the night without a pail of water, although his health was otherwise good. Atkinson in 1856 reported a young man who in childhood was a dirt-eater, though at that time complaining of nothing but excessive thirst. He was active, industrious, enjoyed good health, and was not addicted to alcoholics. His daily ration of water was from eight to twelve gallons. He always placed a tub of water by his bed at night, but this sometimes proved insufficient. He had frequently driven hogs from mudholes to slake his thirst with the water. He married in 1829 and moved into Western Tennessee, and in 1854 he was still drinking the accustomed amount; and at this time he had grown-up children. Ware mentions a young man of twenty who drank six gallons of water daily. He was tormented with thirst, and if he abstained he became weak, sick, and dizzy. Throughout a long life he continued his habit, sometimes drinking a gallon at one draught; he never used spirits. There are three cases of polydipsia reported from London in 1792.

Field describes a boy with bilious remittent fever who would drink until his stomach was completely distended and then call for more. Emesis was followed by cries for more water. Becoming frantic, he would jump from his bed and struggle for the water bucket; failing in this, he ran to the kitchen and drank soapsuds, dishwater, and any other liquid he could find. He had swallowed a mass of mackerel which he had not properly masticated, a fact proved later by ejection of the whole mass. There is a case on record a in which there was intolerable thirst after retiring, lasting for a year. There was apparently no polydipsia during the daytime.

The amount of water drunk by glass-blowers in a day is almost incredible. McElroy has made observations in the glass-factories in his neighborhood, and estimates that in the nine working hours of each day a glass-blower drinks from 50 to 60 pints of water. In addition to this many are addicted to the use of beer and spirits after working hours and at lunch-time. The excreta and urine never seem to be perceptibly increased. When not working these men do not drink more than three or four pints of water. Occasionally a man becomes what is termed "blown-up with water;" that is, the perspiration ceases, the man becomes utterly helpless, has to be carried out, and is disabled until the sweating process is restored by vigorously applied friction. There is little deleterious change noticed in these men; in fact, they are rarely invalids.

Hydroadipsia is a lack of thirst or absence of the normal desire for water. In some of these cases there is a central lesion which accounts for the symptoms. McElroy, among other cases, speaks of one in a patient who was continually dull and listless, eating little, and complaining of much pain after the least food. This, too, will be mentioned under abstinence.

Perverted appetites are of great variety and present many interesting as well as disgusting examples of anomalies. In some cases the tastes of people differ so that an article considered by one race as disgusting would be held as a delicacy by another class. The ancients used asafetida as a seasoning, and what we have called "stercus diaboli," the Asiatics have named the "food of the gods." The inhabitants of Greenland drink the oil of the whale with as much avidity as we would a delicate wine, and they eat blubber the mere smell of which nauseates an European. In some nations of the lower grade, insects, worms, serpents, etc., are considered edible. The inhabitants of the interior of Africa are said to relish the flesh of serpents and eat grubs and worms. The very earliest accounts of the Indians of Florida and Texas show that "for food, they dug roots, and that they ate spiders, ants' eggs, worms, lizards, salamanders, snakes, earth, wood, the dung of deer, and many other things." Gomara, in his "Historia de les Indias," says this loathsome diet was particular to one tribe, the Yagusces of Florida. It is said that a Russian peasant prefers a rotten egg to a fresh one; and there are persons who prefer game partly spoiled.

Bourke recalls that the drinking of human urine has often been a religious rite, and describes the urine-dance of the Zunis of New Mexico, in which the participants drink freely of their urine; he draws an analogy to the Feast of the Fools, a religious custom of Pagan origin which did not disappear in Europe until the time of the Reformation. It is still a practice in some parts of the United States to give children fresh urine for certain diseases. It is said that the ordure of the Grand Lama of Thibet was at one time so venerated that it was collected and worn as amulets.

The disgusting habit of eating human excrement is mentioned by Schurig, who gives numerous examples in epileptics, maniacs, chlorotic young women, pregnant women, children who have soiled their beds and, dreading detection, have swallowed their ejecta, and finally among men and women with abnormal appetites. The Indians of North America consider a broth made from the dung of the hare and caribou a dainty dish, and according to Abbe Domenech, as a means of imparting a flavor, the bands near Lake Superior mix their rice with the excrement of rabbits. De Bry mentions that the negroes of Guinea ate filthy, stinking elephant-meat and buffalo-flesh infested with thousands of maggots, and says that they ravenously devoured dogs' guts raw. Spencer, in his "Descriptive Sociology," describes a "Snake savage" of Australia who devoured the contents of entrails of an animal. Some authors have said that within the last century the Hottentots devoured the flesh and the entrails of wild beasts, uncleansed of their filth and excrement, and whether sound or rotten. In a personal letter to Captain Bourke, the Reverend J. Owen Dorsey reports that while among the Ponkas he saw a woman and child devour the entrails of a beef with their contents. Bourke also cites instances in which human ordure was eaten by East Indian fanatics. Numerous authorities are quoted by Bourke to prove the alleged use of ordure in food by the ancient Israelites. Pages of such reference are to be found in the works on Scatology, and for further reference the reader is referred to books on this subject, of which prominent in English literature is that of Bourke.

Probably the most revolting of all the perverted tastes is that for human flesh. This is called anthropophagy or cannibalism, and is a time-honored custom among some of the tribes of Africa. This custom is often practised more in the spirit of vengeance than of real desire for food. Prisoners of war were killed and eaten, sometimes cooked, and among some tribes raw. In their religious frenzy the Aztecs ate the remains of the human beings who were sacrificed to their idols. At other times cannibalism has been a necessity. In a famine in Egypt, as pictured by the Arab Abdullatif, the putrefying debris of animals, as well as their excrement, was used as food, and finally the human dead were used; then infants were killed and devoured, so great was the distress. In many sieges, shipwrecks, etc., cannibalism has been practiced as a last resort for sustaining life. When supplies have given out several Arctic explorers have had to resort to eating the bodies of their comrades. In the famous Wiertz Museum in Brussels is a painting by this eccentric artist in which he has graphically portrayed a woman driven to insanity by hunger, who has actually destroyed her child with a view to cannibalism. At the siege of Rochelle it is related that, urged by starvation, a father and mother dug up the scarcely cold body of their daughter and ate it. At the siege of Paris by Henry IV the cemeteries furnished food for the starving. One mother in imitation of what occurred at the siege of Jerusalem roasted the limbs of her dead child and died of grief under this revolting nourishment.

St. Jerome states that he saw Scotchmen in the Roman armies in Gaul whose regular diet was human flesh, and who had "double teeth all around."

Cannibalism, according to a prominent New York journal, has been recently made a special study by the Bureau of Ethnology at Washington, D.C. Data on the subject have been gathered from all parts of the world, which are particularly interesting in view of discoveries pointing to the conclusion that this horrible practice is far more widespread than was imagined. Stanley claims that 30,000,000 cannibals dwell in the basin of the Congo to-day—people who relish human flesh above all other meat. Perah, the most peculiar form of cannibalism, is found in certain mountainous districts of northeast Burmah, where there are tribes that follow a life in all important respects like that of wild beasts. These people eat the congealed blood of their enemies. The blood is poured into bamboo reeds, and in the course of time, being corked up, it hardens. The filled reeds are hung under the roofs of the huts, and when a person desires to treat his friends very hospitably the reeds are broken and the contents devoured.

"The black natives of Australia are all professed cannibals. Dr. Carl Lumholtz, a Norwegian scientist, spent many months in studying them in the wilds of the interior. He was alone among these savages, who are extremely treacherous. Wearing no clothing whatever, and living in nearly every respect as monkeys do, they know no such thing as gratitude, and have no feeling that can be properly termed human. Only fear of the traveler's weapons prevented them from slaying him, and more than once he had a narrow escape. One of the first of them whom he employed looked more like a brute than a man. 'When he talked,' says the doctor, 'he rubbed his belly with complacency, as if the sight of me made his mouth water.' This individual was regarded with much respect by his fellows because of his success in procuring human flesh to eat. These aborigines say that the white man's flesh is salt and occasions nausea. A Chinaman they consider as good for eating as a black man, his food being chiefly vegetable.

"The most horrible development of cannibalism among the Australian blacks is the eating of defunct relatives. When a person dies there follows an elaborate ceremony, which terminates with the lowering of the corpse into the grave. In the grave is a man not related to the deceased, who proceeds to cut off the fat adhering to the muscles of the face, thighs, arms, and stomach, and passes it around to be swallowed by some of the near relatives. All those who have eaten of the cadaver have a black ring of charcoal powder and fat drawn around the mouth. The order in which the mourners partake of their dead relatives is duly prescribed. The mother eats of her children and the children of their mother. A man eats of his sister's husband and of his brother's wife. Mothers' brothers, mothers' sisters, sisters' children, mothers' parents, and daughters' children are also eaten by those to whom the deceased person stands in such relation. But the father does not eat of his children, nor the children of their sire.

"The New Zealanders, up to very recent times, were probably the most anthropophagous race that ever existed. As many as 1000 prisoners have been slaughtered by them at one time after a successful battle, the bodies being baked in ovens underground. If the individual consumed had been a redoubtable enemy they dried his head as a trophy and made flutes of his thigh bones.

"Among the Monbuttos of Africa human fat is commonly employed for a variety of purposes. The explorer Schweinfurth speaks of writing out in the evenings his memoranda respecting these people by the light of a little oil-lamp contrived by himself, which was supplied with some questionable-looking grease furnished by the natives. The smell of this grease, he says, could not fail to arouse one's worst suspicions against the negroes. According to his account the Monbuttos are the most confirmed cannibals in Africa. Surrounded as they are by a number of peoples who are blacker than themselves, and who, being inferior to them in culture, are held in contempt, they carry on expeditions of war and plunder which result in the acquisition of a booty especially coveted by them—namely, human flesh. The bodies of all foes who fall in battle are distributed on the field among the victors, and are prepared by drying for transportation. The savages drive their prisoners before them, and these are reserved for killing at a later time. During Schweinfurth's residence at the Court of Munza it was generally understood that nearly every day a little child was sacrificed to supply a meal for the ogre potentate. For centuries past the slave trade in the Congo Basin has been conducted largely for the purpose of furnishing human flesh to consumers. Slaves are sold and bought in great numbers for market, and are fattened for slaughter.

"The Mundurucus of the Upper Amazon, who are exceedingly ferocious, have been accused of cannibalism. It is they who preserve human heads in such a remarkable way. When one of their warriors has killed an enemy he cuts off the head with his bamboo knife, removes the brain, soaks the head in a vegetable oil, takes out bones of the skull, and dries the remaining parts by putting hot pebbles inside of it. At the same time care is taken to preserve all the features and the hair intact. By repeating the process with the hot pebbles many times the head finally becomes shrunken to that of a small doll, though still retaining its human aspect, so that the effect produced is very weird and uncanny. Lastly, the head is decorated with brilliant feathers, and the lips are fastened together with a string, by which the head is suspended from the rafters of the council-house."

Ancient Customs.—According to Herodotus the ancient Lydians and Medes, and according to Plato the islanders in the Atlantic, cemented friendship by drinking human blood. Tacitus speaks of Asian princes swearing allegiance with their own blood, which they drank. Juvenal says that the Scythians drank the blood of their enemies to quench their thirst.

Occasionally a religious ceremony has given sanction to cannibalism. It is said that in the Island of Chios there was a rite by way of sacrifice to Dionysius in which a man was torn limb from limb, and Faber tells us that the Cretans had an annual festival in which they tore a living bull with their teeth. Spencer quotes that among the Bacchic orgies of many of the tribes of North America, at the inauguration of one of the Clallum chiefs on the northwest coast of British America, the chief seized a small dog and began to devour it alive, and also bit the shoulders of bystanders. In speaking of these ceremonies, Boas, quoted by Bourke, says that members of the tribes practicing Hamatsa ceremonies show remarkable scars produced by biting, and at certain festivals ritualistic cannibalism is practiced, it being the duty of the Hamatsa to bite portions of flesh out of the arms, legs, or breast of a man.

Another cause of cannibalism, and the one which deserves discussion here, is genuine perversion or depravity of the appetite for human flesh among civilized persons,—the desire sometimes being so strong as to lead to actual murder. Several examples of this anomaly are on record. Gruner of Jena speaks of a man by the name of Goldschmidt, in the environs of Weimar, who developed a depraved appetite for human flesh. He was married at twenty-seven, and for twenty-eight years exercised his calling as a cow-herd. Nothing extraordinary was noticed in him, except his rudeness of manner and his choleric and gross disposition. In 1771, at the age of fifty-five, he met a young traveler in the woods, and accused him of frightening his cows; a discussion arose, and subsequently a quarrel, in which Goldschmidt killed his antagonist by a blow with a stick which he used. To avoid detection he dragged the body to the bushes, cut it up, and took it home in sections. He then washed, boiled, and ate each piece. Subsequently, he developed a further taste for human flesh, and was finally detected in eating a child which he had enticed into his house and killed. He acknowledged his appetite before his trial.

Hector Boetius says that a Scotch brigand and his wife and children were condemned to death on proof that they killed and ate their prisoners. The extreme youth of one of the girls excused her from capital punishment; but at twelve years she was found guilty of the same crime as her father and suffered capital punishment. This child had been brought up in good surroundings, yet her inherited appetite developed. Gall tells of an individual who, instigated by an irresistible desire to eat human flesh, assassinated many persons; and his daughter, though educated away from him, yielded to the same graving.

At Bicetre there was an individual who had a horribly depraved appetite for decaying human flesh. He would haunt the graveyards and eat the putrefying remains of the recently buried, preferring the intestines. Having regaled himself in a midnight prowl, he would fill his pockets for future use. When interrogated on the subject of his depravity he said it had existed since childhood. He acknowledged the greatest desire to devour children he would meet playing; but he did not possess the courage to kill them.

Prochaska quotes the case of a woman of Milan who attracted children to her home in order that she might slay, salt, and eat them. About 1600, there is the record of a boy named Jean Granier, who had repeatedly killed and devoured several young children before he was discovered. Rodericus a Castro tells of a pregnant woman who so strongly desired to eat the shoulder of a baker that she killed him, salted his body, and devoured it at intervals.

There is a record of a woman who in July, 1817, was discovered in cooking an amputated leg of her little child. Gorget in 1827 reported the celebrated case of Leger the vine dresser, who at the age of twenty-four wandered about a forest for eight days during an attack of depression. Coming across a girl of twelve, he violated her, and then mutilated her genitals, and tore out her heart, eating of it, and drinking the blood. He finally confessed his crime with calm indifference. After Leger's execution Esquirol found morbid adhesions between the brain and the cerebral membranes. Mascha relates a similar instance in a man of fifty-five who violated and killed a young girl, eating of her genitals and mammae. At the trial he begged for execution, saying that the inner impulse that led him to his crime constantly persecuted him.

A modern example of lust-murder and anthropophagy is that of Menesclou, who was examined by Brouardel, Motet, and others, and declared to be mentally sound; he was convicted. This miscreant was arrested with the forearm of a missing child in his pocket, and in his stove were found the head and entrails in a half-burnt condition. Parts of the body were found in the water-closet, but the genitals were missing; he was executed, although he made no confession, saying the deed was an accident. Morbid changes were found in his brain. Krafft-Ebing cites the case of Alton, a clerk in England, who lured a child into a thicket, and after a time returned to his office, where he made an entry in his note-book: "Killed to-day a young girl; it was fine and hot." The child was missed, searched for, and found cut into pieces. Many parts, and among them the genitals, could not be found. Alton did not show the slightest trace of emotion, and gave no explanation of the motive or circumstances of his horrible deed; he was executed.

D'Amador tells of persons who went into slaughter-houses and waste-places to dispute with wolves for the most revolting carrion. It is also mentioned that patients in hospitals have been detected in drinking the blood of patients after venesections, and in other instances frequenting dead-houses and sucking the blood of the recently deceased. Du Saulle quotes the case of a chlorotic girl of fourteen who eagerly drank human blood. She preferred that flowing fresh from a recent wound.

Further Examples of Depraved Appetites.—Bijoux speaks of a porter or garcon at the Jardin des Plantes in Paris who was a prodigious glutton. He had eaten the body of a lion that had died of disease at the menagerie. He ate with avidity the most disgusting things to satiate his depraved appetite. He showed further signs of a perverted mind by classifying the animals of the menagerie according to the form of their excrement, of which he had a collection. He died of indigestion following a meal of eight pounds of hot bread.

Percy saw the famous Tarrare, who died at Versailles, at about twenty-six years of age. At seventeen he weighed 100 pounds. He ate a quarter of beef in twenty-four hours. He was fond of the most revolting things. He particularly relished the flesh of serpents and would quickly devour the largest. In the presence of Lorenze he seized a live cat with his teeth, eventrated it, sucked its blood, and ate it, leaving the bare skeleton only. In about thirty minutes he rejected the hairs in the manner of birds of prey and carnivorous animals. He also ate dogs in the same manner. On one occasion it was said that he swallowed a living eel without chewing it; but he had first bitten off its head. He ate almost instantly a dinner that had been prepared for 15 vigorous workmen and drank the accompanying water and took their aggregate allowance of salt at the same time. After this meal his abdomen was so swollen that it resembled a balloon. He was seen by Courville, a surgeon-major in a military hospital, where he had swallowed a wooden box wrapped in plain white paper. This he passed the next day with the paper intact. The General-in-chief had seen him devour thirty pounds of raw liver and lungs. Nothing seemed to diminish his appetite. He waited around butcher-shops to eat what was discarded for the dogs. He drank the bleedings of the hospital and ate the dead from the dead-houses. He was suspected of eating a child of fourteen months, but no proof could be produced of this. He was of middle height and was always heated and sweating. He died of a purulent diarrhea, all his intestines and peritoneum being in a suppurating condition.

Fulton mentions a girl of six who exhibited a marked taste for feeding on slugs, beetles, cockroaches, spiders, and repulsive insects. This child had been carefully brought up and was one of 13 children, none of whom displayed any similar depravity of appetite. The child was of good disposition and slightly below the normal mental standard for her age. At the age of fourteen her appetite became normal.

In the older writings many curious instances of abnormal appetite are seen. Borellus speaks of individuals swallowing stones, horns, serpents, and toads. Plater mentions snail-eating and eel-eating, two customs still extant. Rhodius is accredited with seeing persons who swallowed spiders and scorpions. Jonston says that Avicenna, Rufus, and Gentilis relate instances of young girls who acquired a taste for poisonous animals and substances, who could ingest them with impunity. Colonia Agrippina was supposed to have eaten spiders with impunity. Van Woensel is said to have seen persons who devoured live eels.

The habit of dirt eating or clay-eating, called pica, is well authenticated in many countries. The Ephemerides contains mention of it; Hunter speaks of the blacks who eat potters' clay; Bartholinus describes dirt-eating as does also a Castro. Properly speaking, dirt-eating should be called geophagism; it is common in the Antilles and South America, among the low classes, and is seen in the negroes and poorest classes of some portions of the Southern United States. It has also been reported from Java, China, Japan, and is said to have been seen in Spain and Portugal. Peat-eating or bog-eating is still seen in some parts of Ireland.

There were a number of people in the sixteenth and seventeenth centuries who had formed the habit of eating small pebbles after each meal. They formed the habit from seeing birds swallowing gravel after eating. A number of such cases are on record.

There is on record the account of a man living in Wurtemberg who with much voracity had eaten a suckling pig, and sometimes devoured an entire sheep. He swallowed dirt, clay, pebbles, and glass, and was addicted to intoxication by brandy. He lived sixty years in this manner and then he became abstemious; he died at seventy-nine. His omentum was very lean, but the liver covered all his abdominal viscera. His stomach was very large and thick, but the intestines were very narrow.

Ely had a patient who was addicted to chalk-eating; this ha said invariably relieved his gastric irritation. In the twenty-five years of the habit he had used over 1/2 ton of chalk; but notwithstanding this he always enjoyed good health. The Ephemerides contains a similar instance, and Verzascha mentions a lime-eater. Adams mentions a child of three who had an instinctive desire to eat mortar. This baby was rickety and had carious teeth. It would pick its preferred diet out of the wall, and if prevented would cry loudly. When deprived of the mortar it would vomit its food until this substance was given to it again. At the time of report part of the routine duties of the sisters of this boy was to supply him with mortar containing a little sand. Lime-water was substituted, but he insisted so vigorously on the solid form of food that it had to be replaced in his diet. He suffered from small-pox; on waking up in the night with a fever, he always cried for a piece of mortar. The quantity consumed in twenty-four hours was about 1/2 teacupful. The child had never been weaned.

Arsenic Eaters.—It has been frequently stated that the peasants of Styria are in the habit of taking from two to five grains of arsenious acid daily for the purpose of improving the health, avoiding infection, and raising the whole tone of the body. It is a well-substantiated fact that the quantities taken habitually are quite sufficient to produce immediate death ordinarily. But the same might be easily said of those addicted to opium and chloral, a subject that will be considered later. Perverted appetites during pregnancy have been discussed on pages 80 and 81.

Glass-eaters, penknife-swallowers, and sword-swallowers, being exhibitionists and jugglers, and not individuals with perverted appetites, will be considered in Chapter XII.

Fasting.—The length of time which a person can live with complete abstinence from food is quite variable. Hippocrates admits the possibility of fasting more than six days without a fatal issue; but Pliny and others allow a much longer time, and both the ancient and modern literature of medicine are replete with examples of abstinence to almost incredible lengths of time. Formerly, and particularly in the Middle Ages when religious frenzy was at its highest pitch, prolonged abstinence was prompted by a desire to do penance and to gain the approbation of Heaven.

In many religions fasting has become a part of worship or religions ceremony, and from the earliest times certain sects have carried this custom to extremes. It is well known that some of the priests and anchorites of the East now subsist on the minimum amount of food, and from the earliest times before the advent of Christianity we find instances of prolonged fasting associated with religious worship. The Assyrians, the Hebrews, the Egyptians, and other Eastern nations, and also the Greeks and Romans, as well as feasting days, had their times of fasting, and some of these were quite prolonged.

At the present day religious fervor accounts for but few of our remarkable instances of abstinence, most of them being due to some form of nervous disorder, varying from hysteria and melancholia to absolute insanity. The ability seen in the Middle Ages to live on the Holy Sacrament and to resist starvation may possibly have its analogy in some of the fasting girls of the present day. In the older times these persons were said to have been nourished by angels or devils; but according to Hammond many cases both of diabolical abstinence from food and of holy fasting exhibited manifest signs of hysteric symptoms. Hammond, in his exhaustive treatise on the subject of "Fasting Girls," also remarks that some of the chronicles detail the exact symptoms of hysteria and without hesitation ascribe them to a devilish agency. For instance, he speaks of a young girl in the valley of Calepino who had all her limbs twisted and contracted and had a sensation in her esophagus as if a ball was sometimes rising in her throat or falling into the stomach—a rather lay description of the characteristic hysteric "lump in the throat," a frequent sign of nervous abstinence.

Abstinence, or rather anorexia, is naturally associated with numerous diseases, particularly of the febrile type; but in all of these the patient is maintained by the use of nutrient enemata or by other means, and the abstinence is never complete.

A peculiar type of anorexia is that striking and remarkable digestive disturbance of hysteria which Sir William Gull has called anorexia nervosa. In this malady there is such annihilation of the appetite that in some cases it seems impossible ever to eat again. Out of it grows an antagonism to food which results at last, and in its worst forms, in spasm on the approach of food, and this in its turn gives rise to some of those remarkable cases of survival for long periods without food. As this goes on there may be an extreme degree of muscular restlessness, so that the patients wander about until exhausted. According to Osler, who reports a fatal case in a girl who, at her death, only weighed 49 pounds, nothing more pitiable is to be seen in medical practice than an advanced case of this malady. The emaciation and exhaustion are extreme, and the patient is as miserable as one with carcinoma of the esophagus, food either not being taken at all or only upon urgent compulsion.

Gull mentions a girl of fourteen, of healthy, plump appearance, who in the beginning of February, 1887, without apparent cause evinced a great repugnance to food and soon afterward declined to take anything but a half cup of tea or coffee. Gull saw her in April, when she was much emaciated; she persisted in walking through the streets, where she was the object of remark of passers-by. At this time her height was five feet four inches, her weight 63 pounds, her temperature 97 degrees F., her pulse 46, and her respiration from 12 to 14. She had a persistent wish to be moving all the time, despite her emaciation and the exhaustion of the nutritive functions.

There is another class of abstainers from food exemplified in the exhibitionists who either for notoriety or for wages demonstrate their ability to forego eating, and sometimes drinking, for long periods. Some have been clever frauds, who by means of artifices have carried on skilful deceptions; others have been really interesting physiologic anomalies.

Older Instances.—Democritus in 323 B.C. is said to have lived forty days by simply smelling honey and hot bread. Hippocrates remarks that most of those who endeavored to abstain five days died within that period, and even if they were prevailed upon to eat and drink before the termination of their fast they still perished. There is a possibility that some of these cases of Hippocrates were instances of pyloric carcinoma or of stenosis of the pylorus. In the older writings there are instances reported in which the period of abstinence has varied from a short time to endurance beyond the bounds of credulity. Hufeland mentions total abstinence from food for seventeen days, and there is a contemporary case of abstinence for forty days in a maniac who subsisted solely on water and tobacco. Bolsot speaks of abstinence for fourteen months, and Consbruch mentions a girl who fasted eighteen months. Muller mentions an old man of forty-five who lived six weeks on cold water. There is an instance of a person living in a cave twenty-four days without food or drink, and another of a man who survived five weeks' burial under ruins. Ramazzini speaks of fasting sixty-six days; Willian, sixty days (resulting in death); von Wocher, thirty-seven days (associated with tetanus); Lantana, sixty days; Hobbes, forty days; Marcardier, six months; Cruikshank, two months; the Ephemerides, thirteen months; Gerard, sixty-nine days (resulting in death); and in 1722 there was recorded an instance of abstinence lasting twenty-five months.

Desbarreaux-Bernard says that Guillaume Granie died in the prison of Toulouse in 1831, after a voluntary suicidal abstinence of sixty-three days.

Haller cites a number of examples of long abstinence, but most extraordinary was that of a girl of Confolens, described by Citois of Poitiers, who published a history of the case in the beginning of the seventeenth century. This girl is said to have passed three entire years, from eleven to fourteen, without taking any kind of aliment. In the "Harleian Miscellanies" is a copy of a paper humbly offered to the Royal Society by John Reynolds, containing a discourse upon prodigious abstinence, occasioned by the twelve months' fasting of a woman named Martha Taylor, a damsel of Derbyshire. Plot gives a great variety of curious anecdotes of prolonged abstinence. Ames refers to "the true and admirable history of the maiden of Confolens," mentioned by Haller. In the Annual Register, vol. i., is an account of three persons who were buried five weeks in the snow; and in the same journal, in 1762, is the history of a girl who is said to have subsisted nearly four years on water. In 1684 four miners were buried in a coal-pit in Horstel, a half mile from Liege, Belgium, and lived twenty-four days without food, eventually making good recoveries. An analysis of the water used during their confinement showed an almost total absence of organic matter and only a slight residue of calcium salts.

Joanna Crippen lay six days in the snow without nutriment, being overcome by the cold while on the way to her house; she recovered despite her exposure. Somis, physician to the King of Sardinia, gives an account of three women of Piedmont, Italy, who were saved from the ruins of a stable where they had been buried by an avalanche of snow, March 19, 1765. thirty-seven days before. Thirty houses and 22 inhabitants were buried in this catastrophe, and these three women, together with a child of two, were sheltered in a stable over which the snow lodged 42 feet deep. They were in a manger 20 inches broad and upheld by a strong arch. Their enforced position was with their backs to the wall and their knees to their faces. One woman had 15 chestnuts, and, fortunately, there were two goats near by, and within reach some hay, sufficient to feed them for a short time. By milking one of the goats which had a kid, they obtained about two pints daily, upon which they subsisted for a time. They quenched their thirst with melted snow liquefied by the heat of their hands. Their sufferings were greatly increased by the filth, extreme cold, and their uncomfortable positions; their clothes had rotted. When they were taken out their eyes were unable to endure the light and their stomachs at first rejected all food.

While returning from Cambridge, February 2, 1799, Elizabeth Woodcock dismounted from her horse, which ran away, leaving her in a violent snowstorm. She was soon overwhelmed by an enormous drift six feet high. The sensation of hunger ceased after the first day and that of thirst predominated, which she quenched by sucking snow. She was discovered on the 10th of February, and although suffering from extensive gangrene of the toes, she recovered. Hamilton says that at a barracks near Oppido, celebrated for its earthquakes, there were rescued two girls, one sixteen and the other eleven; the former had remained under the ruins without food for eleven days. This poor creature had counted the days by a light coming through a small opening. The other girl remained six days under the ruin in a confined and distressing posture, her hands pressing her cheek until they had almost made a hole in it. Two persons were buried under earthquake ruins at Messina for twenty-three and twenty-two days each.

Thomas Creaser gives the history of Joseph Lockier of Bath, who, while going through a woods between 6 and 7 P.M., on the 18th of August, was struck insensible by a violent thunderbolt. His senses gradually returned and he felt excessively cold. His clothes were wet, and his feet so swollen that the power of the lower extremities was totally gone and that of the arms was much impaired. For a long time he was unable to articulate or to summon assistance. Early in September he heard some persons in the wood and, having managed to summon them in a feeble voice, told them his story. They declared him to be an impostor and left him. On the evening of the same day his late master came to his assistance and removed him to Swan Inn. He affirmed that during his exposure in the woods he had nothing to eat; though distressing at first, hunger soon subsided and yielded to thirst, which he appeased by chewing grass having beads of water thereon. He slept during the warmth of the day, but the cold kept him awake at night. During his sleep he dreamt of eating and drinking. On November 17, 1806, several surgeons of Bath made an affidavit, in which they stated that this man was admitted to the Bath City Dispensary on September 15th, almost a month after his reputed stroke, in an extremely emaciated condition, with his legs and thighs shriveled as well as motionless. There were several livid spots on his legs and one toe was gangrenous. After some time they amputated the toe. The power in the lower extremities soon returned.

In relating his travels in the Levant, Hasselquist mentions 1000 Abyssinians who became destitute of provisions while en route to Cairo, and who lived two months on gum arabic alone, arriving at their destination without any unusual sickness or mortality. Dr. Franklin lived on bread and water for a fortnight, at the rate of ten pounds per week, and maintained himself stout and healthy. Sir John Pringle knew a lady of ninety who lived on pure fat meat. Glower of Chelmsford had a patient who lived ten years on a pint of tea daily, only now or then chewing a half dozen raisins or almonds, but not swallowing them. Once in long intervals she took a little bread.

Brassavolus describes a younger daughter of Frederick King of Naples who lived entirely without meat, and could not endure even the taste of it, as often as she put any in her mouth she fell fainting. The monks of Monte Santo (Mount Athos) never touched animal food, but lived on vegetables, olives, end cheese. In 1806 one of them at the age of one hundred and twenty was healthy.

Sometimes in the older writings we find records of incredible abstinence. Jonston speaks of a man in 1460 who, after an unfortunate matrimonial experience, lived alone for fifteen years, taking neither food nor drink. Petrus Aponensis cites the instance of a girl fasting for eight years. According to Jonston, Hermolus lived forty years on air alone. This same author has also collected cases of abstinence lasting eleven, twenty-two, and thirty years and cites Aristotle as an authority in substantiating his instances of fasting girls.

Wadd, the celebrated authority on corpulence, quotes Pennant in mentioning a woman in Rosshire who lived one and three-quarters years without meat or drink. Granger had under observation a woman by the name of Ann Moore, fifty-eight years of age, who fasted for two years. Fabricius Hildanus relates of Apollonia Schreiera that she lived three years without meat or drink. He also tells of Eva Flegen, who began to fast in 1596, and from that time on for sixteen years, lived without meat or drink. According to the Rev. Thos. Steill, Janet Young fasted sixteen years and partially prolonged her abstinence for fifty years. The Edinburgh Medical and Surgical Journal, which contains a mention of the foregoing case, also describes the case of Janet Macleod, who fasted for four years, showing no signs of emaciation. Benjamin Rush speaks of a case mentioned in a letter to St. George Tucker, from J. A. Stuart, of a man who, after receiving no benefit from a year's treatment for hemiplegia, resolved to starve himself to death. He totally abstained from food for sixty days, living on water and chewing apples, but spitting out the pulp; at the expiration of this time he died. Eccles relates the history of a beautiful young woman of sixteen, who upon the death of a most indulgent father refused food for thirty-four days, and soon afterward for fifty-four days, losing all her senses but that of touch.

There is an account of a French adventurer, the Chevalier de Saint-Lubin, who had a loathing for food and abstained from every kind of meat and drink for fifty-eight days. Saint-Sauver, at that time Lieutenant of the Bastille, put a close watch on this man and certified to the verity of the fast. The European Magazine in

1783 contained an account of the Calabria earthquake, at which time a girl of eighteen was buried under ruins for six days. The edge of a barrel fell on her ankle and partly separated it, the dust and mortar effectually stopping the hemorrhage. The foot dropped off and the wound healed without medical assistance, the girl making a complete recovery. There is an account taken from a document in the Vatican of a man living in 1306, in the reign of Pope Clement V, who fasted for two years. McNaughton mentions Rubin Kelsey, a medical student afflicted with melancholia, who voluntarily fasted for fifty-three days, drinking copiously and greedily of water. For the first six weeks he walked about, and was strong to the day of his death.

Hammond has proved many of the reports of "fasting girls" to have been untrustworthy. The case of Miss Faucher of Brooklyn, who was supposed to have taken no food for fourteen years, was fraudulent. He says that Ann Moore was fed by her daughter in several ways; when washing her mother's face she used towels wet with gravy, milk, or strong arrow-root meal. She also conveyed food to her mother by means of kisses. One of the "fasting girls," Margaret Weiss, although only ten years old, had such powers of deception that after being watched by the priest of the parish, Dr. Bucoldianus, she was considered free from juggling, and, to everybody's astonishment, she grew, walked, and talked like other children of her age, still maintaining that she used neither food nor drink. In several other cases reported all attempts to discover imposture failed. As we approach more modern times the detection is more frequent. Sarah Jacobs, the Welsh fasting girl who attained such celebrity among the laity, was taken to Guy's Hospital on December 9, 1869, and after being watched by eight experienced nurses for eight days she died of starvation. A postmortem examination of Anna Garbero of Racconis, in Piedmont, who died on May 19, 1828, after having endured a supposed fast of two years, eight months, and eleven days, revealed remarkable intestinal changes. The serous membranes were all callous and thickened, and the canal of the sigmoid flexure was totally obliterated. The mucous membranes were all soft and friable, and presented the appearance of incipient gangrene.

Modern Cases.—Turning now to modern literature, we have cases of marvelous abstinence well substantiated by authoritative evidence. Dickson describes a man of sixty-two, suffering from monomania, who refused food for four months, but made a successful recovery. Richardson mentions a case, happening in 1848, of a man of thirty-three who voluntarily fasted for fifty-five days. His reason for fasting, which it was impossible to combat, was that he had no gastric juice and that it was utterly useless for him to take any nutrition, as he had no means of digesting it. He lived on water until the day of his death. Richardson gives an interesting account of the changes noticed at the necropsy. There is an account of a religious mendicant of the Jain caste who as a means of penance fasted for ninety-one days. The previous year he had fasted eighty-six days. He had spent his life in strict asceticism, and during his fasting he was always engrossed in prayer.

Collins describes a maiden lady of eighty, always a moderate eater, who was attacked by bronchitis, during which she took food as usual. Two days after her recovery, without any known cause, she refused all food and continued to do so for thirty-three days, when she died. She was delirious throughout this fast and slept daily seven or eight hours. As a rule, she drank about a wineglassful of water each day and her urine was scanty and almost of the consistency of her feces. There is a remarkable case of a girl of seventeen who, suffering with typhoid fever associated with engorgement of the abdomen and suppression of the functions of assimilation, fasted for four months without visible diminution in weight. Pierce reports the history of a woman of twenty-six who fasted for three months and made an excellent recovery.

Grant describes the "Market Harborough fasting-girl," a maiden of nineteen, who abstained from food from April, 1874, until December, 1877, although continually using morphia. Throughout her fast she had periodic convulsions, and voided no urine or feces for twelve months before her death. There was a middle-aged woman in England in 1860 who for two years lived on opium, gin, and water. Her chief symptoms were almost daily sickness and epileptic fits three times a week. She was absolutely constipated, and at her death her abdomen was so distended as to present the appearance of ascites. After death, the distention of the abdomen was found to be due to a coating of fat, four inches thick, in the parietes. There was no obstruction to the intestinal canal and no fecal or other accumulation within it. Christina Marshall, a girl of fourteen, went fifteen and one-half months without taking solid nourishment. She slept very little, seldom spoke, but occasionally asked the time of day. She took sweets and water, with beef tea at intervals, and occasionally a small piece of orange. She died April 18, 1882, after having been confined to her bed for a long while.

King, a surgeon, U.S.A., gives an account of the deprivation of a squad of cavalry numbering 40. While scouting for Indians on the plains they went for eighty-six hours without water; when relieved their mouths and throats were so dry that even brown sugar would not dissolve on their tongues. Many were delirious, and all had drawn fresh blood from their horses. Despite repeated vomiting, some drank their own urine. They were nearly all suffering from overpowering dyspnea, two were dead, and two were missing. The suffering was increased by the acrid atmosphere of the dry plains; the slightest exercise in this climate provoked a thirst. MacLoughlin, the surgeon in charge of the S.S. City of Chester, speaks of a young stowaway found by the stevedores in an insensible condition after a voyage of eleven days. The man was brought on deck and revived sufficiently to be sent to St. Vincent's Hospital, N.Y., about one and one-half hours after discovery, in an extremely emaciated, cold, and nearly pulseless condition. He gave his name as John Donnelly, aged twenty, of Dumbarton, Scotland. On the whole voyage he had nothing to eat or drink. He had found some salt, of which he ate two handfuls, and he had in his pocket a small flask, empty. Into this flask he voided his urine, and afterward drank it. Until the second day he was intensely hungry, but after that time was consumed by a burning thirst; he shouted four or five hours every day, hoping that he might be heard. After this he became insensible and remembered nothing until he awakened in the hospital where, under careful treatment, he finally recovered.

Fodere mentions some workmen who were buried alive fourteen days in a cold, damp cavern under a ruin, and yet all lived. There is a modern instance of a person being buried thirty-two days beneath snow, without food. The Lancet notes that a pig fell off Dover Cliff and was picked up alive one hundred and sixty days after, having been partially imbedded in debris. It was so surrounded by the chalk of the cliff that little motion was possible, and warmth was secured by the enclosing material. This animal had therefore lived on its own fat during the entire period.

Among the modern exhibitionists may be mentioned Merlatti, the fasting Italian, and Succi, both of whom fasted in Paris; Alexander Jacques, who fasted fifty days; and the American, Dr. Tanner, who achieved great notoriety by a fast of forty days, during which time he exhibited progressive emaciation. Merlatti, who fasted in Paris in 1886, lost 22 pounds in a month; during his fast of fifty days he drank only pure filtered water. Prior to the fast his farewell meal consisted of a whole fat goose, including the bones, two pounds of roast beef, vegetables for two, and a plate of walnuts, the latter eaten whole. Alexander Jacques fasted fifty days and Succi fasted forty days. Jacques lost 28 pounds and 4 ounces (from 142 pounds, 8 ounces to 114 pounds, 4 ounces), while Succi's loss was 34 pounds and 3 ounces. Succi diminished in height from 65 3/4 to 64 1/2 inches, while Jacques increased from 64 1/2 to 65 1/2 inches. Jacques smoked cigarettes incessantly, using 700 in the fifty days, although, by professional advice, he stopped the habit on the forty-second day. Three or four times a day he took a powder made of herbs to which he naturally attributed his power of prolonging life without food. Succi remained in a room in which he kept the temperature at a very high point. In speaking of Succi's latest feat a recent report says: "It has come to light in his latest attempt to go for fifty days without food that he privately regaled himself on soup, beefsteak, chocolate, and eggs. It was also discovered that one of the 'committee,' who were supposed to watch and see that the experiment was conducted in a bona fide manner, 'stood in' with the faster and helped him deceive the others. The result of the Vienna experiment is bound to cast suspicion on all previous fasting accomplishments of Signor Succi, if not upon those of his predecessors."

Although all these modern fasters have been accused of being jugglers and deceivers, throughout their fasts they showed constant decrease in weight, and inspection by visitors was welcomed at all times. They invariably invited medical attention, and some were under the closest surveillance; although we may not implicitly believe that the fasts were in every respect bona fide, yet we must acknowledge that these men displayed great endurance in their apparent indifference for food, the deprivation of which in a normal individual for one day only causes intense suffering.

Anomalies of Temperature.—In reviewing the reports of the highest recorded temperatures of the human body, it must be remembered that no matter how good the evidence or how authentic the reference there is always chance for malingering. It is possible to send the index of an ordinary thermometer up to the top in ten or fifteen seconds by rubbing it between the slightly moistened thumb and the finger, exerting considerable pressure at the time. There are several other means of artificially producing enormous temperatures with little risk of detection, and as the sensitiveness of the thermometer becomes greater the easier is the deception.

Mackenzie reports the temperature-range of a woman of forty-two who suffered with erysipelatous inflammation of a stump of the leg. Throughout a somewhat protracted illness, lasting from February 20 to April 22, 1879, the temperature many times registered between 108 degrees and 111 degrees F. About a year later she was again troubled with the stump, and this time the temperature reached as high as 114 degrees. Although under the circumstances, as any rational physician would, Mackenzie suspected fraud, he could not detect any method of deception. Finally the woman confessed that she had produced the temperature artificially by means of hot-water bottles, poultices, etc.

MacNab records a case of rheumatic fever in which the temperature was 111.4 degrees F. as indicated by two thermometers, one in the axilla and the other in the groin. This high degree of temperature was maintained after death. Before the Clinical Society of London, Teale reported a case in which, at different times, there were recorded temperatures from 110 degrees to 120 degrees F. in the mouth, rectum, and axilla. According to a comment in the Lancet, there was no way that the patient could have artificially produced this temperature, and during convalescence the thermometer used registered normal as well as subnormal temperatures. Caesar speaks of a girl of fifteen with enteric fever, whose temperature, on two occasions 110 degrees F., reached the limit of the mercury in the thermometer.

There have been instances mentioned in which, in order to escape duties, prisoners have artificially produced high temperatures, and the same has occasionally been observed among conscripts in the army or navy. There is an account of a habit of prisoners of introducing tobacco into the rectum, thereby reducing the pulse to an alarming degree and insuring their exemption from labor. In the Adelaide Hospital in Dublin there was a case in which the temperature in the vagina and groin registered from 120 degrees to 130 degrees, and one day it reached 130.8 degrees F.; the patient recovered. Ormerod mentions a nervous and hysteric woman of thirty-two, a sufferer with acute rheumatism, whose temperature rose to 115.8 degrees F. She insisted on leaving the hospital when her temperature was still 104 degrees.

Wunderlich mentions a case of tetanus in which the temperature rose to 46.40 degrees C. (115.5 degrees F.), and before death it was as high as 44.75 degrees C. Obernier mentions 108 degrees F. in typhoid fever. Kartulus speaks of a child of five, with typhoid fever, who at different times had temperatures of 107 degrees, 108 degrees, and 108.2 degrees F.; it finally recovered. He also quotes a case of pyemia in a boy of seven, whose temperature rose to 107.6 degrees F. He also speaks of Wunderlich's case of remittent fever, in which the temperature reached 107.8 degrees F. Wilson Fox, in mentioning a case of rheumatic fever, says the temperature reached 110 degrees F.

Philipson gives an account of a female servant of twenty-three who suffered from a neurosis which influenced the vasomotor nervous system, and caused hysteria associated with abnormal temperatures. On the evening of July 9th her temperature was 112 degrees F.; on the 16th, it was 111 degrees; on the 18th, 112 degrees; on the 24th, 117 degrees (axilla); on the 28th, in the left axilla it was 117 degrees, in the right axilla, 114 degrees, and in the mouth, 112 degrees; on the 29th, it was 115 degrees in the right axilla, 110 degrees in the left axilla, and 116 degrees in the mouth The patient was discharged the following September. Steel of Manchester speaks of a hysteric female of twenty, whose temperature was 116.4 degrees. Mahomed mentions a hysteric woman of twenty-two at Guy's Hospital, London, with phthisis of the left lung, associated with marked hectic fevers. Having registered the limit of the ordinary thermometers, the physicians procured one with a scale reaching to 130 degrees F. She objected to using the large thermometers, saying they were "horse thermometers." On October 15, 1879, however, they succeeded in obtaining a temperature of 128 degrees F. with the large thermometer. In March of the following year she died, and the necropsy revealed nothing indicative of a cause for these enormous temperatures. She was suspected of fraud, and was closely watched in Guy's Hospital, but never, in the slightest way, was she detected in using artificial means to elevate the temperature record.

In cases of insolation it is not at all unusual to see a patient whose temperature cannot be registered by an ordinary thermometer. Any one who has been resident at a hospital in which heat-cases are received in the summer will substantiate this. At the Emergency Hospital in Washington, during recent years, several cases have been brought in which the temperatures were above the ordinary registering point of the hospital thermometers, and one of the most extraordinary cases recovered.

At a meeting of the Association of American Physicians in 1895, Jacobi of New York reported a case of hyperthermy reaching 148 degrees F. This instance occurred in a profoundly hysteric fireman, who suffered a rather severe injury as the result of a fall between the revolving rods of some machinery, and was rendered unconscious for four days. Thereafter he complained of various pains, bloody expectoration, and had convulsions at varying intervals, with loss of consciousness, rapid respiration, unaccelerated pulse, and excessively high temperature, the last on one occasion reaching the height of 148 degrees F. The temperature was taken carefully in the presence of a number of persons, and all possible precautions were observed to prevent deception. The thermometer was variously placed in the mouth, anus, axilla, popliteal space, groin, urethra, and different instruments were from time to time employed. The behavior of the patient was much influenced by attention and by suggestion. For a period of five days the temperature averaged continuously between 120 degrees and 125 degrees F.

In the discussion of the foregoing case, Welch of Baltimore referred to a case that had been reported in which it was said that the temperature reached as high as 171 degrees F. These extraordinary elevations of temperature, he said, appear physically impossible when they are long continued, as they are fatal to the life of the animal cell.

In the same connection Shattuck of Boston added that he had observed a temperature of 117 degrees F.; every precaution had been taken to prevent fraud or deception. The patient was a hysteric young woman.

Jacobi closed the discussion by insisting that his observations had been made with the greatest care and precautions and under many different circumstances. He had at first viewed the case with skepticism, but he could not doubt the results of his observation. He added, that although we cannot explain anomalies of this kind, this constitutes no reason why we should deny their occurrence.

Duffy records one of the lowest temperatures on record in a negress of thirty-five who, after an abortion, showed only 84 degrees F. in the mouth and axillae. She died the next day.

The amount of external heat that a human being can endure is sometimes remarkable, and the range of temperature compatible with life is none the less extraordinary. The Esquimaux and the inhabitants of the extreme north at times endure a temperature of—60 degrees F., while some of the people living in equatorial regions are apparently healthy at a temperature as high as 130 degrees F., and work in the sun, where the temperature is far higher. In the engine-rooms of some steamers plying in tropical waters temperatures as high as 150 degrees F. have been registered, yet the engineers and the stokers become habituated to this heat and labor in it without apparent suffering. In Turkish baths, by progressively exposing themselves to graduated temperatures, persons have been able to endure a heat considerably above the boiling point, though having to protect their persons from the furniture and floors and walls of the rooms. The hot air in these rooms is intensely dry, provoking profuse perspiration. Sir Joseph Banks remained some time in a room the temperature of which was 211 degrees F., and his own temperature never mounted above normal.

There have been exhibitionists who claimed particular ability to endure intense heats without any visible disadvantage. These men are generally styled "human salamanders," and must not be confounded with the "fire-eaters," who, as a rule, are simply jugglers. Martinez, the so-called "French Salamander," was born in Havana. As a baker he had exposed himself from boyhood to very high temperatures, and he subsequently gave public exhibitions of his extraordinary ability to endure heat. He remained in an oven erected in the middle of the Gardens of Tivoli for fourteen minutes when the temperature in the oven was 338 degrees F. His pulse on entering was 76 and on coming out 130. He often duplicated this feat before vast assemblages, though hardly ever attaining the same degree of temperature, the thermometer generally varying from 250 degrees F. upward. Chamouni was the celebrated "Russian Salamander," assuming the title of "The Incombustible." His great feat was to enter an oven with a raw leg of mutton, not retiring until the meat was well baked. This person eventually lost his life in the performance of this feat; his ashes were conveyed to his native town, where a monument was erected over them. Since the time of these two contemporaneous salamanders there have been many others, but probably none have attained the same notoriety.

In this connection Tillet speaks of some servant girls to a baker who for fifteen minutes supported a temperature of 270 degrees F.; for ten minutes, 279 degrees F.; and for several minutes, 364 degrees F., thus surpassing Martinez. In the Glasgow Medical Journal, 1859, there is an account of a baker's daughter who remained twelve minutes in an oven at 274 degrees F. Chantrey, the sculptor, and his workman are said to have entered with impunity a furnace of over 320 degrees F.

In some of the savage ceremonies of fire worship the degree of heat endured by the participants is really remarkable, and even if the rites are performed by skilful juggling, nevertheless, the ability to endure intense heat is worthy of comment. A recent report says:—

"The most remarkable ceremonial of fire worship that survives in this country is practiced by the Navajos. They believe in purification by fire, and to this end they literally wash themselves in it. The feats they perform with it far exceed the most wonderful acts of fire-eating and fire-handling accomplished by civilized jugglers. In preparation for the festival a gigantic heap of dry wood is gathered from the desert. At the appointed moment the great pile of inflammable brush is lighted and in a few moments the whole of it is ablaze. Storms of sparks fly 100 feet or more into the air, and ashes fall about like a shower of snow. The ceremony always takes place at night and the effect of it is both weird and impressive.

"Just when the fire is raging at its hottest a whistle is heard from the outer darkness and a dozen warriors, lithe and lean, dressed simply in narrow white breechcloths and moccasins and daubed with white earth so as to look like so many living statues, come bounding through the entrance to the corral that incloses the flaming heap. Yelping like wolves, they move slowly toward the fire, bearing aloft slender wands tipped with balls of eagle-down. Rushing around the fire, always to the left, they begin thrusting their wands toward the fire, trying to burn off the down from the tips. Owing to the intensity of the heat this is difficult to accomplish. One warrior dashes wildly toward the fire and retreats; another lies as close to the ground as a frightened lizard, endeavoring to wriggle himself up to the fire; others seek to catch on their wands the sparks that fly in the air. At last one by one they all succeed in burning the downy balls from the wands. The test of endurance is very severe, the heat of the fire being so great.

"The remarkable feats, however, are performed in connection with another dance that follows. This is heralded by a tremendous blowing of horns. The noise grows louder and louder until suddenly ten or more men run into the corral, each of them carrying two thick bundles of shredded cedar bark.

Four times they run around the fire waving the bundles, which are then lighted. Now begins a wild race around the fire, the rapid running causing the brands to throw out long streamers of flames over the hands and arms of the dancers. The latter apply the brands to their own nude bodies and to the bodies of their comrades in front. A warrior will seize the flaming mass as if it were a sponge, and, keeping close to the man he is pursuing, will rub his back with it as if bathing him. The sufferer in turn catches up with the man in front of him and bathes him in flame. From time to time the dancers sponge their own backs with the flaming brands. When a brand is so far consumed that it can no longer be held it is dropped and the dancers disappear from the corral. The spectators pick up the flaming bunches thus dropped and bathe their own hands in the fire.

"No satisfactory explanation seems to be obtainable as to the means by which the dancers in this extraordinary performance are able to escape injury. Apparently they do not suffer from any burns. Doubtless some protection is afforded by the earth that is applied to their bodies."

Spontaneous combustion of the human body, although doubted by the medical men of this day, has for many years been the subject of much discussion; only a few years ago, among the writers on this subject, there were as many credulous as there were skeptics. There is, however, no reliable evidence to support the belief in the spontaneous combustion of the body. A few apochryphal cases only have been recorded. The opinion that the tissues of drunkards might be so saturated with alcohol as to render the body combustible is disproved by the simple experiment of placing flesh in spirits for a long time and then trying to burn it. Liebig and others found that flesh soaked in alcohol would burn only until the alcohol was consumed. That various substances ignite spontaneously is explained by chemic phenomena, the conditions of which do not exist in the human frame. Watkins in speaking of the inflammability of the human body remarks that on one occasion he tried to consume the body of a pirate given to him by a U. S. Marshal. He built a rousing fire and piled wood on all night, and had not got the body consumed by the forenoon of the following day. Quite a feasible reason for supposed spontaneous human combustion is to be found in several cases quoted by Taylor, in which persons falling asleep, possibly near a fire, have been accidentally ignited, and becoming first stupefied by the smoke, and then suffocated, have been burned to charcoal without awaking. Drunkenness or great exhaustion may also explain certain cases. In substantiation of the possibility of Taylor's instances several prominent physiologists have remarked that persons have endured severe burns during sleep and have never wakened. There is an account of a man who lay down on the top of a lime kiln, which was fired during his sleep, and one leg was burned entirely off without awaking the man, a fact explained by the very slow and gradual increase of temperature.

The theories advanced by the advocates of spontaneous human combustion are very ingenious and deserve mention here. An old authority has said: "Our blood is of such a nature, as also our lymph and bile: all of which, when dried by art, flame like spirit of wine at the approach of the least fire and burn away to ashes." Lord Bacon mentions spontaneous combustion, and Marcellus Donatus says that in the time of Godefroy of Bouillon there were people of a certain locality who supposed themselves to have been burning of an invisible fire in their entrails, and he adds that some cut off a hand or a foot when the burning began, that it should go no further. What may have been the malady with which these people suffered must be a matter of conjecture.

Overton, in a paper on this subject, remarks that in the "Memoirs of the Royal Society of Paris," 1751, there is related an account of a butcher who, opening a diseased beef, was burned by a flame which issued from the maw of the animal; there was first an explosion which rose to a height of five feet and continued to blaze several minutes with a highly offensive odor. Morton saw a flame emanate from beneath the skin of a hog at the instant of making an incision through it. Ruysch, the famous Dutch physician, remarks that he introduced a hollow bougie into a woman's stomach he had just opened, and he observed a vapor issuing from the mouth of the tube, and this lit on contact with the atmosphere. This is probably an exaggeration of the properties of the hydrogen sulphid found in the stomach. There is an account of a man of forty-three, a gross feeder, who was particularly fond of fats and a victim of psoriasis palmaria, who on going to bed one night, after extinguishing the light in the room, was surprised to find himself enveloped in a phosphorescent halo; this continued for several days and recurred after further indiscretions in diet. It is well known that there are insects and other creatures of the lower animal kingdom which possess the peculiar quality of phosphorescence.

There are numerous cases of spontaneous combustion of the human body reported by the older writers. Bartholinus mentions an instance after the person had drunk too much wine. Fouquet mentions a person ignited by lightning. Schrader speaks of a person from whose mouth and fauces after a debauch issued fire. Schurig tells of flames issuing from the vulva, and Moscati records the same occurrence in parturition, Sinibaldust, Borellus, and Bierling have also written on this subject, and the Ephemerides contains a number of instances.

In 1763 Bianchini, Prebendary of Verona, published an account of the death of Countess Cornelia Bandi of Cesena, who in her sixty-second year was consumed by a fire kindled in her own body. In explanation Bianchini said that the fire was caused in the entrails by the inflamed effluvia of the blood, by the juices and fermentation in the stomach, and, lastly, by fiery evaporations which exhaled from the spirits of wine, brandy, etc. In the Gentleman's Magazine, 1763, there is recorded an account of three noblemen who, in emulation, drank great quantities of strong liquor, and two of them died scorched and suffocated by a flame forcing itself from the stomach. There is an account of a poor woman in Paris in the last century who drank plentifully of spirits, for three years taking virtually nothing else. Her body became so combustible that one night while lying on a straw couch she was spontaneously burned to ashes and smoke. The evident cause of this combustion is too plain to be commented on. In the Lancet, 1845, there are two cases reported in which shortly before death luminous breath has been seen to issue from the mouth.

There is an instance reported of a professor of mathematics of thirty-five years of age and temperate, who, feeling a pain in his left leg, discovered a pale flame about the size of a ten-cent piece issuing therefrom. As recent as March, 1850, in a Court of Assizes in Darmstadt during the trial of John Stauff, accused of the murder of the Countess Goerlitz, the counsel for the defense advanced the theory of spontaneous human combustion, and such eminent doctors as von Siebold, Graff, von Liebig, and other prominent members of the Hessian medical fraternity were called to comment on its possibility; principally on their testimony a conviction and life-imprisonment was secured. In 1870 there was a woman of thirty-seven, addicted to alcoholic liquors, who was found in her room with her viscera and part of her limbs consumed by fire, but the hair and clothes intact. According to Walford, in the Scientific American for 1870, there was a case reported by Flowers of Louisiana of a man a hard drinker, who was sitting by a fire surrounded by his Christmas guests, when suddenly flames of a bluish tint burst from his mouth and nostrils and he was soon a corpse. Flowers states that the body remained extremely warm for a much longer period than usual.

Statistics.—From an examination of 28 cases of spontaneous combustion, Jacobs makes the following summary:—

(1) It has always occurred in the human living body.

(2) The subjects were generally old persons.

(3) It was noticed more frequently in women than in men.

(4) All the persons were alone at the time of occurrence.

(5) They all led an idle life.

(6) They were all corpulent or intemperate.

(7) Most frequently at the time of occurrence there was a light and some ignitible substance in the room.

(8) The combustion was rapid and was finished in from one to seven hours.

(9) The room where the combustion took place was generally filled with a thick vapor and the walls covered with a thick, carbonaceous substance.

(10) The trunk was usually the part most frequently destroyed; some part of the head and extremities remained.

(11) With but two exceptions, the combustion occurred in winter and in the northern regions.

Magnetic, Phosphorescent, and Electric Anomalies.—There have been certain persons who have appeared before the public under such names as the "human magnet," the "electric lady," etc. There is no doubt that some persons are supercharged with magnetism and electricity. For instance, it is quite possible for many persons by drawing a rubber comb through the hair to produce a crackling noise, and even produce sparks in the dark. Some exhibitionists have been genuine curiosities of this sort, while others by skilfully arranged electric apparatus are enabled to perform their feats. A curious case was reported in this country many years ago, which apparently emanates from an authoritative source. On the 25th of January, 1837, a certain lady became suddenly and unconsciously charged with electricity. Her newly acquired power was first exhibited when passing her hand over the face of her brother; to the astonishment of both, vivid electric sparks passed from the ends of each finger. This power continued with augmented force from the 25th of January to the last of February, but finally became extinct about the middle of May of the same year.

Schneider mentions a strong, healthy, dark-haired Capuchin monk, the removal of whose head-dress always induced a number of shining, crackling sparks from his hair or scalp. Bartholinus observed a similar peculiarity in Gonzaga, Duke of Mantua. In another case luminous sparks were given out whenever the patient passed urine. Marsh relates two cases of phthisis in which the heads of the patients were surrounded by phosphorescent lights. Kaster mentions an instance in which light was seen in the perspiration and on the body linen after violent exertion. After exertion Jurine, Guyton, and Driessen observed luminous urine passed by healthy persons, and Nasse mentions the same phenomenon in a phthisical patient. Percy and Stokes have observed phosphorescence in a carcinomatous ulcer.

There is a description of a Zulu boy exhibited in Edinburgh in 1882 whose body was so charged with electricity that he could impart a shock to any of his patrons. He was about six-and-a-half years of age, bright, happy, and spoke English thoroughly well. From infancy he had been distinguished for this faculty, variable with the state of the atmosphere. As a rule, the act of shaking hands was generally attended by a quivering sensation like that produced by an electric current, and contact with his tongue gave a still sharper shock.

Sir Charles Bell has made extensive investigation of the subject of human magnetism and is probably the best authority on the subject, but many celebrated scientists have studied it thoroughly. In the Pittsburg Medical Review there is a description of a girl of three and a half, a blonde, and extremely womanly for her age, who possessed a wonderful magnetic power. Metal spoons would adhere to her finger-tips, nose, or chin. The child, however, could not pick up a steel needle, an article generally very sensitive to the magnet; nor would a penny stick to any portion of her body.

Only recently there was exhibited through this country a woman named Annie May Abbott, who styled herself the "Georgia Electric Lady." This person gave exhibitions of wonderful magnetic power, and invited the inspection and discussion of medical men. Besides her chief accomplishment she possessed wonderful strength and was a skilled equilibrist. By placing her hands on the sides of a chair upon which a heavy man was seated, she would raise it without apparent effort. She defied the strongest person in the audience to take from her hand a stick which she had once grasped. Recent reports say that Miss Abbott is amusing herself now with the strong men of China and Japan. The Japanese wrestlers, whose physical strength is celebrated the world over, were unable to raise Miss Abbott from the floor, while with the tips of her fingers she neutralized their most strenuous efforts to lift even light objects, such as a cane, from a table. The possibilities, in this advanced era of electric mechanism, make fraud and deception so easy that it is extremely difficult to pronounce on the genuineness of any of the modern exhibitions of human electricity.

The Effects of Cold.—Gmelin, the famous scientist and investigator of this subject, says that man has lived where the temperature falls as low as -157 degrees F. Habit is a marked factor in this endurance. In Russia men and women work with their breasts and arms uncovered in a temperature many degrees below zero and without attention to the fact. In the most rigorous winter the inhabitants of the Alps work with bare breasts and the children sport about in the snow. Wrapping himself in his pelisse the Russian sleeps in the snow. This influence of habit is seen in the inability of intruders in northern lands to endure the cold, which has no effect on the indigenous people. On their way to besiege a Norwegian stronghold in 1719, 7000 Swedes perished in the snows and cold of their neighboring country. On the retreat from Prague in 1742, the French army, under the rigorous sky of Bohemia, lost 4000 men in ten days. It is needless to speak of the thousands lost in Napoleon's campaign in Russia in 1812.

Pinel has remarked that the insane are less liable to the effects of cold than their normal fellows, and mentions the escape of a naked maniac, who, without any visible after-effect, in January, even, when the temperature was -4 degrees F., ran into the snow and gleefully rubbed his body with ice. In the French journals in 1814 there is the record of the rescue of a naked crazy woman who was found in the Pyrenees, and who had apparently suffered none of the ordinary effects of cold.

Psychologic Effects of Cold.—Lambert says that the mind acts more quickly in cold weather, and that there has been a notion advanced that the emotion of hatred is much stronger in cold weather, a theory exemplified by the assassination of Paul of Russia, the execution of Charles of England, and that of Louis of France. Emotions, such as love, bravery, patriotism, etc., together with diverse forms of excitement, seem to augment the ability of the human body to endure cold.

Cold seems to have little effect on the generative function. In both Sweden, Norway, and other Northern countries the families are as large, if not larger, than in other countries. Cold undoubtedly imparts vigor, and, according to DeThou, Henry III lost his effeminacy and love of pleasure in winter and reacquired a spirit of progress and reformation. Zimmerman has remarked that in a rigorous winter the lubberly Hollander is like the gayest Frenchman. Cold increases appetite, and Plutarch says Brutus experienced intense bulimia while in the mountains, barely escaping perishing. With full rations the Greek soldiers under Xenophon suffered intense hunger as they traversed the snow-clad mountains of Armenia.

Beaupre remarks that those who have the misfortune to be buried under the snow perish less quickly than those who are exposed to the open air, his observations having been made during the retreat of the French army from Moscow. In Russia it is curious to see fish frozen stiff, which, after transportation for great distances, return to life when plunged into cold water.

Sudden death from cold baths and cold drinks has been known for many centuries. Mauriceau mentions death from cold baptism on the head, and Graseccus, Scaliger, Rush, Schenck, and Velschius mention deaths from cold drinks. Aventii, Fabricius Hildanus, the Ephemerides, and Curry relate instances of a fatal issue following the ingestion of cold water by an individual in a superheated condition. Cridland describes a case of sudden insensibility following the drinking of a cold fluid. It is said that Alexander the Great narrowly escaped death from a constrictive spasm, due to the fact that while in a copious sweat he plunged into the river Cydnus. Tissot gives an instance of a man dying at a fountain after a long draught on a hot day. Hippocrates mentions a similar fact, and there are many modern instances.

The ordinary effects of cold on the skin locally and the system generally will not be mentioned here, except to add the remark of Captain Wood that in Greenland, among his party, could be seen ulcerations, blisters, and other painful lesions of the skin. In Siberia the Russian soldiers cover their noses and ears with greased paper to protect them against the cold. The Laplanders and Samoiedes, to avoid the dermal lesions caused by cold (possibly augmented by the friction of the wind and beating of snow), anoint their skins with rancid fish oil, and are able to endure temperatures as low as -40 degrees F. In the retreat of the 10,000 Xenophon ordered all his soldiers to grease the parts exposed to the air.

Effects of Working in Compressed Air.—According to a writer in Cassier's Magazine, the highest working pressures recorded have been close to 50 pounds per square inch, but with extreme care in the selection of men, and corresponding care on the part of the men, it is very probable that this limit may be considerably exceeded. Under average conditions the top limit may be placed at about 45 pounds, the time of working, according to conditions, varying from four to six hours per shift. In the cases in which higher pressures might be used, the shifts for the men should be restricted to two of two hours each, separated by a considerable interval. As an example of heavy pressure work under favorable conditions as to ventilation, without very bad effects on the men, Messrs. Sooysmith &

Company had an experience with a work on which men were engaged in six-hour shifts, separated into two parts by half-hour intervals for lunch. This work was excavation in open, seamy rock, carried on for several weeks under about 45 pounds pressure. The character of the material through which the caisson is being sunk or upon which it may be resting at any time bears quite largely upon the ability of the men to stand the pressure necessary to hold back the water at that point. If the material be so porous as to permit a considerable leakage of air through it, there will naturally result a continuous change of air in the working chamber, and a corresponding relief of the men from the deleterious effects which are nearly always produced by over-used air.

From Strasburg in 1861 Bucuoy reports that during the building of a bridge at Kehl laborers had to work in compressed air, and it was found that the respirations lost their regularity; there were sometimes intense pains in the ears, which after a while ceased. It required a great effort to speak at 2 1/2 atmospheres, and it was impossible to whistle. Perspiration was very profuse. Those who had to work a long time lost their appetites, became emaciated, and congestion of the lung and brain was observed. The movements of the limbs were easier than in normal air, though afterward muscular and rheumatic pains were often observed.

The peculiar and extraordinary development of the remaining special senses when one of the number is lost has always been a matter of great interest. Deaf people have always been remarkable for their acuteness of vision, touch, and smell. Blind persons, again, almost invariably have the sense of hearing, touch, and what might be called the senses of location and temperature exquisitely developed. This substitution of the senses is but; an example of the great law of compensation which we find throughout nature.

Jonston quotes a case in the seventeenth century of a blind man who, it is said, could tell black from white by touch alone; several other instances are mentioned in a chapter entitled "De compensatione naturae monstris facta." It must, however, be held impossible that blind people can thus distinguish colors in any proper sense of the words. Different colored yarns, for example, may have other differences of texture, etc., that would be manifest to the sense of touch. We know of one case in which the different colors were accurately distinguished by a blind girl, but only when located in customary and definite positions. Le Cat speaks of a blind organist, a native of Holland, who still played the organ as well as ever. He could distinguish money by touch, and it is also said that he made himself familiar with colors. He was fond of playing cards, but became such a dangerous opponent, because in shuffling he could tell what cards and hands had been dealt, that he was never allowed to handle any but his own cards.

It is not only in those who are congenitally deficient in any of the senses that the remarkable examples of compensation are seen, but sometimes late in life these are developed. The celebrated sculptor, Daniel de Volterre, became blind after he had obtained fame, and notwithstanding the deprivation of his chief sense he could, by touch alone, make a statue in clay after a model. Le Cat also mentions a woman, perfectly deaf, who without any instruction had learned to comprehend anything said to her by the movements of the lips alone. It was not necessary to articulate any sound, but only to give the labial movements. When tried in a foreign language she was at a loss to understand a single word.

Since the establishment of the modern high standard of blind asylums and deaf-and-dumb institutions, where so many ingenious methods have been developed and are practiced in the education of their inmates, feats which were formerly considered marvelous are within the reach of all those under tuition To-day, those born deaf-mutes are taught to speak and to understand by the movements of the lips alone, and the blind read, become expert workmen, musicians, and even draughtsmen. D. D. Wood of Philadelphia, although one of the finest organists in the country, has been totally blind for years. It is said that he acquires new compositions with almost as great facility as one not afflicted with his infirmity. "Blind Tom," a semi-idiot and blind negro achieved world-wide notoriety by his skill upon the piano.

In some extraordinary cases in which both sight and hearing, and sometimes even taste and smell, are wanting, the individuals in a most wonderful way have developed the sense of touch to such a degree that it almost replaces the absent senses. The extent of this compensation is most beautifully illustrated in the cases of Laura Bridgman and Helen Keller. No better examples could be found of the compensatory ability of differentiated organs to replace absent or disabled ones.

Laura Dewey Bridgman was born December 21, 1829, at Hanover, N.H. Her parents were farmers and healthy people. They were of average height, regular habits, slender build, and of rather nervous dispositions. Laura inherited the physical characteristics of her mother. In her infancy she was subject to convulsions, but at twenty months had improved, and at this time had learned to speak several words. At the age of two years, in common with two of the other children of the family, she had an attack of severe scarlet fever. Her sisters died, and she only recovered after both eyes and ears had suppurated; taste and smell were also markedly impaired. Sight in the left eye was entirely abolished, but she had some sensation for large, bright objects in the right eye up to her eighth year; after that time she became totally blind. After her recovery it was two years before she could sit up all day, and not until she was five years old had she entirely regained her strength. Hearing being lost, she naturally never developed any speech; however, she was taught to sew, knit, braid, and perform several other minor household duties. In 1837 Dr. S. W. Howe, the Director of the Massachusetts Asylum for the Blind, took Laura in charge, and with her commenced the ordinary deaf-mute education. At this time she was seven years and ten months old. Two years later she had made such wonderful progress and shown such ability to learn that, notwithstanding her infirmities, she surpassed any of the pupils of her class. Her advancement was particularly noticed immediately after her realization that an idea could be expressed by a succession of raised letters. In fact, so rapid was her progress, that it was deemed advisable by the authorities to hold her back. By her peculiar sensibility to vibration she could distinguish the difference between a whole and a half note in music, and she struck the notes on the piano quite correctly. During the first years of her education she could not smell at all, but later she could locate the kitchen by this sense. Taste had developed to such an extent that at this time she could distinguish the different degrees of acidity. The sense of touch, however, was exceedingly delicate and acute. As to her moral habits, cleanliness was the most marked. The slightest dirt or rent in her clothes caused her much embarrassment and shame, and her sense of order, neatness, and propriety was remarkable. She seemed quite at home and enjoyed the society of her own sex, but was uncomfortable and distant in the society of males. She quickly comprehended the intellectual capacity of those with whom she was associated, and soon showed an affiliation for the more intelligent of her friends. She was quite jealous of any extra attention shown to her fellow scholars, possibly arising from the fact that she had always been a favorite. She cried only from grief, and partially ameliorated bodily pain by jumping and by other excessive muscular movements. Like most mutes, she articulated a number of noises,—50 or more, all monosyllabic; she laughed heartily, and was quite noisy in her play. At this time it was thought that she had been heard to utter the words doctor, pin, ship, and others. She attached great importance to orientation, and seemed quite ill at ease in finding her way about when not absolutely sure of directions. She was always timid in the presence of animals, and by no persuasion could she be induced to caress a domestic animal. In common with most maidens, at sixteen she became more sedate, reserved and thoughtful; at twenty she had finished her education. In 1878 she was seen by G. Stanley Hall, who found that she located the approach and departure of people through sensation in her feet, and seemed to have substituted the cutaneous sense of vibration for that of hearing. At this time she could distinguish the odors of various fragrant flowers and had greater susceptibility to taste, particularly to sweet and salty substances. She had written a journal for ten years, and had also composed three autobiographic sketches, was the authoress of several poems, and some remarkably clever letters. She died at the Perkins

Institute, May 24, 1889, after a life of sixty years, burdened with infirmities such as few ever endure, and which, by her superior development of the remnants of the original senses left her, she had overcome in a degree nothing less than marvelous. According to a well-known observer, in speaking of her mental development, although she was eccentric she was not defective. She necessarily lacked certain data of thought, but even this feet was not very marked, and was almost counterbalanced by her exceptional power of using what remained.

In the present day there is a girl as remarkable as Laura Bridgman, and who bids fair to attain even greater fame by her superior development. This girl, Helen Keller, is both deaf and blind; she has been seen in all the principal cities of the United States, has been examined by thousands of persons, and is famous for her victories over infirmities. On account of her wonderful power of comprehension special efforts have been made to educate Helen Keller, and for this reason her mind is far more finely developed than in most girls of her age. It is true that she has the advantage over Laura Bridgman in having the senses of taste and smell, both of which she has developed to a most marvelous degree of acuteness. It is said that by odor alone she is always conscious of the presence of another person, no matter how noiseless his entrance into the room in which she may be. She cannot be persuaded to take food which she dislikes, and is never deceived in the taste. It is, however, by the means of what might be called "touch-sight" that the most miraculous of her feats are performed. By placing her hands on the face of a visitor she is able to detect shades of emotion which the normal human eye fails to distinguish, or, in the words of one of her lay observers, "her sense of touch is developed to such an exquisite extent as to form a better eye for her than are yours or mine for us; and what is more, she forms judgments of character by this sight." According to a recent report of a conversation with one of the principals of the school in which her education is being completed, it is said that since the girl has been under his care he has been teaching her to sing with great success. Placing the fingers of her hands on the throat of a singer, she is able to follow notes covering two octaves with her own voice, and sings synchronously with her instructor. The only difference between her voice and that of a normal person is in its resonant qualities. So acute has this sense become, that by placing her hand upon the frame of a piano she can distinguish two notes not more than half a tone apart. Helen is expected to enter the preparatory school for Radcliffe College in the fall of 1896.

At a meeting of the American Association to Promote the Teaching of Speech to the Deaf, in Philadelphia, July, 1896, this child appeared, and in a well-chosen and distinct speech told the interesting story of her own progress. Miss Sarah Fuller, principal of the Horace Mann School for the Deaf, Boston, is credited with the history of Helen Keller, as follows:—

"Helen Keller's home is in Tuscumbia, Ala. At the age of nineteen months she became deaf, dumb, and blind after convulsions lasting three days. Up to the age of seven years she had received no instruction. Her parents engaged Miss Sullivan of the Perkins Institute for the Blind, South Boston, to go to Alabama as her teacher. She was familiar with methods of teaching the blind, but knew nothing about instructing deaf children. Miss Sullivan called upon Miss Fuller for some instruction on the subject. Miss Fuller was at that time experimenting with two little deaf girls to make them speak as hearing children do, and called Miss Sullivan's attention to it. Miss Sullivan left for her charge, and from time to time made reports to Dr. Anagnos the principal of the Perkins School, which mentioned the remarkable mind which she found this little Alabama child possessed. The following year Miss Sullivan brought the child, then eight years old, to Boston, and Mrs. Keller came with her. They visited Miss Fuller's school. Miss Sullivan had taught the child the manual alphabet, and she had obtained much information by means of it. Miss Fuller noticed how quickly she appreciated the ideas given to her in that way.

"It is interesting to note that before any attempt had been made to teach the child to speak or there had been any thought of it, her own quickness of thought had suggested it to her as she talked by hand alphabet to Miss Fuller. Her mother, however, did not approve Miss Fuller's suggestion that an attempt should be made to teach her speech. She remained at the Perkins School, under Miss Sullivan's charge, another year, when the matter was brought up again, this time by little Helen herself, who said she must speak. Miss Sullivan brought her to Miss Fuller's school one day and she received her first lesson, of about two hours' length.

"The child's hand was first passed over Miss Fuller's face, mouth, and neck, then into her mouth, touching the tongue, teeth, lips, and hard palate, to give her an idea of the organs of speech. Miss Fuller then arranged her mouth, tongue, and teeth for the sound of i as in it. She took the child's finger and placed it upon the windpipe so that she might feel the vibration there, put her finger between her teeth to show her how wide apart they were, and one finger in the mouth to feel the tongue, and then sounded the vowel. The child grasped the idea at once. Her fingers flew to her own mouth and throat, and she produced the sound so nearly accurate that it sounded like an echo. Next the sound of ah was made by dropping the jaw a little and letting the child feel that the tongue was soft and lying in the bed of the jaw with the teeth more widely separated. She in the same way arranged her own, but was not so successful as at first, but soon produced the sound perfectly."

Eleven such lessons were given, at intervals of three or four days, until she had acquired all the elements of speech, Miss Sullivan in the meantime practicing with the child on the lessons received. The first word spoken was arm, which was at once associated with her arm; this gave her great delight. She soon learned to pronounce words by herself, combining the elements she had learned, and used them to communicate her simple wants. The first connected language she used was a description she gave Miss Fuller of a visit she had made to Dr. Oliver Wendell Holmes, in all over 200 words. They were, all but two or three, pronounced correctly. She now, six years afterward, converses quite fluently with people who know nothing of the manual alphabet by placing a couple of fingers on the speaker's lips, her countenance showing great intentness and brightening as she catches the meaning. Anybody can understand her answers."

In a beautiful eulogy of Helen Keller in a recent number of Harper's Magazine, Charles Dudley Warner expresses the opinion that she is the purest-minded girl of her age in the world.

Edith Thomas, a little inmate of the Perkins Institute for the Blind, at South Boston, is not only deaf and dumb but also blind. She was a fellow-pupil with Helen Keller, and in a measure duplicated the rapid progress of her former playmate. In commenting on progress in learning to talk the Boston Herald says: "And as the teacher said the word 'Kitty' once or twice she placed the finger-tips of one hand upon the teacher's lips and with the other hand clasped tightly the teacher's throat; then, guided by the muscular action of the throat and the position of the teeth, tongue, and lips, as interpreted by that marvelous and delicate touch of hers, she said the word 'Kitty' over and over again distinctly in a very pretty way. She can be called dumb no longer, and before the summer vacation comes she will have mastered quite a number of words, and such is her intelligence and patience, in spite of the loss of three senses, she may yet speak quite readily.

"Her history is very interesting. She was born in Maplewood, and up to the time of contracting diphtheria and scarlet fever, which occurred when she was four years old, had been a very healthy child of more than ordinary quickness and ability. She had attained a greater command of language than most children of her age. What a contrast between these 'other days,' as she calls them, and the days which followed, when hearing and sight were completely gone, and gradually the senses of speech and smell went, too! After the varied instruction of the blind school the little girl had advanced so far as to make the rest of her study comparatively easy. The extent of her vocabulary is not definitely known, but it numbers at least 700 words. Reading, which was once an irksome task, has become a pleasure to her. Her ideas of locality and the independence of movement are remarkable, and her industry and patience are more noticeable from day to day. She has great ability, and is in every respect a very wonderful child."

According to recent reports, in the vicinity of Rothesay, on the Clyde, there resides a lady totally deaf and dumb, who, in point of intelligence, scholarship, and skill in various ways, far excels many who have all their faculties. Having been educated partly in Paris, she is a good French scholar, and her general composition is really wonderful. She has a shorthand system of her own, and when writing letters, etc., she uses a peculiar machine, somewhat of the nature of a typewriter.

Among the deaf persons who have acquired fame in literature and the arts have been Dibil Alkoffay, an Arabian poet of the eighth century; the tactician, Folard; the German poet, Engelshall; Le Sage; La Condamine, who composed an epigram on his own infirmity; and Beethoven, the famous musician. Fernandez, a Spanish painter of the sixteenth century, was a deaf-mute.

All the world pities the blind, but despite their infirmities many have achieved the highest glory in every profession. Since Homer there have been numerous blind poets. Milton lost none of his poetic power after he had become blind. The Argovienne, Louise Egloff, and Daniel Leopold, who died in 1753, were blind from infancy. Blacklock, Avisse, Koslov, and La Mott-Houdart are among other blind poets. Asconius Pedianus, a grammarian of the first century; Didyme, the celebrated doctor of Alexandria; the Florentine, Bandolini, so well versed in Latin poetry; the celebrated Italian grammarian, Pontanus; the German, Griesinger, who spoke seven languages; the philologist, Grassi, who died in 1831, and many others have become blind at an age more or less advanced in their working lives.

Probably the most remarkable of the blind scientists was the Englishman, Saunderson, who in 1683, in his first year, was deprived of sight after an attack of small-pox. In spite of his complete blindness he assiduously studied the sciences, and graduated with honor at the University of Cambridge in mathematics and optics. His sense of touch was remarkable. He had a collection of old Roman medals, all of which, without mistake, he could distinguish by their impressions. He also seemed to have the ability to judge distance, and was said to have known how far he had walked, and by the velocity he could even tell the distance traversed in a vehicle. Among other blind mathematicians was the Dutchman, Borghes (died in 1652); the French astronomer, the Count de Pagan, who died in 1655; Galileo; the astronomer, Cassini, and Berard, who became blind at twenty-three years, and was for a long time Professor of Mathematics at the College of Briancon.

In the seventeenth century the sculptor, Jean Gonnelli, born in Tuscany, became blind at twenty years; but in spite of his infirmity he afterward executed what were regarded as his masterpieces. It is said that he modeled a portrait of Pope Urban VIII, using as a guide his hand, passed from time to time over the features. Lomazzo, the Italian painter of the eighteenth century, is said to have continued his work after becoming blind.

Several men distinguished for their bravery and ability in the art of war have been blind. Jean de Troczow, most commonly known by the name of Ziska, in 1420 lost his one remaining eye, and was afterward known as the "old blind dog," but, nevertheless, led his troops to many victories. Froissart beautifully describes the glorious death of the blind King of Bohemia at the battle of Crecy in 1346. Louis III, King of Provence; Boleslas III, Duke of Bohemia; Magnus IV, King of Norway, and Bela II, King of Hungary, were blind. Nathaniel Price, a librarian of Norwich in the last century, lost his sight in a voyage to America, which, however, did not interfere in any degree with his duties, for his books were in as good condition and their location as directly under his knowledge, during his blindness as they were in his earlier days. At the present day in New York there is a blind billiard expert who occasionally gives exhibitions of his prowess.

Feats of Memory.—From time to time there have been individuals, principally children, who gave wonderful exhibitions of memory, some for dates, others for names, and some for rapid mental calculation. Before the Anthropological Society in 1880 Broca exhibited a lad of eleven, a Piedmontese, named Jacques Inaudi. This boy, with a trick monkey, had been found earning his livelihood by begging and by solving mentally in a few minutes the most difficult problems in arithmetic. A gentleman residing in Marseilles had seen him while soliciting alms perform most astonishing feats of memory, and brought him to Paris. In the presence of the Society Broca gave him verbally a task in multiplication, composed of some trillions to be multiplied by billions. In the presence of all the members he accomplished his task in less than ten minutes, and without the aid of pencil and paper, solving the whole problem mentally. Although not looking intelligent, and not being able to read or write, he perhaps could surpass any one in the world in his particular feat. It was stated that he proceeded from left to right in his calculations, instead of from right to left in the usual manner. In his personal appearance the only thing indicative of his wonderful abilities was his high forehead.

An infant prodigy named Oscar Moore was exhibited to the physicians of Chicago at the Central Music Hall in 1888, and excited considerable comment at the time. The child was born of mulatto parents at Waco, Texas, on August 19,

1885, and when only thirteen months old manifested remarkable mental ability and precocity. S. V. Clevenger, a physician of Chicago, has described the child as follows:—

"Oscar was born blind and, as frequently occurs in such cases, the touch-sense compensatingly developed extraordinarily. It was observed that after touching a person once or twice with his stubby baby fingers, he could thereafter unfailingly recognize and call by name the one whose hand he again felt. The optic sense is the only one defective, for tests reveal that his hearing, taste, and smell are acute, and the tactile development surpasses in refinement. But his memory is the most remarkable peculiarity, for when his sister conned her lessons at home, baby Oscar, less than two years old, would recite all he heard her read. Unlike some idiot savants, in which category he is not to be included, who repeat parrot-like what they have once heard, baby Oscar seems to digest what he hears, and requires at least more than one repetition of what he is trying to remember, after which he possesses the information imparted and is able to yield it at once when questioned. It is not necessary for him to commence at the beginning, as the possessors of some notable memories were compelled to do, but he skips about to any required part of his repertoire.

"He sings a number of songs and counts in different languages, but it is not supposable that he understands every word he utters. If, however, his understanding develops as it promises to do, he will become a decided polyglot. He has mastered an appalling array of statistics, such as the areas in square miles of hundreds of countries, the population of the world's principal cities, the birthdays of all the Presidents, the names of all the cities of the United States of over 10,000 inhabitants, and a lot of mathematical data. He is greatly attracted by music, and this leads to the expectation that when more mature he may rival Blind Tom.

"In disposition he is very amiable, but rather grave beyond his years. He shows great affection for his father, and is as playful and as happy as the ordinary child. He sleeps soundly, has a good childish appetite, and appears to be in perfect health. His motions are quick but not nervous, and are as well coordinated as in a child of ten. In fact, he impresses one as having the intelligence of a much older child than three years (now five years), but his height, dentition, and general appearance indicate the truthfulness of the age assigned. An evidence of his symmetrical mental development appears in his extreme inquisitiveness. He wants to understand the meaning of what he is taught, and some kind of an explanation must be given him for what he learns. Were his memory alone abnormally great and other faculties defective, this would hardly be the case; but if so, it cannot at present be determined.

"His complexion is yellow, with African features, flat nose, thick lips but not prognathous, superciliary ridges undeveloped, causing the forehead to protrude a little. His head measures 19 inches in circumference, on a line with the upper ear-tips, the forehead being much narrower than the occipitoparietal portion, which is noticeably very wide. The occiput protrudes backward, causing a forward sweep of the back of the neck. From the nose-root to the nucha over the head he measures 13 1/2 inches, and between upper ear- tips across and over the head 11 inches, which is so close to the eight-and ten-inch standard that he may be called mesocephalic. The bulging in the vicinity of the parietal region accords remarkably with speculations upon the location of the auditory memory in that region, such as those in the American Naturalist, July, 1888, and the fact that injury of that part of the brain may cause loss of memory of the meaning of words. It may be that the premature death of the mother's children has some significance in connection with Oscar's phenomenal development. There is certainly a hypernutrition of the parietal brain with atrophy of the optic tract, both of which conditions could arise from abnormal vascular causes, or the extra growth of the auditory memory region may have deprived of nutrition, by pressure, the adjacent optic centers in the occipital brain. The otherwise normal motion of the eyes indicates the nystagmus to be functional.

"Sudden exaltation of the memory is often the consequence of grave brain disease, and in children this symptom is most frequent. Pritchard, Rush, and other writers upon mental disorders record interesting instances of remarkable memory-increase before death, mainly in adults, and during fever and insanity. In simple mania the memory is often very acute. Romberg tells of a young girl who lost her sight after an attack of small-pox, but acquired an extraordinary memory. He calls attention to the fact that the scrofulous and rachitic diatheses in childhood are sometimes accompanied by this disorder. Winslow notes that in the incipient state of the brain disease of early life connected with fevers, disturbed conditions of the cerebral circulation and vessels, and in affections of advanced life, there is often witnessed a remarkable exaltation of the memory, which may herald death by apoplexy.

"Not only has the institution of intelligence in idiots dated from falls upon the head, but extra mentality has been conferred by such an event Pritchard tells of three idiot brothers, one of whom, after a severe head injury, brightened up and became a barrister, while his brothers remained idiotic. 'Father Mabillon,' says Winslow, 'is said to have been an idiot until twenty- six years of age, when he fractured his skull against a stone staircase. He was trepanned. After recovering, his intellect fully developed itself in a mind endowed with a lively imagination, an amazing memory, and a zeal for study rarely equaled.' Such instances can be accounted for by the brain having previously been poorly nourished by a defective blood supply, which defect was remedied by the increased circulation afforded by the head-injury.

"It is a commonly known fact that activity of the brain is attended with a greater head-circulation than when the mind is dull, within certain limits. Anomalous development of the brain through blood-vessels, affording an extra nutritive supply to the mental apparatus, can readily be conceived as occurring before birth, just as aberrant nutrition elsewhere produces giants from parents of ordinary size.

"There is but one sense-defect in the child Oscar, his eyesight-absence, and that is atoned for by his hearing and touch-acuteness, as it generally is in the blind. Spitzka and others demonstrate that in such cases other parts of the brain enlarge to compensate for the atrophic portion which is connected with the functionless nerves. This, considered with his apparently perfect, mental and physical health, leaves no reason to suppose that Oscar's extravagant memory depends upon disease any more than we can suspect all giants of being sickly, though the anomaly is doubtless due to pathologic conditions. Of course, there is no predicting what may develop later in his life, but in any event science will be benefited.

"It is a popular idea that great vigor of memory is often associated with low-grade intelligence, and cases such as Blind Tom and other 'idiot savants,' who could repeat the contents of a newspaper after a single reading, justify the supposition. Fearon, on 'Mental Vigor,' tells of a man who could remember the day that every person had been buried in the parish for thirty-five years, and could repeat with unvarying accuracy the name and age of the deceased and the mourners at the funeral. But he was a complete fool. Out of the line of burials he had not one idea, could not give an intelligible reply to a single question, nor be trusted even to feed himself. While memory-development is thus apparent in some otherwise defective intellects, it has probably as often or oftener been observed to occur in connection with full or great intelligence. Edmund Burke, Clarendon, John Locke, Archbishop Tillotson, and Dr. Johnson were all distinguished for having great strength of memory. Sir W. Hamilton observed that Grotius, Pascal, Leibnitz, and Euler were not less celebrated for their intelligence than for their memory. Ben Jonson could repeat all that he had written and whole books he had read. Themistocles could call by name the 20,000 citizens of Athens. Cyrus is said to have known the name of every soldier in his army. Hortensius, a great Roman orator, and Seneca had also great memories. Niebuhr, the Danish historian, was remarkable for his acuteness of memory. Sir James Mackintosh, Dugald Stewart, and Dr. Gregory had similar reputations.

"Nor does great mental endowment entail physical enfeeblement; for, with temperance, literary men have reached extreme old age, as in the cases of Klopstock, Goethe, Chaucer, and the average age attained by all the signers of the American Declaration of Independence was sixty-four years, many of them being highly gifted men intellectually. Thus, in the case of the phenomenal Oscar it cannot be predicted that he will not develop, as he now promises to do, equal and extraordinary powers of mind, even though it would be rare in one of his racial descent, and in the face of the fact that precocity gives no assurance of adult brightness, for it can be urged that John Stuart Mill read Greek when four years of age.

"The child is strumous, however, and may die young. His exhibitors, who are coining him into money, should seek the best medical care for him and avoid surcharging his memory with rubbish. Proper cultivation of his special senses, especially the tactile, by competent teachers, will give Oscar the best chance of developing intellectually and acquiring an education in the proper sense of the word."

By long custom many men of letters have developed wonderful feats of memory; and among illiterate persons, by means of points of association, the power of memory has been little short of marvelous. At a large hotel in Saratoga there was at one time a negro whose duty was to take charge of the hats and coats of the guests as they entered the dining-room and return to each his hat after the meal. It was said that, without checks or the assistance of the owners, he invariably returned the right articles to the right persons on request, and no matter how large the crowd, his limit of memory never seemed to be reached. Many persons have seen expert players at draughts and chess who, blindfolded, could carry on numerous games with many competitors and win most of the matches. To realize what a wonderful feat of memory this performance is, one need only see the absolute exhaustion of one of these men after a match. In whist, some experts have been able to detail the succession of the play of the cards so many hands back that their competitors had long since forgotten it.

There is reported to be in Johnson County, Missouri, a mathematical wonder by the name of Rube Fields. At the present day he is between forty and fifty years of age, and his external appearance indicates poverty as well as indifference. His temperament is most sluggish; he rarely speaks unless spoken to, and his replies are erratic.

The boyhood of this strange character was that of an overgrown country lout with boorish manners and silly mind. He did not and would not go to school, and he asserts now that if he had done so he "would have become as big a fool as other people." A shiftless fellow, left to his own devices, he performed some wonderful feats, and among the many stories connected with this period of his life is one which describes how he actually ate up a good-sized patch of sugar cane, simply because he found it good to his taste.

Yet from this clouded, illiterate mind a wonderful mathematical gift shines. Just when he began to assert his powers is not known; but his feats have been remembered for twenty years by his neighbors. A report says:—

"Give Rube Fields the distance by rail between any two points, and the dimensions of a car-wheel, and almost as soon as the statement has left your lips he will tell you the number of revolutions the wheel will make in traveling over the track. Call four or five or any number of columns of figures down a page, and when you have reached the bottom he will announce the sum. Given the number of yards or pounds of articles and the price, and at once he will return the total cost—and this he will do all day long, without apparent effort or fatigue.

"A gentleman relates an instance of Fields' knowledge of figures. After having called several columns of figures for addition, he went back to the first column, saying that it was wrong, and repeating it, purposely miscalling the next to the last figure. At once Fields threw up his hand, exclaiming: 'You didn't call it that way before.'

"Fields' answers come quick and sharp, seemingly by intuition. Calculations which would require hours to perform are made in less time than it takes to state the question. The size of the computations seems to offer no bar to their rapid solution, and answers in which long lines of figures are reeled off come with perfect ease. In watching the effort put forth in reaching an answer, there would seem to be some process going on in the mind, and an incoherent mumbling is often indulged in, but it is highly probable that Fields does not himself know how he derives his answers. Certain it is that he is unable to explain the process, nor has any one ever been able to draw from him anything concerning it. Almost the only thing he knows about the power is that he possesses it, and, while he is not altogether averse to receiving money for his work, he has steadily refused to allow himself to be exhibited." In reviewing the peculiar endowment of Fields, the Chicago Record says:—

"How this feat is performed is as much a mystery as the process by which he solves a problem in arithmetic. He answers no questions. Rapid mathematicians, men of study, who by intense application and short methods have become expert, have sought to probe these two mysteries, but without results. Indeed, the man's intelligence is of so low an order as to prevent him from aiding those who seek to know. With age, too, he grows more surly. Of what vast value this 'gift' might be to the world of science, if coupled with average intelligence, is readily imagined. That it will ever be understood is unlikely. As it is, the power staggers belief and makes modern psychology, with its study of brain-cells, stand aghast. As to poor Fields himself, he excites only sympathy. Homeless, unkempt, and uncouth, traveling aimlessly on a journey which he does not understand, he hugs to his heart a marvelous power, which he declares to be a gift from God. To his weak mind it lifts him above his fellow-men, and yet it is as useless to the world as a diamond in a dead man's hand."

Wolf-Children.—It is interesting to know to what degree a human being will resemble a beast when deprived of the association with man. We seem to get some insight to this question in the investigation of so called cases of "wolf-children."

Saxo Grammaticus speaks of a bear that kidnapped a child and kept it a long time in his den. The tale of the Roman she-wolf is well known, and may have been something more than a myth, as there have been several apparently authentic cases reported in which a child has been rescued from its associations with a wolf who had stolen it some time previously. Most of the stories of wolf-children come from India. According to Oswald in Ball's "Jungle Life in India," there is the following curious account of two children in the Orphanage of Sekandra, near Agra, who had been discovered among wolves: "A trooper sent by a native Governor of Chandaur to demand payment of some revenue was passing along the bank of the river about noon when he saw a large female wolf leave her den, followed by three whelps and a little boy. The boy went on all-fours, and when the trooper tried to catch him he ran as fast as the whelps, and kept up with the old one. They all entered the den, but were dug out by the people and the boy was secured. He struggled hard to rush into every hole or gully they came near. When he saw a grown-up person he became alarmed, but tried to fly at children and bite them. He rejected cooked meat with disgust, but delighted in raw flesh and bones, putting them under his paws like a dog." The other case occurred at Chupra, in the Presidency of Bengal. In March, 1843, a Hindoo mother went out to help her husband in the field, and while she was cutting rice her little boy was carried off by a wolf. About a year afterward a wolf, followed by several cubs and a strange, ape-like creature, was seen about ten miles from Chupra. After a lively chase the nondescript was caught and recognized (by the mark of a burn on his knee) as the Hindoo boy that had disappeared in the rice-field. This boy would not eat anything but raw flesh, and could never be taught to speak, but expressed his emotions in an inarticulate mutter. His elbows and the pans of his knees had become horny from going on all-fours with his foster mother. In the winter of 1850 this boy made several attempts to regain his freedom, and in the following spring he escaped for good and disappeared in the jungle-forest of Bhangapore.

The Zoologist for March, 1888, reproduced a remarkable pamphlet printed at Plymouth in 1852, which had been epitomized in the Lancet. This interesting paper gives an account of wolves nurturing small children in their dens. Six cases are given of boys who have been rescued from the maternal care of wolves. In one instance the lad was traced from the moment of his being carried off by a lurking wolf while his parents were working in the field, to the time when, after having been recovered by his mother six years later, he escaped from her into the jungle. In all these cases certain marked features reappear. In the first, the boy was very inoffensive, except when teased, and then he growled surlily. He would eat anything thrown to him, but preferred meat, which he devoured with canine voracity. He drank a pitcher of buttermilk at one gulp, and could not be induced to wear clothing even in the coldest weather. He showed the greatest fondness for bones, and gnawed them contentedly, after the manner of his adopted parents. This child had coarse features, a repulsive countenance, was filthy in his habits, and could not articulate a word.

In another case the child was kidnapped at three and recovered at nine. He muttered, but could not articulate. As in the other case, he could not be enticed to wear clothes. From constantly being on all-fours the front of this child's knees and his elbows had become hardened. In the third case the father identified a son who had been carried away at the age of six, and was found four years afterward. The intellectual deterioration was not so marked. The boy understood signs, and his hearing was exceedingly acute; when directed by movements of the hands to assist the cultivators in turning out cattle, he readily comprehended what was asked of him; yet this lad, whose vulpine career was so short, could neither talk nor utter any decidedly articulate sound.

The author of the pamphlet expressed some surprise that there was no case on record in which a grown man had been found in such association. This curious collection of cases of wolf-children is attributed to Colonel Sleeman, a well-known officer, who is known to have been greatly interested in the subject, and who for a long time resided in the forests of India. A copy, now a rarity, is in the South Kensington Museum.

An interesting case of a wolf-child was reported many years ago in Chambers' Journal. In the Etwah district, near the banks of the river Jumna, a boy was captured from the wolves. After a time this child was restored to his parents, who, however, "found him very difficult to manage, for he was most fractious and troublesome—in fact, just a caged wild beast. Often during the night for hours together he would give vent to most unearthly yells and moans, destroying the rest and irritating the tempers of his neighbors and generally making night hideous. On one occasion his people chained him by the waist to a tree on the outskirts of the village. Then a rather curious incident occurred. It was a bright moonlight night, and two wolf cubs (undoubtedly those in whose companionship he had been captured), attracted by his cries while on the prowl, came to him, and were distinctly seen to gambol around him with as much familiarity and affection as if they considered him quite one of themselves. They only left him on the approach of morning, when movement and stir again arose in the village. This boy did not survive long. He never spoke, nor did a single ray of human intelligence ever shed its refining light over his debased features."

Recently a writer in the Badmington Magazine, in speaking of the authenticity of wolf-children, says:—

"A jemidar told me that when he was a lad he remembered going, with others, to see a wolf-child which had been netted. Some time after this, while staying at an up-country place called Shaporeooundie, in East Bengal, it was my fortune to meet an Anglo-Indian gentleman who had been in the Indian civil service for upward of thirty years, and had traveled about during most of that time; from him I learned all I wanted to know of wolf-children, for he not only knew of several cases, but had actually seen and examined, near Agra, a child which had been recovered from the wolves. The story of Romulus and Remus, which all schoolboys and the vast majority of grown people regard as a myth, appears in a different light when one studies the question of wolf-children, and ascertains how it comes to pass that boys are found living on the very best terms with such treacherous and rapacious animals as wolves, sleeping with them in their dens, sharing the raw flesh of deer and kids which the she-wolf provides, and, in fact, leading in all essentials the actual life of a wolf.

"A young she-wolf has a litter of cubs, and after a time her instinct tells her that they will require fresh food. She steals out at night in quest of prey. Soon she espies a weak place in the fence (generally constructed of thatching grass and bamboos) which encloses the compound, or 'unguah,' of a poor villager. She enters, doubtless, in the hope of securing a kid; and while prowling about inside looks into a hut where a woman and infant are soundly sleeping. In a moment she has pounced on the child, and is out of reach before its cries can attract the villagers. Arriving safely at her den under the rocks, she drops the little one among her cubs. At this critical time the fate of the child hangs in the balance. Either it will be immediately torn to pieces and devoured, or in a most wonderful way remain in the cave unharmed. In the event of escape, the fact may be accounted for in several ways. Perhaps the cubs are already gorged when the child is thrown before them, or are being supplied with solid food before their carnivorous instinct is awakened, so they amuse themselves by simply licking the sleek, oily body (Hindoo mothers daily rub their boy babies with some native vegetable oil) of the infant, and thus it lies in the nest, by degrees getting the odor of the wolf cubs, after which the mother wolf will not molest it. In a little time the infant begins to feel the pangs of hunger, and hearing the cubs sucking, soon follows their example. Now the adoption is complete, all fear of harm to the child from wolves has gone, and the foster-mother will guard and protect it as though it were of her own flesh and blood.

"The mode of progression of these children is on all fours—not, as a rule, on the hands and feet, but on the knees and elbows. The reason the knees are used is to be accounted for by the fact that, owing to the great length of the human leg and thigh in proportion to the length of the arm, the knee would naturally be brought to the ground, and the instep and top of the toes would be used instead of the sole and heel of the almost inflexible foot. Why the elbow should be employed instead of the hand is less easy to understand, but probably it is better suited to give support to the head and fore-part of the body.

"Some of these poor waifs have been recovered after spending ten or more years in the fellowship of wolves, and, though wild and savage at first, have in time become tractable in some degree. They are rarely seen to stand upright, unless to look around, and they gnaw bones in the manner of a dog, holding one end between the forearms and hands, while snarling and snapping at everybody who approaches too near. The wolf-child has little except his outward form to show that it is a human being with a soul. It is a fearful and terrible thing, and hard to understand, that the mere fact of a child's complete isolation from its own kind should bring it to such a state of absolute degradation. Of course, they speak no language, though some, in time, have learned to make known their wants by signs. When first taken they fear the approach of adults, and, if possible, will slink out of sight; but should a child of their own size, or smaller, come near, they will growl, and even snap and bite at it. On the other hand, the close proximity of "pariah" dogs or jackals is unresented, in some cases welcomed; for I have heard of them sharing their food with these animals, and even petting and fondling them. They have in time been brought to a cooked-meat diet, but would always prefer raw flesh. Some have been kept alive after being reclaimed for as long as two years, but for some reason or other they all sicken and die, generally long before that time. One would think, however, that, having undoubtedly robust constitutions, they might be saved if treated in a scientific manner and properly managed."

Rudyard Kipling, possibly inspired by accounts of these wolf-children in India, has ingeniously constructed an interesting series of fabulous stories of a child who was brought up by the beasts of the jungles and taught their habits and their mode of communication. The ingenious way in which the author has woven the facts together and interspersed them with his intimate knowledge of animal-life commends his "Jungle-Book" as a legitimate source of recreation to the scientific observer.

Among observers mentioned in the "Index Catalogue" who have studied this subject are Giglioli, Mitra, and Ornstein.

The artificial manufacture of "wild men" or "wild boys" in the Chinese Empire is shown by recent reports. Macgowan says the traders kidnap a boy and skin him alive bit by bit, transplanting on the denuded surfaces the hide of a bear or dog. This process is most tedious and is by no means complete when the hide is completely transplanted, as the subject must be rendered mute by destruction of the vocal cords, made to use all fours in walking, and submitted to such degradation as to completely blight all reason. It is said that the process is so severe that only one in five survive. A "wild boy" exhibited in Kiangse had the entire skin of a dog substituted and walked on all fours. It was found that he had been kidnapped. His proprietor was decapitated on the spot. Macgowan says that parasitic monsters are manufactured in China by a similar process of transplantation. He adds that the deprivation of light for several years renders the child a great curiosity, if in conjunction its growth is dwarfed by means of food and drugs, and its vocal apparatus destroyed. A certain priest subjected a kidnapped boy to this treatment and exhibited him as a sacred deity. Macgowan mentions that the child looked like wax, as though continually fed on lardaceous substances. He squatted with his palms together and was a driveling idiot. The monk was discovered and escaped, but his temple was razed.

Equilibrists.—Many individuals have cultivated their senses so acutely that by the eye and particularly by touch they are able to perform almost incredible feats of maintaining equilibrium under the most difficult circumstances Professional rope-walkers have been known in all times. The Greeks had a particular passion for equilibrists, and called them "neurobates," "oribates," and "staenobates." Blondin would have been one of the latter. Antique medals showing equilibrists making the ascent of an inclined cord have been found. The Romans had walkers both of the slack-rope and tight-rope Many of the Fathers of the Church have pronounced against the dangers of these exercises. Among others, St. John Chrysostom speaks of men who execute movements on inclined ropes at unheard-of heights. In the ruins of Herculaneum there is still visible a picture representing an equilibrist executing several different exercises, especially one in which he dances on a rope to the tune of a double flute, played by himself. The Romans particularly liked to witness ascensions on inclined ropes, and sometimes these were attached to the summits of high hills, and while mounting them the acrobats performed different pantomimes. It is said that under Charles VI a Genoese acrobat, on the occasion of the arrival of the Queen of France, carried in each hand an illuminated torch while descending a rope stretched from the summit of the towers of Notre Dame to a house on the Pont au Change. According to Guyot-Daubes, a similar performance was seen in London in 1547. In this instance the rope was attached to the highest pinnacle of St. Paul's Cathedral. Under Louis XII an acrobat named Georges Menustre, during a passage of the King through Macon, executed several performances on a rope stretched from the grand tower of the Chateau and the clock of the Jacobins, at a height of 156 feet. A similar performance was given at Milan before the French Ambassadors, and at Venice under the Doges and the Senate on each St. Mark's Day, rope-walkers performed at high altitudes. In 1649 a man attempted to traverse the Seine on a rope placed between the Tour de Nesles and the Tour du Grand-Prevost. The performance, however, was interrupted by the fall of the mountebank into the Seine. At subsequent fairs in France other acrobats have appeared. At the commencement of this century there was a person named Madame Saqui who astonished the public with her nimbleness and extraordinary skill in rope walking. Her specialty was military maneuvers. On a cord 20 meters from the ground she executed all sorts of military pantomimes without assistance, shooting off pistols, rockets, and various colored fires. Napoleon awarded her the title of the first acrobat of France. She gave a performance as late as 1861 at the Hippodrome of Paris.

In 1814 there was a woman called "La Malaga," who, in the presence of the allied sovereigns at Versailles, made an ascension on a rope 200 feet above the Swiss Lake.

In the present generation probably the most famous of all the equilibrists was Blondin. This person, whose real name was Emile Gravelet, acquired a universal reputation; about 1860 he traversed the Niagara Falls on a cable at an elevation of nearly 200 feet. Blondin introduced many novelties in his performances. Sometimes he would carry a man over on his shoulders; again he would eat a meal while on his wire; cook and eat an omelet, using a table and ordinary cooking utensils, all of which he kept balanced. In France Blondin was almost the patron saint of the rope-walkers; and at the present day the performers imitate his feats, but never with the same grace and perfection.

In 1882 an acrobat bearing the natural name of Arsens Blondin traversed one river after another in France on a wire stretched at high altitudes. With the aid of a balancing-rod he walked the rope blindfolded; with baskets on his feet; sometimes he wheeled persons over in a wheelbarrow. He was a man of about thirty, short, but wonderfully muscled and extremely supple.

It is said that a negro equilibrist named Malcom several times traversed the Meuse at Sedan on a wire at about a height of 100 feet. Once while attempting this feat, with his hands and feet shackled with iron chains, allowing little movement, the support on one side fell, after the cable had parted, and landed on the spectators, killing a young girl and wounding many others. Malcom was precipitated into the river, but with wonderful presence of mind and remarkable strength he broke his bands and swam to the shore, none the worse for his high fall; he immediately helped in attention to his wounded spectators. A close inspection of all the exhibitionists of this class will show that they are of superior physique and calm courage. They only acquire their ability after long gymnastic exercise, as well as actual practice on the rope. Most of these persons used means of balancing themselves, generally a long and heavy pole; but some used nothing but their outstretched arms. In 1895, at the Royal Aquarium in London, there was an individual who slowly mounted a long wire reaching to the top of this huge structure, and, after having made the ascent, without the aid of any means of balancing but his arms, slid the whole length of the wire, landing with enormous velocity into an outstretched net.

The equilibrists mentioned thus far have invariably used a tightly stretched rope or wire; but there are a number of persons who perform feats, of course not of such magnitude, on a slack wire, in which they have to defy not only the force of gravity, but the to-and-fro motion of the cable as well. It is particularly with the Oriental performers that we see this exhibition. Some use open parasols, which, with their Chinese or Japanese costumes, render the performance more picturesque; while others seem to do equally well without such adjuncts. There have been performers of this class who play with sharp daggers while maintaining themselves on thin and swinging wires.

Another class of equilibrists are those who maintain the upright position resting on their heads with their feet in the air. At the Hippodrome in Paris some years since there was a man who remained in this position seven minutes and ate a meal during the interval. There were two clowns at the Cirque Franconi who duplicated this feat, and the program called their dinner "Un dejouner en tete-a-tete." Some other persons perform wonderful feats of a similar nature on an oscillating trapeze, and many similar performances have been witnessed by the spectators of our large circuses.

The "human pyramids" are interesting, combining, as they do, wonderful power of maintaining equilibrium with agility and strength. The rapidity with which they are formed and are tumbled to pieces is marvelous they sometimes include as many as 16 persons men, women, and children.

The exhibitions given by the class of persons commonly designated as "jugglers" exemplify the perfect control that by continual practice one may obtain over his various senses and muscles. The most wonderful feats of dexterity are thus reduced into mere automatic movements. Either standing, sitting, mounted on a horse, or even on a wire, they are able to keep three four, five, and even six balls in continual motion in the air. They use articles of the greatest difference in specific gravity in the same manner. A juggler called "Kara," appearing in London and Paris in the summer of 1895, juggled with an open umbrella, an eye-glass, and a traveling satchel, and received each after its course in the air with unerring precision. Another man called "Paul Cinquevalli," well known in this country, does not hesitate to juggle with lighted lamps or pointed knives. The tricks of the clowns with their traditional pointed felt hats are well known. Recently there appeared in Philadelphia a man who received six such hats on his head, one on top of the other, thrown by his partner from the rear of the first balcony of the theater. Others will place a number of rings on their fingers, and with a swift and dexterous movement toss them all in the air, catching them again all on one finger. Without resorting to the fabulous method of Columbus, they balance eggs on a table, and in extraordinary ways defy all the powers of gravity.

In India and China we see the most marvelous of the knife-jugglers.

With unerring skill they keep in motion many pointed knives, always receiving them at their fall by the handles. They throw their implements with such precision that one often sees men, who, placing their partner against a soft board, will stand at some distance and so pen him in with daggers that he cannot move until some are withdrawn, marking a silhouette of his form on the board,—yet never once does one as much as graze the skin. With these same people the foot-jugglers are most common. These persons, both made and female, will with their feet juggle substances and articles that it requires several assistants to raise.

A curious trick is given by Rousselet in his magnificent work entitled "L'Inde des Rajahs," and quoted by Guyot-Daubes. It is called in India the "dance of the eggs." The dancer, dressed in a rather short skirt, places on her head a large wheel made of light wood, and at regular intervals having hanging from it pieces of thread, at the ends of which are running knots kept open by beads of glass. She then brings forth a basket of eggs, and passes them around for inspection to assure her spectators of their genuineness. The monotonous music commences and the dancer sets the wheel on her head in rapid motion; then, taking an egg, with a quick movement she puts it on one of the running knots and increases the velocity of the revolution of the wheel by gyrations until the centrifugal force makes each cord stand out in an almost horizontal line with the circumference of the wheel. Then one after another she places the eggs on the knots of the cord, until all are flying about her head in an almost horizontal position. At this moment the dance begins, and it is almost impossible to distinguish the features of the dancer. She continues her dance, apparently indifferent to the revolving eggs. At the velocity with which they revolve the slightest false movement would cause them to knock against one another and surely break. Finally, with the same lightning-like movements, she removes them one by one, certainly the most delicate part of the trick, until they are all safely laid away in the basket from which they came, and then she suddenly brings the wheel to a stop; after this wonderful performance, lasting possibly thirty minutes, she bows herself out.

A unique Japanese feat is to tear pieces of paper into the form of butterflies and launch them into the air about a vase full of flowers; then with a fan to keep them in motion, making them light on the flowers, fly away, and return, after the manner of several living butterflies, without allowing one to fall to the ground.

Marksmen.—It would be an incomplete paper on the acute development of the senses that did not pay tribute to the men who exhibit marvelous skill with firearms. In the old frontier days in the Territories, the woodsmen far eclipsed Tell with his bow or Robin Hood's famed band by their unerring aim with their rifles. It is only lately that there disappeared in this country the last of many woodsmen, who, though standing many paces away and without the aid of the improved sights of modern guns, could by means of a rifle-ball, with marvelous precision, drive a nail "home" that had been placed partly in a board. The experts who shoot at glass balls rarely miss, and when we consider the number used each year, the proportion of inaccurate shots is surprisingly small. Ira Paine, Doctor Carver, and others have been seen in their marvelous performances by many people of the present generation. The records made by many of the competitors of the modern army-shooting matches are none the less wonderful, exemplifying as they do the degree of precision that the eye may attain and the control which may be developed over the nerves and muscles. The authors know of a countryman who successfully hunted squirrels and small game by means of pebbles thrown with his hand.

Physiologic wonders are to be found in all our modern sports and games. In billiards, base-ball, cricket, tennis, etc., there are experts who are really physiologic curiosities. In the trades and arts we see development of the special senses that is little less than marvelous. It is said that there are workmen in Krupp's gun factory in Germany who have such control over the enormous trip hammers that they can place a watch under one and let the hammer fall, stopping it with unerring precision just on the crystal. An expert tool juggler in one of the great English needle factories, in a recent test of skill, performed one of the most delicate mechanical feats imaginable. He took a common sewing needle of medium size (length 1 5/8 inches) and drilled a hole through its entire length from eye to point—the opening being just large enough to admit the passage of a very fine hair. Another workman in a watch-factory of the United States drilled a hole through a hair of his beard and ran a fiber of silk through it.

Ventriloquists, or "two-voiced men," are interesting anomalies of the present day; it is common to see a person who possesses the power of speaking with a voice apparently from the epigastrium. Some acquire this faculty, while with others it is due to a natural resonance, formed, according to Dupont, in the space between the third and fourth ribs and their cartilaginous union and the middle of the first portion of the sternum. Examination of many of these cases proves that the vibration is greatest here. It is certain that ventriloquists have existed for many centuries. It is quite possible that some of the old Pagan oracles were simply the deceptions of priests by means of ventriloquism.

Dupont, Surgeon-in-chief of the French Army about a century since, examined minutely an individual professing to be a ventriloquist. With a stuffed fox on his lap near his epigastrium, he imitated a conversation with the fox. By lying on his belly, and calling to some one supposed to be below the surface of the ground, he would imitate an answer seeming to come from the depths of the earth. With his belly on the ground he not only made the illusion more complete, but in this way he smothered "the epigastric voice."

He was always noticed to place the inanimate objects with which he held conversations near his umbilicus.

Ventriloquists must not be confounded with persons who by means of skilful mechanisms, creatures with movable fauces, etc., imitate ventriloquism. The latter class are in no sense of the word true ventriloquists, but simulate the anomaly by quickly changing the tones of their voice in rapid succession, and thus seem to make their puppets talk in many different voices. After having acquired the ability to suddenly change the tone of their voice, they practice imitations of the voices of the aged, of children, dialects, and feminine tones, and, with a set of mechanical puppets, are ready to appear as ventriloquists. By contraction of the pharyngeal and laryngeal muscles they also imitate tones from a distance. Some give their performance with little labial movement, but close inspection of the ordinary performer of this class shows visible movements of his lips. The true ventriloquist pretends only to speak from the belly and needs no mechanical assistance.

The wonderful powers of mimicry displayed by expert ventriloquists are marvelous; they not only imitate individuals and animals, but do not hesitate to imitate a conglomeration of familiar sounds and noises in such a manner as to deceive their listeners into believing that they hear the discussions of an assemblage of people. The following description of an imitation of a domestic riot by a Chinese ventriloquist is given by the author of "The Chinaman at Home" and well illustrates the extent of their abilities: "The ventriloquist was seated behind a screen, where there were only a chair, a table, a fan, and a ruler. With this ruler he rapped on the table to enforce silence, and when everybody had ceased speaking there was suddenly heard the barking of a dog. Then we heard the movements of a woman. She had been waked by the dog and was shaking her husband. We were just expecting to hear the man and wife talking together when a child began to cry. To pacify it the mother gave it food; we could hear it drinking and crying at the same time. The mother spoke to it soothingly and then rose to change its clothes. Meanwhile another child had wakened and was beginning to make a noise. The father scolded it, while the baby continued crying. By-and-by the whole family went back to bed and fell asleep. The patter of a mouse was heard. It climbed up some vase and upset it. We heard the clatter of the vase as it fell. The woman coughed in her sleep. Then cries of "Fire! fire!" were heard. The mouse had upset the lamp; the bed curtains were on fire. The husband and wife waked up, shouted, and screamed, the children cried, people came running and shouting. Children cried, dogs barked, squibs and crackers exploded. The fire brigade came racing up. Water was pumped up in torrents and hissed in the flames. The representation was so true to life that every one rose to his feet and was starting away when a second blow of the ruler on the table commanded silence. We rushed behind the screen, but there was nothing there except the ventriloquist, his table, his chair, and his ruler."

Athletic Feats.—The ancients called athletes those who were noted for their extraordinary agility, force, and endurance. The history of athletics is not foreign to that of medicine, but, on the contrary, the two are in many ways intimately blended. The instances of feats of agility and endurance are in every sense of the word examples of physiologic and functional anomalies, and have in all times excited the interest and investigation of capable physicians.

The Greeks were famous for their love of athletic pastimes; and classical study serves powerfully to strengthen the belief that no institution exercised greater influence than the public contests of Greece in molding national character and producing that admirable type of personal and intellectual beauty that we see reflected in her art and literature. These contests were held at four national festivals, the Olympian, the Pythian, the Nemean, and the Isthmean games. On these occasions every one stopped labor, truce was declared between the States, and the whole country paid tribute to the contestants for the highly-prized laurels of these games. Perhaps the enthusiasm shown in athletics and interest in physical development among the Greeks has never been equaled by any other people. Herodotus and all the Greek writers to Plutarch have elaborated on the glories of the Greek athlete, and tell us of the honors rendered to the victors by the spectators and the vanquished, dwelling with complacency on the fact that in accepting the laurel they cared for nothing but honor. The Romans in "ludi publici," as they called their games, were from first to last only spectators; but in Greece every eligible person was an active participant. In the regimen of diet and training the physicians from the time of Hippocrates, and even before, have been the originators and professional advisers of the athlete. The change in the manner of living of athletes, if we can judge from the writings of Hippocrates, was anterior to his time; for in Book V of the "Epidemics" we read of Bias, who, "suapte nature vorax, in choleram-morbum incidit ex carnium esu, praecipueque suillarum crudarum, etc."

From the time of the well-known fable of the hero who, by practicing daily from his birth, was able to lift a full-grown bull, thus gradually accustoming himself to the increased weight, physiologists and scientists have collaborated with the athlete in evolving the present ideas and system of training. In his aphorisms Hippocrates bears witness to the dangers of over- exercise and superabundant training, and Galen is particularly averse to an art which so preternaturally develops the constitution and nature of man; many subsequent medical authorities believed that excessive development of the human frame was necessarily followed by a compensatory shortening of life.

The foot-race was the oldest of the Greek institutions, and in the first of the Olympiads the "dromos," a course of about 200 yards, was the only contest; but gradually the "dialos," in which the course was double that of the dromos, was introduced, and, finally, tests of endurance as well as speed were instituted in the long-distance races and the contests of racing in heavy armor, which were so highly commended by Plato as preparation for the arduous duties of a soldier. Among the Greeks we read of Lasthenes the Theban, who vanquished a horse in the course; of Polymnestor, who chased and caught a hare; and Philonides, the courier of Alexander the Great, who in nine hours traversed the distance between the Greek cities Sicyone and Elis, a distance of over 150 miles. We read of the famous soldier of Marathon, who ran to announce the victory to the Magistrates of Athens and fell dead at their feet. In the Olympian games at Athens in 1896 this distance (about 26 miles) was traversed in less than three hours.

It is said of Euchidas, who carried the fire necessary for the sacrifices which were to replace those which the Persians had spoiled, that he ran a thousand stadia (about 125 miles) and fell dead at the end of his mission. The Roman historians have also recited the extraordinary feats of the couriers of their times. Pliny speaks of an athlete who ran 235 kilometers (almost 150 miles) without once stopping. He also mentions a child who ran almost half this distance.

In the Middle Ages the Turks had couriers of almost supernatural agility and endurance. It is said that the distance some of them would traverse in twenty-four hours was 120 miles, and that it was common for them to make the round trip from Constantinople to Adrianople, a distance of 80 leagues, in two days. They were dressed very lightly, and by constant usage the soles of their feet were transformed into a leathery consistency. In the last century in the houses of the rich there were couriers who preceded the carriages and were known as "Basques," who could run for a very long time without apparent fatigue. In France there is a common proverb, "Courir comme un Basque." Rabelais says: "Grand-Gousier depeche le Basque son laquais pour querir Gargantua en toute hate."

In the olden times the English nobility maintained running footmen who, living under special regimen and training, were enabled to traverse unusual distances without apparent fatigue. There is an anecdote of a nobleman living in a castle not far from Edinburgh, who one evening charged his courier to carry a letter to that city. The next morning when he arose he found this valet sleeping in his antechamber. The nobleman waxed wroth, but the courier gave him a response to the letter. He had traveled 70 miles during the night. It is said that one of the noblemen under Charles II in preparing for a great dinner perceived that one of the indispensable pieces of his service was missing. His courier was dispatched in great haste to another house in his domain, 15 miles distant, and returned in two hours with the necessary article, having traversed a distance of over 30 miles. It is also said that a courier carrying a letter to a London physician returned with the potion prescribed within twenty-four hours, having traversed 148 miles. There is little doubt of the ability of these couriers to tire out any horse. The couriers who accompany the diligences in Spain often fatigue the animals who draw the vehicles.

At the present time in this country the Indians furnish examples of marvelous feats of running. The Tauri-Mauri Indians, who live in the heart of the Sierra Madre Mountains, are probably the most wonderful long-distance runners in the world. Their name in the language of the mountain Mexicans means foot-runners; and there is little doubt that they perform athletic feats which equal the best in the days of the Olympian games. They are possibly the remnants of the wonderful runners among the Indian tribes in the beginning of this century. There is an account of one of the Tauri-Mauri who was mail carrier between Guarichic and San Jose de los Cruces, a distance of 50 miles of as rough, mountainous road as ever tried a mountaineer's lungs and limbs. Barehearted and barelegged, with almost no clothing, this man made this trip each day, and, carrying on his back a mail-pouch weighing 40 pounds, moved gracefully and easily over his path, from time to time increasing his speed as though practicing, and then again more slowly to smoke a cigarette. The Tauri-Mauri are long-limbed and slender, giving the impression of being above the average height. There is scarcely any flesh on their puny arms, but their legs are as muscular as those of a greyhound. In short running they have the genuine professional stride, something rarely seen in other Indian racers. In traversing long distances they leap and bound like deer.

"Deerfoot," the famous Indian long-distance runner, died on the Cattaraugus Reservation in January, 1896. His proper name was Louis Bennett, the name "Deerfoot" having been given to him for his prowess in running. He was born on the reservation in 1828. In 1861 he went to England, where he defeated the English champion runners. In April, 1863, he ran 11 miles in London in fifty-six minutes fifty-two seconds, and 12 miles in one hour two minutes and two and one-half seconds, both of which have stood as world's records ever since.

In Japan, at the present day, the popular method of conveyance, both in cities and in rural districts, is the two-wheeled vehicle, looking like a baby-carriage, known to foreigners as the jinrickisha, and to the natives as the kuruma. In the city of Tokio there is estimated to be 38,000 of these little carriages in use. They are drawn by coolies, of whose endurance remarkable stories are told. These men wear light cotton breeches and a blue cotton jacket bearing the license number, and the indispensable umbrella hat. In the course of a journey in hot weather the jinrickisha man will gradually remove most of his raiment and stuff it into the carriage. In the rural sections he is covered with only two strips of cloth, one wrapped about his head and the other about his loins. It is said that when the roadway is good, these "human horses" prefer to travel bare-footed; when working in the mud they wrap a piece of straw about each big toe, to prevent slipping and to give them a firmer grip. For any of these men a five-mile spurt on a good road without a breathing spell is a small affair. A pair of them will roll a jinrickisha along a country road at the rate of four miles an hour, and they will do this eight hours a day. The general average of the distance traversed in a day is 25 miles. Cockerill, who has recently described these men, says that the majority of them die early. The terrible physical strain brings on hypertrophy and valvular diseases of the heart, and many of them suffer from hernia. Occasionally one sees a veteran jinrickisha man, and it is interesting to note how tenderly he is helped by his confrѐres. They give him preference as regards wages, help push his vehicle up heavy grades, and show him all manner of consideration.

Figure 180 represents two Japanese porters and their usual load, which is much more difficult to transport than a jinrickisha carriage. In other Eastern countries, palanquins and other means of conveyance are still borne on the shoulders of couriers, and it is not so long since our ancestors made their calls in Sedan-chairs borne by sturdy porters.

Some of the letter-carriers of India make a daily journey of 30 miles. They carry in one hand a stick, at the extremity of which is a ring containing several little plates of iron, which, agitated during the course, produce a loud noise designed to keep off ferocious beasts and serpents. In the other hand they carry a wet cloth, with which they frequently refresh themselves by wiping the countenance. It is said that a regular Hindustanee carrier, with a weight of 80 pounds on his shoulder,—carried, of course, in two divisions, hung on his neck by a yoke,—will, if properly paid, lope along over 100 miles in twenty-four hours—a feat which would exhaust any but the best trained runners.

The "go-as-you-please" pedestrians, whose powers during the past years have been exhibited in this country and in England, have given us marvelous examples of endurance, over 600 miles having been accomplished in a six-days' contest. Hazael, the professional pedestrian, has run over 450 miles in ninety-nine hours, and Albert has traveled over 500 miles in one hundred and ten hours. Rowell, Hughes, and Fitzgerald have astonishingly high records for long-distance running, comparing favorably with the older, and presumably mythical, feats of this nature. In California, C. A. Harriman of Truckee in April, 1883, walked twenty-six hours without once resting, traversing 122 miles.

For the purpose of comparison we give the best modern records for running:—

100 Yards.—9 3/5 seconds, made by Edward Donavan, at Natick, Mass., September 2, 1895.

220 Yards.—21 3/5 seconds, made by Harry Jewett, at Montreal, September 24, 1892.

Quarter-Mile.—47 3/4 seconds, made by W. Baker, at Boston, Mass., July 1, 1886.

Half-Mile.—1 minute 53 2/3 seconds, made by C. J. Kirkpatrick, at Manhattan Field, New York, September 21, 1895.

1 Mile.—4 minutes 12 3/4 seconds, made by W. G. George, at London, England, August 23, 1886.

5 Miles.—24 minutes 40 seconds, made by J. White, in England, May 11, 1863.

10 Miles.—51 minutes 6 3/5 seconds, made by William Cummings, at London, England, September 18, 1895.

25 Miles.—2 hours 33 minutes 44 seconds, made by G. A. Dunning, at London, England, December 26, 1881.

50 Miles.—5 hours 55 minutes 4 1/2 seconds, made by George Cartwright, at London, England, February 21, 1887.

75 Miles.—8 hours 48 minutes 30 seconds, made by George Littlewood, at London, England, November 24, 1884.

100 Miles.—13 hours 26 minutes 30 seconds, made by Charles Rowell at New York, February 27, 1882.

In instances of long-distance traversing, rapidity is only a secondary consideration, the remarkable fact being in the endurance of fatigue and the continuity of the exercise. William Gale walked 1500 miles in a thousand consecutive hours, and then walked 60 miles every twenty-four hours for six weeks on the Lillie Bridge cinder path. He was five feet five inches tall, forty-nine years of age, and weighed 121 pounds, and was but little developed muscularly. He was in good health during his feat; his diet for the twenty-four hours was 16 pounds of meat, five or six eggs, some cocoa, two quarts of milk, a quart of tea, and occasionally a glass of bitter ale, but never wine nor spirits. Strange to say, he suffered from constipation, and took daily a compound rhubarb pill. He was examined at the end of his feat by Gant. His pulse was 75, strong, regular, and his heart was normal. His temperature was 97.25 degrees F., and his hands and feet warm; respirations were deep and averaged 15 a minute. He suffered from frontal headache and was drowsy. During the six weeks he had lost only seven pounds, and his appetite maintained its normal state.

Zeuner of Cincinnati refers to John Snyder of Dunkirk, whose walking-feats were marvelous. He was not an impostor. During forty-eight hours he was watched by the students of the Ohio Medical College, who stated that he walked constantly; he assured them that it did not rest him to sit down, but made him uncomfortable. The celebrated Weston walked 5000 miles in one hundred days, but Snyder was said to have traveled 25,000 miles in five hundred days and was apparently no more tired than when he began.

Recently there was a person who pushed a wheelbarrow from San Francisco to New York in one hundred and eighteen days. In 1809 the celebrated Captain Barclay wagered that he could walk 1000 miles in one thousand consecutive hours, and gained his bet with some hours to spare. In 1834 Ernest Mensen astonished all Europe by his pedestrian exploits. He was a Norwegian sailor, who wagered that he could walk from Paris to Moscow in fifteen days. On June 25, 1834, at ten o'clock A.M., he entered the Kremlin, after having traversed 2500 kilometers (1550 miles) in fourteen days and eighteen hours. His performances all over Europe were so marvelous as to be almost incredible. In 1836, in the service of the East India Company, he was dispatched from Calcutta to Constantinople, across Central Asia. He traversed the distance in fifty-nine days, accomplishing 9000 kilometers (5580 miles) in one-third less time than the most rapid caravan. He died while attempting to discover the source of the Nile, having reached the village of Syang.

A most marvelous feat of endurance is recorded in England in the first part of this century. It is said that on a wager Sir Andrew Leith Hay and Lord Kennedy walked two days and a night under pouring rain, over the Grampian range of mountains, wading all one day in a bog. The distance traversed was from a village called Banchory on the river Dee to Inverness. This feat was accomplished without any previous preparation, both men starting shortly after the time of the wager.

Riders.—The feats of endurance accomplished by the couriers who ride great distances with many changes of horses are noteworthy. According to a contemporary medical journal there is, in the Friend of India, an account of the Thibetan couriers who ride for three weeks with intervals of only half an hour to eat and change horses. It is the duty of the officials at the Dak bungalows to see that the courier makes no delay, and even if dying he is tied to his horse and sent to the next station. The celebrated English huntsman, "Squire" Osbaldistone, on a wager rode 200 miles in seven hours ten minutes and four seconds. He used 28 horses; and as one hour twenty-two minutes and fifty-six seconds were allowed for stoppages, the whole time, changes and all, occupied in accomplishing this wonderful feat was eight hours and forty-two minutes. The race was ridden at the Newmarket Houghton Meeting over a four-mile course. It is said that a Captain Horne of the Madras Horse Artillery rode 200 miles on Arab horses in less than ten hours along the road between Madras and Bangalore. When we consider the slower speed of the Arab horses and the roads and climate of India, this performance equals the 200 miles in the shorter time about an English race track and on thoroughbreds. It is said that this wonderful horseman lost his life in riding a horse named "Jumping Jenny" 100 miles a day for eight days. The heat was excessive, and although the horse was none the worse for the performance, the Captain died from the exposure he encountered. There is a record of a Mr. Bacon of the Bombay Civil Service, who rode one camel from Bombay to Allygur (perhaps 800 miles) in eight days.

As regards the physiology of the runners and walkers, it is quite interesting to follow the effects of training on the respiration, whereby in a measure is explained the ability of these persons to maintain their respiratory function, although excessively exercising. A curious discussion, persisted in since antiquity, is as to the supposed influence of the spleen on the ability of couriers. For ages runners have believed that the spleen was a hindrance to their vocation, and that its reduction was followed by greater agility on the course. With some, this opinion is perpetuated to the present day. In France there is a proverb, "Courir comme un derate." To reduce the size of the spleen, the Greek athletes used certain beverages, the composition of which was not generally known; the Romans had a similar belief and habit Pliny speaks of a plant called equisetum, a decoction of which taken for three days after a fast of twenty-four hours would effect absorption of the spleen. The modern pharmacopeia does not possess any substance having a similar virtue, although quinin has been noticed to diminish the size of the spleen when engorged in malarial fevers. Strictly speaking, however, the facts are not analogous. Hippocrates advises a moxa of mushrooms applied over the spleen for melting or dissolving it. Godefroy Moebius is said to have seen in the village of Halberstadt a courier whose spleen had been cauterized after incision; and about the same epoch (seventeenth century) some men pretended to be able to successfully extirpate the spleen for those who desired to be couriers. This operation we know to be one of the most delicate in modern surgery, and as we are progressing with our physiologic knowledge of the spleen we see nothing to justify the old theory in regard to its relations to agility and coursing.

Swimming.—The instances of endurance that we see in the aquatic sports are equally as remarkable as those that we find among the runners and walkers. In the ancient days the Greeks, living on their various islands and being in a mild climate, were celebrated for their prowess as swimmers. Socrates relates the feats of swimming among the inhabitants of Delos. The journeys of Leander across the Hellespont are well celebrated in verse and prose, but this feat has been easily accomplished many times since, and is hardly to be classed as extraordinary. Herodotus says that the Macedonians were skilful swimmers; and all the savage tribes about the borders of waterways are found possessed of remarkable dexterity and endurance in swimming.

In 1875 the celebrated Captain Webb swam from Dover to Calais. On landing he felt extremely cold, but his body was as warm as when he started. He was exhausted and very sleepy, falling in deep slumber on his way to the hotel. On getting into bed his temperature was 98 degrees F. and his pulse normal. In five hours he was feverish, his temperature rising to 101 degrees F. During the passage he was blinded from the salt water in his eyes and the spray beating against his face. He strongly denied the newspaper reports that he was delirious, and after a good rest was apparently none the worse for the task. In 1876 he again traversed this passage with the happiest issue. In 1883 he was engaged by speculators to swim the rapids at Niagara, and in attempting this was overcome by the powerful currents, and his body was not recovered for some days after. The passage from Dover to Calais has been duplicated.

In 1877 Cavill, another Englishman, swam from Cape Griz-Nez to South Forland in less than thirteen hours. In 1880 Webb swam and floated at Scarborough for seventy-four consecutive hours—of course, having no current to contend with and no point to reach. This was merely a feat of staying in the water. In London in 1881, Beckwith, swimming ten hours a day over a 32-lap course for six days, traversed 94 miles. Since the time of Captain Webb, who was the pioneer of modern long-distance swimming, many men have attempted and some have duplicated his feats; but these foolhardy performances have in late years been diminishing, and many of the older feats are forbidden by law.

Jumpers and acrobatic tumblers have been popular from the earliest time. By the aid of springing boards and weights in their hands, the old jumpers covered great distances. Phayllus of Croton is accredited with jumping the incredible distance of 55 feet, and we have the authority of Eustache and Tzetzes that this jump is genuine. In the writings of many Greek and Roman historians are chronicled jumps of about 50 feet by the athletes; if they are true, the modern jumpers have greatly degenerated. A jump of over 20 feet to-day is considered very clever, the record being 29 feet seven inches with weights, and 23 feet eight inches without weights, although much greater distances have been jumped with the aid of apparatus, but never an approximation to 50 feet. The most surprising of all these athletes are the tumblers, who turn somersaults over several animals arranged in a row. Such feats are not only the most amusing sights of a modern circus, but also the most interesting as well. The agility of these men is marvelous, and the force with which they throw themselves in the air apparently enables them to defy gravity. In London, Paris, or New York one may see these wonderful tumblers and marvel at the capabilities of human physical development.

In September, 1895, M. F. Sweeney, an American amateur, at Manhattan Field in New York jumped six feet 5 5/8 inches high in the running high jump without weights. With weights, J. H. Fitzpatrick at Oak Island, Mass., jumped six feet six inches high. The record for the running high kick is nine feet eight inches, a marvelous performance, made by C. C. Lee at New Haven, Conn., March 19, 1887.

Extraordinary physical development and strength has been a grand means of natural selection in the human species. As Guyot-Daubes remarks, in prehistoric times, when our ancestors had to battle against hunger, savage beasts, and their neighbors, and when the struggle for existence was so extremely hard, the strong man alone resisted and the weak succumbed. This natural selection has been perpetuated almost to our day; during the long succession of centuries, the chief or the master was selected on account of his being the strongest, or the most valiant in the combat. Originally, the cavaliers, the members of the nobility, were those who were noted for their courage and strength, and to them were given the lands of the vanquished. Even in times other than those of war, disputes of succession were settled by jousts and tourneys. This fact is seen in the present day among the lower animals, who in their natural state live in tribes; the leader is usually the strongest, the wisest, and the most courageous.

The strong men of all times have excited the admiration of their fellows and have always been objects of popular interest. The Bible celebrates the exploits of Samson of the tribe of Dan. During his youth he, single handed, strangled a lion; with the jaw-bone of an ass he is said to have killed 1000 Philistines and put the rest to flight. At another time during the night he transported from the village of Gaza enormous burdens and placed them on the top of a mountain. Betrayed by Delilah, he was delivered into the hands of his enemies and employed in the most servile labors. When old and blind he was attached to the columns of an edifice to serve as an object of public ridicule; with a violent effort he overturned the columns, destroying himself and 3000 Philistines.

In the Greek mythology we find a great number of heroes, celebrated for their feats of strength and endurance. Many of them have received the name of Hercules; but the most common of these is the hero who was supposed to be the son of Jupiter and Alemena. He was endowed with prodigious strength by his father, and was pursued with unrelenting hatred by Juno. In his infancy he killed with his hands the serpents which were sent to devour him. The legends about him are innumerable. He was said to have been armed with a massive club, which only he was able to carry. The most famous of his feats were the twelve labors, with which all readers of mythology are familiar. Hercules, personified, meant to the Greeks physical force as well as strength, generosity, and bravery, and was equivalent to the Assyrian Hercules. The Gauls had a Hercules-Pantopage, who, in addition to the ordinary qualities attributed to Hercules, had an enormous appetite.

As late as the sixteenth century, and in a most amusing and picturesque manner, Rabelais has given us the history of Gargantua, and even to this day, in some regions, there are groups of stones which are believed by ignorant people to have been thrown about by Gargantua in his play. In their citations the older authors often speak of battles, and in epic ballads of heroes with marvelous strength. In the army of Charlemagne, after Camerarius, and quoted by Guyot-Daubes (who has made an extensive collection of the literature on this subject and to whom the authors are indebted for much information), there was found a giant named Oenother, a native of a village in Suabia, who performed marvelous feats of strength. In his history of Bavaria Aventin speaks of this monster. To Roland, the nephew of Charlemagne, the legends attributed prodigious strength; and, dying in the valley of Roncesveaux, he broke his good sword "Durandal" by striking it against a rock, making a breach, which is stilled called the "Breche de Roland." Three years before his death, on his return from Palestine, Christopher, Duke of Bavaria, was said to have lifted to his shoulders a stone which weighed more than 340 pounds. Louis de Boufflers, surnamed the "Robust," who lived in 1534, was noted for his strength and agility. When he placed his feet together, one against the other, he could find no one able to disturb them. He could easily bend and break a horseshoe with his hands, and could seize an ox by the tail and drag it against its will. More than once he was said to have carried a horse on his shoulders. According to Guyot-Daubes there was, in the last century, a Major Barsaba who could seize the limb of a horse and fracture its bone. There was a tale of his lifting an iron anvil, in a blacksmith's forge, and placing it under his coat.

To the Emperor Maximilian I was ascribed enormous strength; even in his youth, when but a simple patriot, he vanquished, at the games given by Severus, 16 of the most vigorous wrestlers, and accomplished this feat without stopping for breath. It is said that this feat was the origin of his fortune. Among other celebrated persons in history endowed with uncommon strength were Edmund "Ironsides," King of England; the Caliph Mostasem-Billah; Baudouin, "Bras-de-Fer," Count of Flanders; William IV, called by the French "Fier-a-Bras," Duke of

Aquitaine; Christopher, son of Albert the Pious, Duke of Bavaria; Godefroy of Bouillon; the Emperor Charles IV; Scanderbeg; Leonardo da Vinci; Marshal Saxe; and the recently deceased Czar of Russia, Alexander III.

Turning now to the authentic modern Hercules, we have a man by the name of Eckeberg, born in Anhalt, and who traveled under the name of "Samson." He was exhibited in London, and performed remarkable feats of strength. He was observed by the celebrated Desaguliers (a pupil of Newton) in the commencement of the last century, who at that time was interested in the physiologic experiments of strength and agility. Desaguliers believed that the feats of this new Samson were more due to agility than strength. One day, accompanied by two of his confreres, although a man of ordinary strength, he duplicated some of Samson's feats, and followed his performance by a communication to the Royal Society. One of his tricks was to resist the strength of five or six men or of two horses. Desaguliers claimed that this was entirely due to the position taken. This person would lift a man by one foot, and bear a heavy weight on his chest when resting with his head and two feet on two chairs. By supporting himself with his arms he could lift a piece of cannon attached to his feet.

A little later Desaguliers studied an individual in London named Thomas Topham, who used no ruse in his feats and was not the skilful equilibrist that the German Samson was, his performances being merely the results of abnormal physical force. He was about thirty years old, five feet ten inches in height and well proportioned, and his muscles well developed, the strong ligaments showing under the skin. He ignored entirely the art of appearing supernaturally strong, and some of his feats were rendered difficult by disadvantageous positions. In the feat of the German—resisting the force of several men or horses—Topham exhibited no knowledge of the principles of physics, like that of his predecessor, but, seated on the ground and putting his feet against two stirrups, he was able to resist the traction of a single horse; when he attempted the same feat against two horses he was severely strained and wounded about the knees. According to Desaguliers, if Topham had taken the advantageous positions of the German Samson, he could have resisted not only two, but four horses. On another occasion, with the aid of a bridle passed about his neck, he lifted three hogsheads full of water, weighing 1386 pounds. If he had utilized the force of his limbs and his loins, like the German, he would have been able to perform far more difficult feats. With his teeth he could lift and maintain in a horizontal position a table over six feet long, at the extremity of which he would put some weight. Two of the feet of the table he rested on his knees. He broke a cord five cm. in diameter, one part of which was attached to a post and the other to a strap passed under his shoulder. He was able to carry in his hands a rolling-pin weighing 800 pounds, about twice the weight a strong man is considered able to lift.

Tom Johnson was another strong man who lived in London in the last century, but he was not an exhibitionist, like his predecessors. He was a porter on the banks of the Thames, his duty being to carry sacks of wheat and corn from the wharves to the warehouses. It was said that when one of his comrades was ill, and could not provide support for his wife and children, Johnson assumed double duty, carrying twice the load. He could seize a sack of wheat, and with it execute the movements of a club-swinger, and with as great facility. He became quite a celebrated boxer, and, besides his strength, he soon demonstrated his powers of endurance, never seeming fatigued after a lively bout. The porters of Paris were accustomed to lift and carry on their shoulders bags of flour weighing 159 kilograms (350 pounds) and to mount stairs with them. Johnson, on hearing this, duplicated the feat with three sacks, and on one occasion attempted to carry four, and resisted this load some little time. These four sacks weighed 1400 pounds.

Some years since there was a female Hercules who would get on her hands and knees under a carriage containing six people, and, forming an arch with her body, she would lift it off the ground, an attendant turning the wheels while in the air to prove that they were clear from the ground.

Guyot-Daubes considers that one of the most remarkable of all the men noted for their strength was a butcher living in the mountains of Margeride, known as Lapiada (the extraordinary). This man, whose strength was legendary in the neighboring country, one day seized a mad bull that had escaped from his stall and held him by the horns until his attendants could bind him. For amusement he would lie on his belly and allow several men to get on his back; with this human load he would rise to the erect position. One of Lapiada's great feats was to get under a cart loaded with hay and, forming an arch with his body, raise it from the ground, then little by little he would mount to his haunches, still holding the cart and hay. Lapiada terminated his Herculean existence in attempting a mighty effort. Having charged himself alone with the task of placing a heavy tree-trunk in a cart, he seized it, his muscles stiffened, but the blood gushed from his mouth and nostrils, and he fell, overcome at last. The end of Lapiada presents an analogue to that of the celebrated athlete, Polydamas, who was equally the victim of too great confidence in his muscular force, and who died crushed by the force that he hoped to maintain. Figures 181 and 183 portray the muscular development of an individual noted for his feats of strength, and who exhibited not long since.

In recent years we have had Sebastian Miller, whose specialty was wrestling and stone-breaking; Samson, a recent English exhibitionist, Louis Cyr, and Sandow, who, in addition to his remarkable strength and control over his muscles, is a very clever gymnast. Sandow gives an excellent exposition of the so-called "checkerboard "arrangement of the muscular fibers of the lower thoracic and abdominal regions, and in a brilliant light demonstrates his extraordinary power over his muscles, contracting muscles ordinarily involuntary in time with music, a feat really more remarkable than his exhibition of strength. Figures 182 and 184 show the beautiful muscular development of this remarkable man.

Joseph Pospischilli, a convict recently imprisoned in the Austrian fortress of Olen, surprised the whole Empire by his wonderful feats of strength. One of his tricks was to add a fifth leg to a common table (placing the useless addition in the exact center) and then balance it with his teeth while two full-grown gipsies danced on it, the music being furnished by a violinist seated in the middle of the well-balanced platform. One day when the prison in which this Hercules was confined was undergoing repairs, he picked up a large carpenter's bench with his teeth and held it balanced aloft for nearly a minute. Since being released from the Olen prison, Pospischilli and his cousin, another local "strong man" named Martenstine, have formed a combination and are now starring Southern Europe, performing all kinds of startling feats of strength. Among other things they have had a 30-foot bridge made of strong timbers, which is used in one of their great muscle acts. This bridge has two living piers—Pospischilli acting as one and Martenstine the other. Besides supporting this monstrous structure (weight, 1866 pounds) upon their shoulders, these freaks of superhuman strength allow a team of horses and a wagon loaded with a ton of cobble-stones to be driven across it.

It is said that Selig Whitman, known as "Ajax," a New York policeman, has lifted 2000 pounds with his hands and has maintained 450 pounds with his teeth. This man is five feet 8 1/2 inches tall and weighs 162 pounds. His chest measurement is 40 inches, the biceps 17 inches, that of his neck 16 1/2 inches, the forearm 11, the wrist 9 1/2, the thigh 23, and the calf 17.

One of the strongest of the "strong women" is Madame Elise, a Frenchwoman, who performs with her husband. Her greatest feat is the lifting of eight men weighing altogether about 1700 pounds. At her performances she supports across her shoulders a 700-pound dumb-bell, on each side of which a person is suspended.

Miss Darnett, the "singing strong lady," extends herself upon her hands and feet, face uppermost, while a stout platform, with a semicircular groove for her neck, is fixed upon her chest, abdomen, and thighs by means of a waist-belt which passes through brass receivers on the under side of the board. An ordinary upright piano is then placed on the platform by four men; a performer mounts the platform and plays while the "strong lady" sings a love song while supporting possibly half a ton.

Strength of the Jaws.—There are some persons who exhibit extraordinary power of the jaw. In the curious experiments of Regnard and Blanchard at the Sorbonne, it was found that a crocodile weighing about 120 pounds exerted a force between its jaws at a point corresponding to the insertion of the masseter muscles of 1540 pounds; a dog of 44 pounds exerted a similar force of 363 pounds.

It is quite possible that in animals like the tiger and lion the force would equal 1700 or 1800 pounds. The anthropoid apes can easily break a cocoanut with their teeth, and Guyot-Daubes thinks that possibly a gorilla has a jaw-force of 200 pounds. A human adult is said to exert a force of from 45 to 65 pounds between his teeth, and some individuals exceed this average as much as 100 pounds. In Buffon's experiments he once found a Frenchman who could exert a force of 534 pounds with his jaws.

In several American circuses there have been seen women who hold themselves by a strap between their teeth while they are being hauled up to a trapeze some distance from the ground. A young mulatto girl by the name of "Miss Kerra" exhibited in the Winter Circus in Paris; suspended from a trapeze, she supported a man at the end of a strap held between her teeth, and even permitted herself to be turned round and round.

She also held a cannon in her teeth while it was fired. This feat has been done by several others. According to Guyot-Daubes, at Epernay in 1882, while a man named Bucholtz, called "the human cannon," was performing this feat, the cannon, which was over a yard long and weighed nearly 200 pounds, burst and wounded several of the spectators.

There was another Hercules in Paris, who with his teeth lifted and held a heavy cask of water on which was seated a man and varying weights, according to the size of his audience, at the same time keeping his hands occupied with other weights. Figure 185 represents a well-known modern exhibitionist lifting with his teeth a cask on which are seated four men. The celebrated Mlle. Gauthier, an actress of the Comedie-Francais, had marvelous power of her hands, bending coins, rolling up silver plate, and performing divers other feats. Major Barsaba had enormous powers of hand and fingers. He could roll a silver plate into the shape of a goblet. Being challenged by a Gascon, he seized the hand of his unsuspecting adversary in the ordinary manner of salutation and crushed all the bones of the fingers, thus rendering unnecessary any further trial of strength.

It is said that Marshal Saxe once visited a blacksmith ostensibly to have his horse shod, and seeing no shoe ready he took a bar of iron, and with his hands fashioned it into a horseshoe. There are Japanese dentists who extract teeth with their wonderfully developed fingers. There are stories of a man living in the village of Cantal who received the sobriquet of "La Coupia" (The Brutal). He would exercise his function as a butcher by strangling with his fingers the calves and sheep, instead of killing them in the ordinary manner. It is said that one day, by placing his hands on the shoulders of the strong man of a local fair, he made him faint by the pressure exerted by his fingers.

Manual strangulation is a well-known crime and is quite popular in some countries. The Thugs of India sometimes murdered their victims in this way. Often such force is exerted by the murderer's fingers as to completely fracture the cricoid cartilage.

In viewing the feats of strength of the exhibitionist we must bear in consideration the numerous frauds perpetrated. A man of extraordinary strength sometimes finds peculiar stone, so stratified that he is able to break it with the force he can exert by a blow from the hand alone, although a man of ordinary strength would try in vain. In most of these instances, if one were to take a piece of the exhibitionist's stone, he would find that a slight tap of the hammer would break it. Again, there are many instances in which the stone has been found already separated and fixed quite firmly together, placing it out of the power of an ordinary man to break, but which the exhibitionist finds within his ability. This has been the solution of the feats of many of the individuals who invite persons to send them marked stones to use at their performances. By skilfully arranging stout twine on the hands, it is surprising how easily it is broken, and there are many devices and tricks to deceive the public, all of which are more or less used by "strong men."

The recent officially recorded feats of strength that stand unequaled in the last decade are as follows:—

Weight-lifting.—Hands alone 1571 1/4 pounds, done by C. G. Jefferson, an amateur, at Clinton, Mass December 10, 1890; with harness, 3239 pounds, by W B. Curtis, at New York December 20 1868; Louis Cyr, at Berthierville, Can., October 1, 1888, pushed up 3536 pounds of pig-iron with his back, arms, and legs.

Dumb-bells.—H. Pennock, in New York, 1870, put up a 10-pound dumb-bell 8431 times in four hours thirty-four minutes; by using both hands to raise it to the shoulder, and then using one hand alone, R. A. Pennell, in New York, January 31, 1874, managed to put up a bell weighing 201 pounds 5 ounces; and Eugene Sandow, at London, February 11, 1891, surpassed this feat with a 250-pound bell.

Throwing 16-pound hammer.—J. S. Mitchell, at Travers Island, N. Y., October 8, 1892, made a record-throw of 145 feet 3/4 inch.

Putting 16-pound Shot.—George R. Gray, at Chicago, September 16, 1893, made the record of 47 feet.

Throwing 50-pound Weight.—J. S. Mitchell, at New York, September 22, 1894, made the distance record of 35 feet 10 inches; and at Chicago, September 16, 1893, made the height record of 15 feet 4 1/2 inches.

The class of people commonly known as contortionists by the laxity of their muscles and ligaments are able to dislocate or preternaturally bend their joints. In entertainments of an arena type and even in what are now called "variety performances" are to be seen individuals of this class. These persons can completely straddle two chairs, and do what they call "the split;" they can place their foot about their neck while maintaining the upright position; they can bend almost double at the waist in such a manner that the back of the head will touch the calves, while the legs are perpendicular with the ground; they can bring the popliteal region over their shoulders and in this position walk on their hands; they can put themselves in a narrow barrel; eat with a fork attached to a heel while standing on their hands, and perform divers other remarkable and almost incredible feats. Their performances are genuine, and they are real physiologic curiosities. Plate 6 represents two well-known contortionists in their favorite feats.

Wentworth, the oldest living contortionist, is about seventy years of age, but seems to have lost none of his earlier sinuosity. His chief feat is to stow himself away in a box 23 X 29 X 16 inches. When inside, six dozen wooden bottles of the same size and shape as those which ordinarily contain English soda water are carefully stowed away, packed in with him, and the lid slammed down. He bestows upon this act the curious and suggestive name of "Packanatomicalization."

Another class of individuals are those who can either partially or completely dislocate the major articulations of the body. Many persons exhibit this capacity in their fingers. Persons vulgarly called "double jointed" are quite common.

Charles Warren, an American contortionist, has been examined by several medical men of prominence and descriptions of him have appeared from time to time in prominent medical journals. When he was but a child he was constantly tumbling down, due to the heads of the femurs slipping from the acetabula, but reduction was always easy. When eight years old he joined a company of acrobats and strolling performers, and was called by the euphonious title of "the Yankee dish-rag." His muscular system was well-developed, and, like Sandow, he could make muscles act in concert or separately.

He could throw into energetic single action the biceps, the supinator longus, the radial extensors, the platysma myoides, and many other muscles. When he "strings," as he called it, the sartorius, that ribbon muscle shows itself as a tight cord, extending from the front of the iliac spine to the inner side of the knee. Another trick was to leave flaccid that part of the serratus magnus which is attached to the inferior angle of the scapula whilst he roused energetic contraction in the rhomboids. He could displace his muscles so that the lower angles of the scapulae projected and presented the appearance historically attributed to luxation of the scapula.

Warren was well informed on surgical landmarks and had evidently been a close student of Sir Astley Cooper's classical illustrations of dislocations. He was able so to contract his abdominal muscles that the aorta could be distinctly felt with the fingers. In this feat nearly all the abdominal contents were crowded beneath the diaphragm. On the other hand, he could produce a phantom abdominal tumor by driving the coils of the intestine within a peculiar grasp of the rectus and oblique muscles. The "growth" was rounded, dull on percussion, and looked as if an exploratory incision or puncture would be advisable for diagnosis.

By extraordinary muscular power and extreme laxity of his ligaments, he simulated all the dislocations about the hip joint. Sometimes he produced actual dislocation, but usually he said he could so distort his muscles as to imitate in the closest degree the dislocations. He could imitate the various forms of talipes, in such a way as to deceive an expert. He dislocated nearly every joint in the body with great facility. It was said that he could contract at will both pillars of the fauces. He could contract his chest to 34 inches and expand it to 41 inches.

Warren weighed 150 pounds, was a total abstainer, and was the father of two children, both of whom could readily dislocate their hips.

In France in 1886 there was shown a man who was called "l'homme protee," or protean man. He had an exceptional power over his muscles. Even those muscles ordinarily involuntary he could exercise at will. He could produce such rigidity of stature that a blow by a hammer on his body fell as though on a block of stone. By his power over his abdominal muscles he could give himself different shapes, from the portly alderman to the lean and haggard student, and he was even accredited with assuming the shape of a "living skeleton." Quatrefages, the celebrated French scientist, examined him, and said that he could shut off the blood from the right side and then from the left side of the body, which feat he ascribed to unilateral muscular action.

In 1893 there appeared in Washington, giving exhibitions at the colleges there and at the Emergency Hospital, a man named Fitzgerald, claiming to reside in Harrisburg, Pa., who made his living by exhibiting at medical colleges over the country. He simulated all the dislocations, claiming that they were complete, using manual force to produce and reduce them. He exhibited a thorough knowledge of the pathology of dislocations and of the anatomy of the articulations. He produced the different forms of talipes, as well as all the major hip-dislocations. When interrogated as to the cause of his enormous saphenous veins, which stood out like huge twisted cords under the skin and were associated with venous varicosity on the leg, he said he presumed they were caused by his constantly compressing the saphenous vein at the hip in giving his exhibitions, which in some large cities were repeated several times a day.

Endurance of Pain.—The question of the endurance of pain is, necessarily, one of comparison. There is little doubt that in the lower classes the sensation of pain is felt in a much less degree than in those of a highly intellectual and nervous temperament. If we eliminate the element of fear, which always predominates in the lower classes, the result of general hospital observation will show this distinction. There are many circumstances which have a marked influence on pain. Patriotism, enthusiasm, and general excitement, together with pride and natural obstinacy, prove the power of the mind over the body. The tortures endured by prisoners of war, religious martyrs and victims, exemplify the power of a strong will excited by deep emotion over the sensation of pain. The flagellants, persons who expiated their sins by voluntarily flaying themselves to the point of exhaustion, are modern examples of persons who in religious enthusiasm inflict pain on themselves. In the ancient times in India the frenzied zealots struggled for positions from which they could throw themselves under the car of the Juggernaut, and their intense emotions turned the pains of their wounds into a pleasure. According to the reports of her Majesty's surgeons, there are at the present time in India native Brahmins who hang themselves on sharp hooks placed in the flesh between the scapulae, and remain in this position without the least visible show of pain. In a similar manner they pierce the lips and cheeks with long pins and bore the tongue with a hot iron. From a reliable source the authors have an account of a man in Northern India who as a means of self-inflicted penance held his arm aloft for the greater part of each day, bending the fingers tightly on the palms. After a considerable time the nails had grown or been forced through the palms of the hands, making their exit on the dorsal surfaces. There are many savage rites and ceremonies calling for the severe infliction of pain on the participants which have been described from time to time by travelers. The Aztecs willingly sacrificed even their lives in the worship of their Sun-god.

By means of singing and dancing the Aissaoui, in the Algerian town of Constantine, throw themselves into an ecstatic state in which their bodies seem to be insensible even to severe wounds. Hellwald says they run sharp-pointed irons into their heads, eyes, necks, and breasts without apparent pain or injury to themselves. Some observers claim they are rendered insensible to pain by self-induced hypnotism.

An account by Carpenter of the Algerian Aissaoui contained the following lucid description of the performances of these people:—

"The center of the court was given up to the Aissaoui. These were 12 hollow-checked men, some old and some young, who sat cross-legged in an irregular semicircle on the floor. Six of them had immense flat drums or tambours, which they presently began to beat noisily. In front of them a charcoal fire burned in a brazier, and into it one of them from time to time threw bits of some sort of incense, which gradually filled the place with a thin smoke and a mildly pungent odor.

"For a long time—it seemed a long time—this went on with nothing to break the silence but the rhythmical beat of the drums. Gradually, however, this had become quicker, and now grew wild and almost deafening, and the men began a monotonous chant which soon was increased to shouting. Suddenly one of the men threw himself with a howl to the ground, when he was seized by another, who stripped him of part of his garments and led him in front of the fire. Here, while the pounding of the drums and the shouts of the men became more and more frantic, he stood swaying his body backward and forward, almost touching the ground in his fearful contortions, and wagging his head until it seemed as if he must dislocate it from his shoulders. All at once he drew from the fire a red-hot bar of iron, and with a yell of horror, which sent a shiver down one's back, held it up before his eyes. More violently than ever he swayed his body and wagged his head, until he had worked himself up to a climax of excitement, when he passed the glowing iron several times over the palm of each hand and then licked it repeatedly with his tongue. He next took a burning coal from the fire, and, placing it between his teeth, fanned it by his breath into a white heat. He ended his part of the performance by treading on red-hot coals scattered on the floor after which he resumed his place with the rest. Then the next performer with a yell as before, suddenly sprang to his feet and began again the same frantic contortions, in the midst of which he snatched from the fire an iron rod with a ball on one end, and after winding one of his eyelids around it until the eyeball was completely exposed, he thrust its point in behind the eye, which was forced far out on his cheek. It was held there for a moment when it was withdrawn, the eye released, and then rubbed vigorously a few times with the balled end of the rod.

"The drums all the time had been beaten lustily, and the men had kept up their chant, which still went unceasingly on. Again a man sprang to his feet and went through the same horrid motions. This time the performer took from the fire a sharp nail and, with a piece of the sandy limestone common to this region, proceeded with a series of blood-curdling howls to hammer it down into the top of his head, where it presently stuck upright, while he tottered dizzily around until it was pulled out with apparent effort and with a hollow snap by one of the other men.

"The performance had now fairly begun, and, with short intervals and always in the same manner, the frenzied contortions first, another ate up a glass lamp-chimney, which he first broke in pieces in his hands and then crunched loudly with his teeth. He then produced from a tin box a live scorpion, which ran across the floor with tail erect, and was then allowed to attach itself to the back of his hand and his face, and was finally taken into his mouth, where it hung suspended from the inside of his cheek and was finally chewed and swallowed. A sword was next produced, and after the usual preliminaries it was drawn by the same man who had just given the scorpion such unusual opportunities several times back and forth across his throat and neck, apparently deeply imbedded in the flesh. Not content with this, he bared his body at his waist, and while one man held the sword, edge upward, by the hilt and another by the point, about which a turban had been wrapped, he first stood upon it with his bare feet and then balanced himself across it on his naked stomach, while still another of the performers stood upon his back, whither he had sprung without any attempt to mollify the violence of the action. With more yells and genuflections, another now drew from the fire several iron skewers, some of which he thrust into the inner side of his cheeks and others into his throat at the larynx, where they were left for a while to hang.

"The last of the actors in this singular entertainment was a stout man with a careworn face, who apparently regarded his share as a melancholy duty which he was bound to perform, and the last part of it, I have no doubt, was particularly painful. He first took a handful of hay, and, having bared the whole upper part of his body, lighted the wisp at the brazier and then passed the blazing mass across his chest and body and over his arms and face. This was but a preliminary, and presently he began to sway backward and forward until one grew dazed with watching him. The drums grew noisier and noisier and the chant louder and wilder. The man himself had become maudlin, his tongue hung from his mouth, and now and then he ejaculated a sound like the inarticulate cry of an animal. He could only totter to the fire, out of which he snatched the balled instrument already described, which he thereupon thrust with a vicious stab into the pit of his stomach, where it was left to hang. A moment after he pulled it out again, and, picking up the piece of stone used before, he drove it with a series of resounding blows into a new place, where it hung, drawing the skin downward with its weight, until a companion pulled it out and the man fell in a heap on the floor."

To-day it is only through the intervention of the United States troops that some of the barbarous ceremonies of the North American Indians are suppressed. The episode of the "Ghost-dance" is fresh in every mind. Instances of self-mutilation, although illustrating this subject, will be discussed at length in Chapter XIV.

Malingerers often endure without flinching the most arduous tests. Supraorbital pressure is generally of little avail, and pinching, pricking, and even incision are useless with these hospital impostors. It is reported that in the City Hospital of St. Louis a negro submitted to the ammonia-test, inhaling this vapor for several hours without showing any signs of sensibility, and made his escape the moment his guard was absent. A contemporary journal says:—

"The obstinacy of resolute impostors seems, indeed, capable of emulating the torture-proof perseverance of religious enthusiasts and such martyrs of patriotism as Mueius Scaevola or Grand Master Ruediger of the Teutonic Knights, who refused to reveal the hiding place of his companion even when his captors belabored him with red-hot irons.

"One Basil Rohatzek, suspected of fraudulent enlistment (bounty-jumping, as our volunteers called it), pretended to have been thrown by his horse and to have been permanently disabled by a paralysis of the lower extremities. He dragged himself along in a pitiful manner, and his knees looked somewhat bruised, but he was known to have boasted his ability to procure his discharge somehow or other. One of his tent mates had also seen him fling himself violently and repeatedly on his knees (to procure those questionable bruises), and on the whole there seemed little doubt that the fellow was shamming. All the surgeons who had examined him concurred in that view, and the case was finally referred to his commanding officer, General Colloredo. The impostor was carried to a field hospital in a little Bohemian border town and watched for a couple of weeks, during which he had been twice seen moving his feet in his sleep. Still, the witnesses were not prepared to swear that those changes of position might not have been effected by a movement of the whole body. The suspect stuck to his assertion, and Colloredo, in a fit of irritation, finally summoned a surgeon, who actually placed the feet of the professed paralytic in "aqua fortis," but even this rigorous method availed the cruel surgeon nothing, and he was compelled to advise dismissal from the service.

"The martyrdom of Rohatzek, however, was a mere trifle compared with the ordeal by which the tribunal of Paris tried in vain to extort a confession of the would-be regicide, Damiens. Robert Damiens, a native of Arras, had been exiled as an habitual criminal, and returning in disguise made an attempt upon the life of Louis XV, January 5, 1757. His dagger pierced the mantle of the King, but merely grazed his neck. Damiens, who had stumbled, was instantly seized and dragged to prison, where a convocation of expert torturers exhausted their ingenuity in the attempt to extort a confession implicating the Jesuits, a conspiracy of Huguenots, etc. But Damiens refused to speak. He could have pleaded his inability to name accomplices who did not exist, but he stuck to his resolution of absolute silence. They singed off his skin by shreds, they wrenched out his teeth and finger-joints, they dragged him about at the end of a rope hitched to a team of stout horses, they sprinkled him from head to foot with acids and seething oil, but Damiens never uttered a sound till his dying groan announced the conclusion of the tragedy."

The apparent indifference to the pain of a major operation is sometimes marvelous, and there are many interesting instances on record. When at the battle of Dresden in 1813 Moreau, seated beside the Emperor Alexander, had both limbs shattered by a French cannon-ball, he did not utter a groan, but asked for a cigar and smoked leisurely while a surgeon amputated one of his members. In a short time his medical attendants expressed the danger and questionability of saving his other limb, and consulted him. In the calmest way the heroic General instructed them to amputate it, again remaining unmoved throughout the operation.

Crompton records a case in which during an amputation of the leg not a sound escaped from the patient's lips, and in three weeks, when it was found necessary to amputate the other leg, the patient endured the operation without an anesthetic, making no show of pain, and only remarking that he thought the saw did not cut well. Crompton quotes another case, in which the patient held a candle with one hand while the operator amputated his other arm at the shoulder-joint. Several instances of self-performed major operations are mentioned in Chapter XIV.

Supersensitiveness to Pain.—Quite opposite to the foregoing instances are those cases in which such influences as expectation, naturally inherited nervousness, and genuine supersensitiveness make the slightest pain almost unendurable. In many of these instances the state of the mind and occasionally the time of day have a marked influence. Men noted for their sagacity and courage have been prostrated by fear of pain. Sir Robert Peel, a man of acknowledged superior physical and intellectual power, could not even bear the touch of Brodie's finger to his fractured clavicle. The authors know of an instance of a pugilist who had elicited admiration by his ability to stand punishment and his indomitable courage in his combats, but who fainted from the puncture of a small boil on his neck.

The relation of pain to shock has been noticed by many writers. Before the days of anesthesia, such cases as the following, reported by Sir Astley Cooper, seem to have been not unusual: A brewer's servant, a man of middle age and robust frame, suffered much agony for several days from a thecal abscess, occasioned by a splinter of wood beneath the thumb. A few seconds after the matter was discharged by an incision, the man raised himself by a convulsive effort from his bed and instantly expired.

It is a well-known fact that powerful nerve-irritation, such as produces shock, is painless, and this accounts for the fact that wounds received during battle are not painful.

Leyden of Berlin showed to his class at the Charite Hospital a number of hysteric women with a morbid desire for operation without an anesthetic. Such persons do not seem to experience pain, and, on the contrary, appear to have genuine pleasure in pain. In illustration, Leyden showed a young lady who during a hysteric paroxysm had suffered a serious fracture of the jaw, injuring the facial artery, and necessitating quite an extensive operation. The facial and carotid arteries had to be ligated and part of the inferior maxilla removed, but the patient insisted upon having the operations performed without an anesthetic, and afterward informed the operator that she had experienced great pleasure throughout the whole procedure.

Pain as a Means of Sexual Enjoyment.—There is a form of sexual perversion in which the pervert takes delight in being subjected to degrading, humiliating, and cruel acts on the part of his or her associate. It was named masochism from Sacher-Masoch, an Austrian novelist, whose works describe this form of perversion. The victims are said to experience peculiar pleasure at the sight of a rival who has obtained the favor of their mistress, and will even receive blows and lashes from the rival with a voluptuous mixture of pain and pleasure. Masochism corresponds to the passivism of Stefanowski, and is the opposite of sadism, in which the pleasure is derived from inflicting pain on the object of affection. Krafft-Ebing cites several instances of masochism.

Although the enjoyment and frenzy of flagellation are well known, its pleasures are not derived from the pain but by the undoubted stimulation offered to the sexual centers by the castigation. The delight of the heroines of flagellation, Maria Magdalena of Pazzi and Elizabeth of Genton, in being whipped on the naked loins, and thus calling up sensual and lascivious fancies, clearly shows the significance of flagellation as a sexual excitant. It is said that when Elizabeth of Genton was being whipped she believed herself united with her ideal and would cry out in the loudest tones of the joys of love.

There is undoubtedly a sympathetic communication between the ramifying nerves of the skin of the loins and the lower portion of the spinal cord which contains the sexual centers. Recently, in cases of dysmenorrhea, amenorrhea dysmenorrhagia, and like sexual disorders, massage or gentle flagellation of the parts contiguous with the genitalia and pelvic viscera has been recommended. Taxil is the authority for the statement that just before the sexual act rakes sometimes have themselves flagellated or pricked until the blood flows in order to stimulate their diminished sexual power. Rhodiginus, Bartholinus, and other older physicians mention individuals in whom severe castigation was a prerequisite of copulation. As a ritual custom flagellation is preserved to the present day by some sects.

Before leaving the subject of flagellation it should be stated that among the serious after-results of this practice as a disciplinary means, fatal emphysema, severe hemorrhage, and shock have been noticed. There are many cases of death from corporal punishment by flogging. Ballingal records the death of a soldier from flogging; Davidson has reported a similar case, and there is a death from the same cause cited in the Edinburgh Medical and Surgical Journal for 1846.

Idiosyncrasy is a peculiarity of constitution whereby an individual is affected by external agents in a different manner from others. Begin defines idiosyncrasy as the predominance of an organ, of a viscus, or a system of organs. This definition does not entirely grasp the subject. An idiosyncrasy is something inherent in the organization of the individual, of which we only see the manifestation when proper causes are set in action. We do not attempt to explain the susceptibility of certain persons to certain foods and certain exposures. We know that such is the fact. According to Begin's idea, there is scarcely any separation between idiosyncrasy and temperament, whereas from what would appear to be sound reasoning, based on the physiology of the subject, a very material difference exists.

Idiosyncrasies may be congenital, hereditary, or acquired, and, if acquired, may be only temporary. Some, purely of mental origin, are often readily cured. One individual may synchronously possess an idiosyncrasy of the digestive, circulatory, and nervous systems. Striking examples of transitory or temporary idiosyncrasies are seen in pregnant women.

There are certain so-called antipathies that in reality are idiosyncrasies, and which are due to peculiarities of the ideal and emotional centers. The organ of sense in question and the center that takes cognizance of the image brought to it are in no way disordered. In some cases the antipathy or the idiosyncrasy develops to such an extent as to be in itself a species of monomania. The fear-maladies, or "phobias," as they are called, are examples of this class, and, belonging properly under temporary mental derangements, the same as hallucinations or delusions, will be spoken of in another chapter.

Possibly the most satisfactory divisions under which to group the material on this subject collected from literature are into examples of idiosyncrasies in which, although the effect is a mystery, the sense is perceptible and the cause distinctly defined and known, and those in which sensibility is latent. The former class includes all the peculiar antipathies which are brought about through the special senses, while the latter groups all those strange instances in which, without the slightest antipathy on the part of the subject, a certain food or drug, after ingestion, produces an untoward effect.

The first examples of idiosyncrasies to be noticed will be those manifested through the sense of smell. On the authority of Spigelius, whose name still survives in the nomenclature of the anatomy of the liver, Mackeuzie quotes an extraordinary case in a Roman Cardinal, Oliver Caraffa, who could not endure the smell of a rose. This is confirmed from personal observation by another writer, Pierius, who adds that the Cardinal was obliged every year to shut himself up during the rose season, and guards were stationed at the gates of his palace to stop any visitors who might be wearing the dreadful flower. It is, of course, possible that in this case the rose may not have caused the disturbance, and as it is distinctly stated that it was the smell to which the Cardinal objected, we may fairly conclude that what annoyed him was simply a manifestation of rose-fever excited by the pollen. There is also an instance of a noble Venetian who was always confined to his palace during the rose season. However, in this connection Sir Kenelm Digby relates that so obnoxious was a rose to Lady Heneage, that she blistered her cheek while accidentally lying on one while she slept. Ledelius records the description of a woman who fainted before a red rose, although she was accustomed to wear white ones in her hair. Cremer describes a Bishop who died of the smell of a rose from what might be called "aromatic pain."

The organ of smell is in intimate relation with the brain and the organs of taste and sight; and its action may thus disturb that of the esophagus, the stomach, the diaphragm, the intestines, the organs of generation, etc. Odorous substances have occasioned syncope, stupor, nausea, vomiting, and sometimes death. It is said that the Hindoos, and some classes who eat nothing but vegetables, are intensely nauseated by the odors of European tables, and for this reason they are incapable of serving as dining-room servants.

Fabricius Hildanus mentions a person who fainted from the odor of vinegar. The Ephemerides contains an instance of a soldier who fell insensible from the odor of a peony. Wagner knew a man who was made ill by the odor of bouillon of crabs. The odors of blood, meat, and fat are repugnant to herbivorous animals. It is a well-known fact that horses detest the odor of blood.

Schneider, the father of rhinology, mentions a woman in whom the odor of orange-flowers produced syncope. Odier has known a woman who was affected with aphonia whenever exposed to the odor of musk, but who immediately recovered after taking a cold bath. Dejean has mentioned a man who could not tolerate an atmosphere of cherries. Highmore knew a man in whom the slightest smell of musk caused headache followed by epistaxis. Lanzonius gives an account of a valiant soldier who could neither bear the sight nor smell of an ordinary pink. There is an instance on record in which the odor coming from a walnut tree excited epilepsy. It is said that one of the secretaries of Francis I was forced to stop his nostrils with bread if apples were on the table. He would faint if one was held near his nose Schenck says that the noble family of Fystates in Aquitaine had a similar peculiarity—an innate hatred of apples. Bruyerinus knew a girl of sixteen who could not bear the smell of bread, the slightest particle of which she would detect by its odor. She lived almost entirely on milk. Bierling mentions an antipathy to the smell of musk, and there is a case on record in which it caused convulsions. Boerhaave bears witness that the odor of cheese caused nasal hemorrhage. Whytt mentions an instance in which tobacco became repugnant to a woman each time she conceived, but after delivery this aversion changed to almost an appetite for tobacco fumes. Panaroli mentions an instance of sickness caused by the smell of sassafras, and there is also a record of a person who fell helpless at the smell of cinnamon. Wagner had a patient who detested the odor of citron. Ignorant of this repugnance, he prescribed a potion in which there was water of balm-mint, of an odor resembling citron. As soon as the patient took the first dose he became greatly agitated and much nauseated, and this did not cease until Wagner repressed the balm-mint. There is reported the case of a young woman, rather robust, otherwise normal, who always experienced a desire to go to stool after being subjected to any nasal irritation sufficient to excite sneezing.

It has already been remarked that individuals and animals have their special odors, certain of which are very agreeable to some people and extremely unpleasant to others. Many persons are not able to endure the emanations from cats, rats, mice, etc., and the mere fact of one of these animals being in their vicinity is enough to provoke distressing symptoms. Mlle. Contat, the celebrated French actress, was not able to endure the odor of a hare. Stanislaus, King of Poland and Duke of Lorraine, found it impossible to tolerate the smell of a cat. The Ephemerides mentions the odor of a little garden-frog as causing epilepsy. Ab Heers mentions a similar anomaly, fainting caused by the smell of eels. Habit had rendered Haller insensible to the odor of putrefying cadavers, but according to Zimmerman the odor of the perspiration of old people, not perceptible to others, was intolerable to him at a distance of ten or twelve paces. He also had an extreme aversion for cheese. According to Dejan, Gaubius knew a man who was unable to remain in a room with women, having a great repugnance to the female odor. Strange as it may seem, some individuals are incapable of appreciating certain odors. Blumenbach mentions an Englishman whose sense of smell was otherwise very acute, but he was unable to perceive the perfume of the mignonette.

The impressions which come to us through the sense of hearing cause sensations agreeable or disagreeable, but even in this sense we see marked examples of idiosyncrasies and antipathies to various sounds and tones. In some individuals the sensations in one ear differ from those of the other. Everard Home has cited several examples, and Heidmann of Vienna has treated two musicians, one of whom always perceived in the affected ear, during damp weather, tones an octave lower than in the other ear. The other musician perceived tones an octave higher in the affected ear. Cheyne is quoted as mentioning a case in which, when the subject heard the noise of a drum, blood jetted from the veins with considerable force. Sauvages has seen a young man in whom intense headache and febrile paroxysm were only relieved by the noise from a beaten drum. Esparron has mentioned an infant in whom an ataxic fever was established by the noise of this instrument. Ephemerides contains an account of a young man who became nervous and had the sense of suffocation when he heard the noise made by sweeping. Zimmerman speaks of a young girl who had convulsions when she heard the rustling of oiled silk. Boyle, the father of chemistry, could not conquer an aversion he had to the sound of water running through pipes. A gentleman of the Court of the Emperor Ferdinand suffered epistaxis when he heard a cat mew. La Mothe Le Vayer could not endure the sounds of musical instruments, although he experienced pleasurable sensations when he heard a clap of thunder. It is said that a chaplain in England always had a sensation of cold at the top of his head when he read the 53d chapter of Isaiah and certain verses of the Kings. There was an unhappy wight who could not hear his own name pronounced without being thrown into convulsions. Marguerite of Valois, sister of Francis I, could never utter the words "mort" or "petite verole," such a horrible aversion had she to death and small-pox. According to Campani, the Chevalier Alcantara could never say "lana," or words pertaining to woolen clothing. Hippocrates says that a certain Nicanor had the greatest horror of the sound of the flute at night, although it delighted him in the daytime. Rousseau reports a Gascon in whom incontinence of urine was produced by the sound of a bagpipe. Frisch, Managetta, and Rousse speak of a man in whom the same effect was produced by the sound of a hurdy-gurdy. Even Shakespeare alludes to the effects of the sound of bagpipes. Tissot mentions a case in which music caused epileptic convulsions, and Forestus mentions a beggar who had convulsions at the sound of a wooden trumpet similar to those used by children in play. Rousseau mentions music as causing convulsive laughter in a woman. Bayle mentions a woman who fainted at the sound of a bell. Paullini cites an instance of vomiting caused by music, and Marcellus Donatus mentions swooning from the same cause. Many people are unable to bear the noise caused by the grating of a pencil on a slate, the filing of a saw, the squeak of a wheel turning about an axle, the rubbing of pieces of paper together, and certain similar sounds. Some persons find the tones of music very disagreeable, and some animals, particularly dogs, are unable to endure it. In Albinus the younger the slightest perceptible tones were sufficient to produce an inexplicable anxiety. There was a certain woman of fifty who was fond of the music of the clarionet and flute, but was not able to listen to the sound of a bell or tambourine. Frank knew a man who ran out of church at the beginning of the sounds of an organ, not being able to tolerate them. Pope could not imagine music producing any pleasure. The harmonica has been noticed to produce fainting in females. Fischer says that music provokes sexual frenzy in elephants. Gutfeldt speaks of a peculiar idiosyncrasy of sleep produced by hearing music. Delisle mentions a young person who during a whole year passed pieces of ascarides and tenia, during which time he could not endure music.

Autenreith mentions the vibrations of a loud noise tickling the fauces to such an extent as to provoke vomiting. There are some emotional people who are particularly susceptible to certain expressions. The widow of Jean Calas always fell in a faint when she heard the words of the death-decree sounded on the street. There was a Hanoverian officer in the Indian war against Typoo-Saib, a good and brave soldier, who would feel sick if he heard the word "tiger" pronounced. It was said that he had experienced the ravages of this beast.

The therapeutic value of music has long been known. For ages warriors have been led to battle to the sounds of martial strains. David charmed away Saul's evil spirit with his harp. Horace in his 32d Ode Book 1, concludes his address to the lyre:—

"O laborum
Dulce lenimen mihicumque calve,
Rite vocanti;"

Or, as Kiessling of Berlin interprets:—

"O laborum,
Dulce lenimen medieumque, salve,
Rite vocanti."

—"O, of our troubles the sweet, the healing sedative, etc."

Homer, Plutarch, Theophrastus, and Galen say that music cures rheumatism, the pests, and stings of reptiles, etc. Diemerbroeck, Bonet, Baglivi, Kercher, and Desault mention the efficacy of melody in phthisis, gout, hydrophobia, the bites of venomous reptiles, etc. There is a case in the Lancet of a patient in convulsions who was cured in the paroxysm by hearing the tones of music. Before the French Academy of Sciences in 1708, and again in 1718, there was an instance of a dancing-master stricken with violent fever and in a condition of delirium, who recovered his senses and health on hearing melodious music. There is little doubt of the therapeutic value of music, but particularly do we find its value in instances of neuroses. The inspiration offered by music is well-known, and it is doubtless a stimulant to the intellectual work. Bacon, Milton, Warburton, and Alfieri needed music to stimulate them in their labors, and it is said that Bourdaloue always played an air on the violin before preparing to write.

According to the American Medico-Surgical Bulletin, "Professor Tarchanoff of Saint Petersburg has been investigating the influence of music upon man and other animals. The subject is by no means a new one. In recent times Dagiel and Fere have investigated the effect of music upon the respirations, the pulse, and the muscular system in man. Professor Tarchanoff made use of the ergograph of Mosso, and found that if the fingers were completely fatigued, either by voluntary efforts or by electric excitation, to the point of being incapable of making any mark except a straight line on the registering cylinder, music had the power of making the fatigue disappear, and the finger placed in the ergograph again commenced to mark lines of different heights, according to the amount of excitation. It was also found that music of a sad and lugubrious character had the opposite effect, and could check or entirely inhibit the contractions. Professor Tarchanoff does not profess to give any positive explanation of these facts, but he inclines to the view that 'the voluntary muscles, being furnished with excitomotor and depressant fibers, act in relation to the music similarly to the heart—that is to say, that joyful music resounds along the excitomotor fibers, and sad music along the depressant or inhibitory fibers.' Experiments on dogs showed that music was capable of increasing the elimination of carbonic acid by 16.7 per cent, and of increasing the consumption of oxygen by 20.1 per cent. It was also found that music increased the functional activity of the skin. Professor Tarchanoff claims as the result of these experiments that music may fairly be regarded as a serious therapeutic agent, and that it exercises a genuine and considerable influence over the functions of the body. Facts of this kind are in no way surprising, and are chiefly of interest as presenting some physiologic basis for phenomena that are sufficiently obvious. The influence of the war-chant upon the warrior is known even to savage tribes. We are accustomed to regard this influence simply as an ordinary case of psychic stimuli producing physiologic effects.

"Professor Tarchanoff evidently prefers to regard the phenomena as being all upon the same plane, namely, that of physiology; and until we know the difference between mind and body, and the principles of their interaction, it is obviously impossible to controvert this view successfully. From the immediately practical point of view we should not ignore the possible value of music in some states of disease. In melancholia and hysteria it is probably capable of being used with benefit, and it is worth bearing in mind in dealing with insomnia. Classical scholars will not forget that the singing of birds was tried as a remedy to overcome the insomnia of Maecenas. Music is certainly a good antidote to the pernicious habit of introspection and self-analysis, which is often a curse both of the hysteric and of the highly cultured. It would seem obviously preferable to have recourse to music of a lively and cheerful character."

Idiosyncrasies of the visual organs are generally quite rare. It is well-known that among some of the lower animals, e.g., the turkey-cocks, buffaloes, and elephants, the color red is unendurable. Buchner and Tissot mention a young boy who had a paroxysm if he viewed anything red. Certain individuals become nauseated when they look for a long time on irregular lines or curves, as, for examples, in caricatures. Many of the older examples of idiosyncrasies of color are nothing more than instances of color-blindness, which in those times was unrecognized. Prochaska knew a woman who in her youth became unconscious at the sight of beet-root, although in her later years she managed to conquer this antipathy, but was never able to eat the vegetable in question. One of the most remarkable forms of idiosyncrasy on record is that of a student who was deprived of his senses by the very sight of an old woman. On one occasion he was carried out from a party in a dying state, caused, presumably, by the abhorred aspect of the chaperons The Count of Caylus was always horror-stricken at the sight of a Capuchin friar. He cured himself by a wooden image dressed in the costume of this order placed in his room and constantly before his view. It is common to see persons who faint at the sight of blood. Analogous are the individuals who feel nausea in an hospital ward.

All Robert Boyle's philosophy could not make him endure the sight of a spider, although he had no such aversion to toads, venomous snakes, etc. Pare mentions a man who fainted at the sight of an eel, and another who had convulsions at the sight of a carp. There is a record of a young lady in France who fainted on seeing a boiled lobster. Millingen cites the case of a man who fell into convulsions whenever he saw a spider. A waxen one was made, which equally terrified him. When he recovered, his error was pointed out to him, and the wax figure was placed in his hand without causing dread, and henceforth the living insect no longer disturbed him. Amatus Lusitanus relates the case of a monk who fainted when he beheld a rose, and never quitted his cell when that flower was in bloom. Scaliger, the great scholar, who had been a soldier a considerable portion of his life, confesses that he could not look on a water-cress without shuddering, and remarks: "I, who despise not only iron, but even thunderbolts, who in two sieges (in one of which I commanded) was the only one who did not complain of the food as unfit and horrible to eat, am seized with such a shuddering horror at the sight of a water-cress that I am forced to go away." One of his children was in the same plight as regards the inoffensive vegetable, cabbage. Scaliger also speaks of one of his kinsmen who fainted at the sight of a lily. Vaughheim, a great huntsman of Hanover, would faint at the sight of a roasted pig. Some individuals have been disgusted at the sight of eggs. There is an account of a sensible man who was terrified at the sight of a hedgehog, and for two years was tormented by a sensation as though one was gnawing at his bowels. According to Boyle, Lord Barrymore, a veteran warrior and a person of strong mind, swooned at the sight of tansy. The Duke d'Epernon swooned on beholding a leveret, although a hare did not produce the same effect. Schenck tells of a man who swooned at the sight of pork. The Ephemerides contains an account of a person who lost his voice at the sight of a crab, and also cites cases of antipathy to partridges, a white hen, to a serpent, and to a toad. Lehman speaks of an antipathy to horses; and in his observations Lyser has noticed aversion to the color purple. It is a strange fact that the three greatest generals of recent years, Wellington, Napoleon, and Roberts, could never tolerate the sight of a cat, and Henry III of France could not bear this animal in his room. We learn of a Dane of herculean frame who had a horror of cats. He was asked to a supper at which, by way of a practical joke, a live cat was put on the table in a covered dish. The man began to sweat and shudder without knowing why, and when the cat was shown he killed his host in a paroxysm of terror. Another man could not even see the hated form even in a picture without breaking into a cold sweat and feeling a sense of oppression about the heart. Quercetanus and Smetius mention fainting at the sight of cats. Marshal d'Abret was supposed to be in violent fear of a pig.

As to idiosyncrasies of the sense of touch, it is well known that some people cannot handle velvet or touch the velvety skin of a peach without having disagreeable and chilly sensations come over them. Prochaska knew a man who vomited the moment he touched a peach, and many people, otherwise very fond of this fruit, are unable to touch it. The Ephemerides speaks of a peculiar idiosyncrasy of skin in the axilla of a certain person, which if tickled would provoke vomiting. It is occasionally stated in the older writings that some persons have an idiosyncrasy as regards the phases of the sun and moon. Baillou speaks of a woman who fell unconscious at sunset and did not recover till it reappeared on the horizon. The celebrated Chancellor Bacon, according to Mead, was very delicate, and was accustomed to fall into a state of great feebleness at every moon-set without any other imaginable cause. He never recovered from his swooning until the moon reappeared.

Nothing is more common than the idiosyncrasy which certain people display for certain foods. The trite proverb, "What is one man's meat is another man's poison," is a genuine truth, and is exemplified by hundreds of instances. Many people are unable to eat fish without subsequent disagreeable symptoms. Prominent among the causes of urticaria are oysters, crabs, and other shell fish, strawberries, raspberries, and other fruits. The abundance of literature on this subject makes an exhaustive collection of data impossible, and only a few of the prominent and striking instances can be reported.

Amatus Lusitanus speaks of vomiting and diarrhea occurring each time a certain Spaniard ate meat. Haller knew a person who was purged violently by syrup of roses. The son of one of the friends of Wagner would vomit immediately after the ingestion of any substance containing honey. Bayle has mentioned a person so susceptible to honey that by a plaster of this substance placed upon the skin this untoward effect was produced. Whytt knew a woman who was made sick by the slightest bit of nutmeg. Tissot observed vomiting in one of his friends after the ingestion of the slightest amount of sugar. Ritte mentions a similar instance. Roose has seen vomiting produced in a woman by the slightest dose of distilled water of linden. There is also mentioned a person in whom orange-flower water produced the same effect. Dejean cites a case in which honey taken internally or applied externally acted like poison. It is said that the celebrated Haen would always have convulsions after eating half a dozen strawberries. Earle and Halifax attended a child for kidney-irritation produced by strawberries, and this was the invariable result of the ingestion of this fruit. The authors personally know of a family the male members of which for several generations could not eat strawberries without symptoms of poisoning. The female members were exempt from the idiosyncrasy. A little boy of this family was killed by eating a single berry. Whytt mentions a woman of delicate constitution and great sensibility of the digestive tract in whom foods difficult of digestion provoked spasms, which were often followed by syncopes. Bayle describes a man who vomited violently after taking coffee. Wagner mentions a person in whom a most insignificant dose of manna had the same effect. Preslin speaks of a woman who invariably had a hemorrhage after swallowing a small quantity of vinegar. According to Zimmerman, some people are unable to wash their faces on account of untoward symptoms. According to Ganbius, the juice of a citron applied to the skin of one of his acquaintances produced violent rigors.

Brasavolus says that Julia, wife of Frederick, King of Naples, had such an aversion to meat that she could not carry it to her mouth without fainting. The anatomist Gavard was not able to eat apples without convulsions and vomiting. It is said that Erasmus was made ill by the ingestion of fish; but this same philosopher, who was cured of a malady by laughter, expressed his appreciation by an elegy on the folly. There is a record of a person who could not eat almonds without a scarlet rash immediately appearing upon the face. Marcellus Donatus knew a young man who could not eat an egg without his lips swelling and purple spots appearing on his face. Smetius mentions a person in whom the ingestion of fried eggs was often followed by syncope. Brunton has seen a case of violent vomiting and purging after the slightest bit of egg. On one occasion this person was induced to eat a small morsel of cake on the statement that it contained no egg, and, although fully believing the words of his host, he subsequently developed prominent symptoms, due to the trace of egg that was really in the cake. A letter from a distinguished litterateur to Sir Morell Mackenzie gives a striking example of the idiosyncrasy to eggs transmitted through four generations. Being from such a reliable source, it has been deemed advisable to quote the account in full: "My daughter tells me that you are interested in the ill-effects which the eating of eggs has upon her, upon me, and upon my father before us. I believe my grandfather, as well as my father, could not eat eggs with impunity. As to my father himself, he is nearly eighty years old; he has not touched an egg since he was a young man; he can, therefore, give no precise or reliable account of the symptoms the eating of eggs produce in him. But it was not the mere 'stomach-ache' that ensued, but much more immediate and alarming disturbances. As for me, the peculiarity was discovered when I was a spoon-fed child. On several occasions it was noticed (that is my mother's account) that I felt ill without apparent cause; afterward it was recollected that a small part of a yolk of an egg had been given to me. Eclaircissement came immediately after taking a single spoonful of egg. I fell into such an alarming state that the doctor was sent for. The effect seems to have been just the same that it produces upon my daughter now,—something that suggested brain-congestion and convulsions. From time to time, as a boy and a young man, I have eaten an egg by way of trying it again, but always with the same result—a feeling that I had been poisoned; and yet all the while I liked eggs. Then I never touched them for years. Later I tried again, and I find the ill-effects are gradually wearing off. With my daughter it is different; she, I think, becomes more susceptible as time goes on, and the effect upon her is more violent than in my case at any time. Sometimes an egg has been put with coffee unknown to her, and she has been seen immediately afterward with her face alarmingly changed—eyes swollen and wild, the face crimson, the look of apoplexy. This is her own account: 'An egg in any form causes within a few minutes great uneasiness and restlessness, the throat becomes contracted and painful, the face crimson, and the veins swollen. These symptoms have been so severe as to suggest that serious consequences might follow.' To this I may add that in her experience and my own, the newer the egg, the worse the consequences."

Hutchinson speaks of a Member of Parliament who had an idiosyncrasy as regards parsley. After the ingestion of this herb in food he always had alarming attacks of sickness and pain in the abdomen, attended by swelling of the tongue and lips and lividity of the face. This same man could not take the smallest quantity of honey, and certain kinds of fruit always poisoned him. There was a collection of instances of idiosyncrasy in the British Medical Journal, 1859, which will be briefly given in the following lines: One patient could not eat rice in any shape without extreme distress. From the description given of his symptoms, spasmodic asthma seemed to be the cause of his discomfort. On one occasion when at a dinner-party he felt the symptoms of rice-poisoning come on, and, although he had partaken of no dish ostensibly containing rice, was, as usual, obliged to retire from the table. Upon investigation it appeared that some white soup with which he had commenced his meal had been thickened with ground rice. As in the preceding case there was another gentleman who could not eat rice without a sense of suffocation. On one occasion he took lunch with a friend in chambers, partaking only of simple bread and cheese and bottled beer. On being seized with the usual symptoms of rice-poisoning he informed his friend of his peculiarity of constitution, and the symptoms were explained by the fact that a few grains of rice had been put into each bottle of beer for the purpose of exciting a secondary fermentation. The same author speaks of a gentleman under treatment for stricture who could not eat figs without experiencing the most unpleasant formication of the palate and fauces. The fine dust from split peas caused the same sensation, accompanied with running at the nose; it was found that the father of the patient suffered from hay-fever in certain seasons. He also says a certain young lady after eating eggs suffered from swelling of the tongue and throat, accompanied by "alarming illness," and there is recorded in the same paragraph a history of another young girl in whom the ingestion of honey, and especially honey-comb, produced swelling of the tongue, frothing of the mouth, and blueness of the fingers. The authors know of a gentleman in whom sneezing is provoked on the ingestion of chocolate in any form. There was another instance—in a member of the medical profession—who suffered from urticaria after eating veal. Veal has the reputation of being particularly indigestible, and the foregoing instance of the production of urticaria from its use is doubtless not an uncommon one.

Overton cites a striking case of constitutional peculiarity or idiosyncrasy in which wheat flour in any form, the staff of life, an article hourly prayed for by all Christian nations as the first and most indispensable of earthly blessings, proved to one unfortunate individual a prompt and dreadful poison. The patient's name was David Waller, and he was born in Pittsylvania County, Va., about the year 1780. He was the eighth child of his parents, and, together with all his brothers and sisters, was stout and healthy. At the time of observation Waller was about fifty years of age. He had dark hair, gray eyes, dark complexion, was of bilious and irascible temperament, well formed, muscular and strong, and in all respects healthy as any man, with the single exception of his peculiar idiosyncrasy. He had been the subject of but few diseases, although he was attacked by the epidemic of 1816. From the history of his parents and an inquiry into the health of his ancestry, nothing could be found which could establish the fact of heredity in his peculiar disposition. Despite every advantage of stature, constitution, and heredity, David Waller was through life, from his cradle to his grave, the victim of what is possibly a unique idiosyncrasy of constitution. In his own words he declared: "Of two equal quantities of tartar and wheat flour, not more than a dose of the former, he would rather swallow the tartar than the wheat flour." If he ate flour in any form or however combined, in the smallest quantity, in two minutes or less he would have painful itching over the whole body, accompanied by severe colic and tormina in the bowels, great sickness in the stomach, and continued vomiting, which he declared was ten times as distressing as the symptoms caused by the ingestion of tartar emetic. In about ten minutes after eating the flour the itching would be greatly intensified, especially about the head, face, and eyes, but tormenting all parts of the body, and not to be appeased. These symptoms continued for two days with intolerable violence, and only declined on the third day and ceased on the tenth. In the convalescence, the lungs were affected, he coughed, and in expectoration raised great quantities of phlegm, and really resembled a phthisical patient. At this time he was confined to his room with great weakness, similar to that of a person recovering from an asthmatic attack. The mere smell of wheat produced distressing symptoms in a minor degree, and for this reason he could not, without suffering, go into a mill or house where the smallest quantity of wheat flour was kept. His condition was the same from the earliest times, and he was laid out for dead when an infant at the breast, after being fed with "pap" thickened with wheat flour. Overton remarks that a case of constitutional peculiarity so little in harmony with the condition of other men could not be received upon vague or feeble evidence, and it is therefore stated that Waller was known to the society in which he lived as an honest and truthful man. One of his female neighbors, not believing in his infirmity, but considering it only a whim, put a small quantity of flour in the soup which she gave him to eat at her table, stating that it contained no flour, and as a consequence of the deception he was bed-ridden for ten days with his usual symptoms. It was also stated that Waller was never subjected to militia duty because it was found on full examination of his infirmity that he could not live upon the rations of a soldier, into which wheat flour enters as a necessary ingredient. In explanation of this strange departure from the condition of other men, Waller himself gave a reason which was deemed equivalent in value to any of the others offered. It was as follows: His father being a man in humble circumstances in life, at the time of his birth had no wheat with which to make flour, although his mother during gestation "longed" for wheat-bread. The father, being a kind husband and responsive to the duty imposed by the condition of his wife, procured from one of his opulent neighbors a bag of wheat and sent it to the mill to be ground. The mother was given much uneasiness by an unexpected delay at the mill, and by the time the flour arrived her strong appetite for wheat-bread had in a great degree subsided. Notwithstanding this, she caused some flour to be immediately baked into bread and ate it, but not so freely as she had expected The bread thus taken caused intense vomiting and made her violently and painfully ill, after which for a considerable time she loathed bread. These facts have been ascribed as the cause of the lamentable infirmity under which the man labored, as no other peculiarity or impression in her gestation was noticed. In addition it may be stated that for the purpose of avoiding the smell of flour Waller was in the habit of carrying camphor in his pocket and using snuff, for if he did not smell the flour, however much might be near him, it was as harmless to him as to other men.

The authors know of a case in which the eating of any raw fruit would produce in a lady symptoms of asthma; cooked fruit had no such effect.

Food-Superstitions.—The superstitious abhorrence and antipathy to various articles of food that have been prevalent from time to time in the history of the human race are of considerable interest and well deserve some mention here. A writer in a prominent journal has studied this subject with the following result:—

"From the days of Adam and Eve to the present time there has been not only forbidden fruit, but forbidden meats and vegetables. For one reason or another people have resolutely refused to eat any and all kinds of flesh, fish, fowl, fruits, and plants. Thus, the apple, the pear, the strawberry, the quince, the bean, the onion, the leek, the asparagus, the woodpecker, the pigeon, the goose, the deer, the bear, the turtle, and the eel—these, to name only a few eatables, have been avoided as if unwholesome or positively injurious to health and digestion.

"As we all know, the Jews have long had an hereditary antipathy to pork. On the other hand, swine's flesh was highly esteemed by the ancient Greeks and Romans. This fact is revealed by the many references to pig as a dainty bit of food. At the great festival held annually in honor of Demeter, roast pig was the piece de resistance in the bill of fare, because the pig was the sacred animal of Demeter. Aristophanes in 'The Frogs' makes one of the characters hint that some of the others 'smell of roast pig.' These people undoubtedly had been at the festival (known as the Thesmophoria) and had eaten freely of roast pig, Those who took part in another Greek mystery or festival (known as the Eleusinia) abstained from certain food, and above all from beans.

"Again, as we all know, mice are esteemed in China and in some parts of India. But the ancient Egyptians, Greeks, and Jews abhorred mice and would not touch mouse-meat. Rats and field-mice were sacred in Old Egypt, and were not to be eaten on this account. So, too, in some parts of Greece, the mouse was the sacred animal of Apollo, and mice were fed in his temples. The chosen people were forbidden to eat 'the weasel, and the mouse, and the tortoise after his kind.' These came under the designation of unclean animals, which were to be avoided.

"But people have abstained from eating kinds of flesh which could not be called unclean. For example, the people of Thebes, as Herodotus tells us, abstained from sheep. Then, the ancients used to abstain from certain vegetables. In his 'Roman

Questions' Plutarch asks: 'Why do the Latins abstain strictly from the flesh of the woodpecker?' In order to answer Plutarch's question correctly it is necessary to have some idea of the peculiar custom and belief called 'totemism.' There is a stage of society in which people claim descent from and kinship with beasts, birds, vegetables, and other objects. This object, which is a 'totem,' or family mark, they religiously abstain from eating. The members of the tribe are divided into clans or stocks, each of which takes the name of some animal, plant, or object, as the bear, the buffalo, the woodpecker, the asparagus, and so forth. No member of the bear family would dare to eat bear-meat, but he has no objection to eating buffalo steak. Even the marriage law is based on this belief, and no man whose family name is Wolf may marry a woman whose family name is also Wolf.

"In a general way it may be said that almost all our food prohibitions spring from the extraordinary custom generally called totemism. Mr. Swan, who was missionary for many years in the Congo Free State, thus describes the custom: 'If I were to ask the Yeke people why they do not eat zebra flesh, they would reply, 'Chijila,' i.e., 'It is a thing to which we have an antipathy;' or better, 'It is one of the things which our fathers taught us not to eat.' So it seems the word 'Bashilang' means 'the people who have an antipathy to the leopard;' the 'Bashilamba,' 'those who have an antipathy to the dog,' and the 'Bashilanzefu,' 'those who have an antipathy to the elephant.' In other words, the members of these stocks refuse to eat their totems, the zebra, the leopard, or the elephant, from which they take their names.

"The survival of antipathy to certain foods was found among people as highly civilized as the Egyptians, the Greeks, and the Romans. Quite a list of animals whose flesh was forbidden might be drawn up. For example, in Old Egypt the sheep could not be eaten in Thebes, nor the goat in Mendes, nor the cat in Bubastis, nor the crocodile at Ombos, nor the rat, which was sacred to Ra, the sun-god. However, the people of one place had no scruples about eating the forbidden food of another place. And this often led to religious disputes.

"Among the vegetables avoided as food by the Egyptians may be mentioned the onion, the garlic, and the leek. Lucian says that the inhabitants of Pelusium adored the onion. According to Pliny the Egyptians relished the leek and the onion. Juvenal exclaims: 'Surely a very religious nation, and a blessed place, where every garden is overrun with gods!' The survivals of totemism among the ancient Greeks are very interesting. Families named after animals and plants were not uncommon. One Athenian gens, the Ioxidae, had for its ancestral plant the asparagus. One Roman gens, the Piceni, took a woodpecker for its totem, and every member of this family refused, of course, to eat the flesh of the woodpecker. In the same way as the nations of the Congo Free State, the Latins had an antipathy to certain kinds of food. However, an animal or plant forbidden in one place was eaten without any compunction in another place. 'These local rites in Roman times,' says Mr. Lang, 'caused civil brawls, for the customs of one town naturally seemed blasphemous to neighbors with a different sacred animal. Thus when the people of dog-town were feeding on the fish called oxyrrhyncus, the citizens of the town which revered the oxyrrhyncus began to eat dogs. Hence arose a riot.' The antipathy of the Jews to pork has given rise to quite different explanations. The custom is probably a relic of totemistic belief. That the unclean animals—animals not to be eaten—such as the pig, the mouse, and the weasel, were originally totems of the children of Israel, Professor Robertson Smith believes is shown by various passages in the Old Testament.

"When animals and plants ceased to be held sacred they were endowed with sundry magical or mystic properties. The apple has been supposed to possess peculiar virtues, especially in the way of health. 'The relation of the apple to health,' says Mr. Conway, 'is traceable to Arabia. Sometimes it is regarded as a bane. In Hessia it is said an apple must not be eaten on New Year's Day, as it will produce an abscess. But generally it is curative. In Pomerania it is eaten on Easter morning against fevers; in Westphalia (mixed with saffron) against jaundice; while in Silesia an apple is scraped from top to stalk to cure diarrhea, and upward to cure costiveness.' According to an old English fancy, if any one who is suffering from a wound in the head should eat strawberries it will lead to fatal results. In the South of England the folk say that the devil puts his cloven foot upon the blackberries on Michaelmas Day, and hence none should be gathered or eaten after that day. On the other hand, in Scotland the peasants say that the devil throws his cloak over the blackberries and makes them unwholesome after that day, while in Ireland he is said to stamp on the berries. Even that humble plant, the cabbage, has been invested with some mystery. It was said that the fairies were fond of its leaves, and rode to their midnight dances on cabbage-stalks. The German women used to say that 'Babies come out of the cabbage-heads.' The Irish peasant ties a cabbage-leaf around the neck for sore throat. According to Gerarde, the Spartans ate watercress with their bread, firmly believing that it increased their wit and wisdom. The old proverb is, 'Eat cress to learn more wit.'

"There is another phase to food-superstitions, and that is the theory that the qualities of the eaten pass into the eater. Mr. Tylor refers to the habit of the Dyak young men in abstaining from deer-meat lest it should make them timid, while the warriors of some South American tribes eat the meat of tigers, stags, and boars for courage and speed. He mentions the story of an English gentleman at Shanghai who at the time of the Taeping attack met his Chinese servant carrying home the heart of a rebel, which he intended to eat to make him brave. There is a certain amount of truth in the theory that the quality of food does affect the mind and body. Buckle in his 'History of Civilization' took this view, and tried to prove that the character of a people depends on their diet."

Idiosyncrasies to Drugs.—In the absorption and the assimilation of drugs idiosyncrasies are often noted; in fact, they are so common that we can almost say that no one drug acts in the same degree or manner on different individuals. In some instances the untoward action assumes such a serious aspect as to render extreme caution necessary in the administration of the most inert substances. A medicine ordinarily so bland as cod-liver oil may give rise to disagreeable eruptions. Christison speaks of a boy ten years old who was said to have been killed by the ingestion of two ounces of Epsom salts without inducing purgation; yet this common purge is universally used without the slightest fear or caution. On the other hand, the extreme tolerance exhibited by certain individuals to certain drugs offers a new phase of this subject. There are well-authenticated cases on record in which death has been caused in children by the ingestion of a small fraction of a grain of opium. While exhibiting especial tolerance from peculiar disposition and long habit, Thomas De Quincey, the celebrated English litterateur, makes a statement in his "Confessions" that with impunity he took as much as 320 grains of opium a day, and was accustomed at one period of his life to call every day for "a glass of laudanum negus, warm, and without sugar," to use his own expression, after the manner a toper would call for a "hot-Scotch."

The individuality noted in the assimilation and the ingestion of drugs is functional as well as anatomic. Numerous cases have been seen by all physicians. The severe toxic symptoms from a whiff of cocain-spray, the acute distress from the tenth of a grain of morphin, the gastric crises and profuse urticarial eruptions following a single dose of quinin,—all are proofs of it. The "personal equation" is one of the most important factors in therapeutics, reminding us of the old rule, "Treat the patient, not the disease."

The idiosyncrasy may be either temporary or permanent, and there are many conditions that influence it. The time and place of administration; the degree of pathologic lesion in the subject; the difference in the physiologic capability of individual organs of similar nature in the same body; the degree of human vitality influencing absorption and resistance; the peculiar epochs of life; the element of habituation, and the grade and strength of the drug, influencing its virtue,—all have an important bearing on untoward action and tolerance of poisons.

It is not in the province of this work to discuss at length the explanations offered for these individual idiosyncrasies. Many authors have done so, and Lewin has devoted a whole volume to this subject, of which, fortunately, an English translation has been made by Mulheron, and to these the interested reader is referred for further information. In the following lines examples of idiosyncrasy to the most common remedial substances will be cited, taking the drugs up alphabetically.

Acids.—Ordinarily speaking, the effect of boric acid in medicinal doses on the human system is nil, an exceptionally large quantity causing diuresis. Binswanger, according to Lewin, took eight gm. in two doses within an hour, which was followed by nausea, vomiting, and a feeling of pressure and fulness of the stomach which continued several hours. Molodenkow mentions two fatal cases from the external employment of boric acid as an antiseptic. In one case the pleural cavity was washed out with a five per cent solution of boric acid and was followed by distressing symptoms, vomiting, weak pulse, erythema, and death on the third day. In the second case, in a youth of sixteen, death occurred after washing out a deep abscess of the nates with the same solution. The autopsy revealed no change or signs indicative of the cause of death. Hogner mentions two instances of death from the employment of 2 1/2 per cent solution of boric acid in washing out a dilated stomach The symptoms were quite similar to those mentioned by Molodenkow.

In recent years the medical profession has become well aware that in its application to wounds it is possible for carbolic acid or phenol to exercise exceedingly deleterious and even fatal consequences. In the earlier days of antisepsis, when operators and patients were exposed for some time to an atmosphere saturated with carbolic spray, toxic symptoms were occasionally noticed. Von Langenbeck spoke of severe carbolic-acid intoxication n a boy in whom carbolic paste had been used in the treatment of abscesses. The same author reports two instances of death following the employment of dry carbolized dressings after slight operations. Kohler mentions the death of a man suffering from scabies who had applied externally a solution containing about a half ounce of phenol. Rose spoke of gangrene of the finger after the application of carbolized cotton to a wound thereon. In some cases phenol acts with a rapidity equal to any poison. Taylor speaks of a man who fell unconscious ten seconds after an ounce of phenol had been ingested, and in three minutes was dead. There is recorded an account of a man of sixty-four who was killed by a solution containing slightly over a dram of phenol. A half ounce has frequently caused death; smaller quantities have been followed by distressing symptoms, such as intoxication (which Olshausen has noticed to follow irrigation of the uterus), delirium, singultus, nausea, rigors, cephalalgia, tinnitus aurium, and anasarca. Hind mentions recovery after the ingestion of nearly six ounces of crude phenol of 14 per cent strength. There was a case at the Liverpool Northern Hospital in which recovery took place after the ingestion with suicidal intent of four ounces of crude carbolic acid. Quoted by Lewin, Busch accurately describes a case which may be mentioned as characteristic of the symptoms of carbolism. A boy, suffering from abscess under the trochanter, was operated on for its relief. During the few minutes occupied by the operation he was kept under a two per cent carbolic spray, and the wound was afterward dressed with carbolic gauze. The day following the operation he was seized with vomiting, which was attributed to the chloroform used as an anesthetic. On the following morning the bandages were removed under the carbolic spray; during the day there was nausea, in the evening there was collapse, and carbolic acid was detected in the urine. The pulse became small and frequent and the temperature sank to 35.5 degrees C. The frequent vomiting made it impossible to administer remedies by the stomach, and, in spite of hypodermic injections and external application of analeptics, the boy died fifty hours after operation.

Recovery has followed the ingestion of an ounce of officinal hydrochloric acid. Black mentions a man of thirty-nine who recovered after swallowing 1 1/2 ounces of commercial hydrochloric acid. Johnson reports a case of poisoning from a dram of hydrochloric acid. Tracheotomy was performed, but death resulted.

Burman mentions recovery after the ingestion of a dram of dilute hydrocyanic acid of Scheele's strength (2.4 am. of the acid). In this instance insensibility did not ensue until two minutes after taking the poison, the retarded digestion being the means of saving life.

Quoting Taafe, in 1862 Taylor speaks of the case of a man who swallowed the greater part of a solution containing an ounce of potassium cyanid. In a few minutes the man was found insensible in the street, breathing stertorously, and in ten minutes after the ingestion of the drug the stomach-pump was applied. In two hours vomiting began, and thereafter recovery was rapid.

Mitscherlich speaks of erosion of the gums and tongue with hemorrhage at the slightest provocation, following the long administration of dilute nitric acid. This was possibly due to the local action.

According to Taylor, the smallest quantity of oxalic acid causing death is one dram. Ellis describes a woman of fifty who swallowed an ounce of oxalic acid in beer. In thirty minutes she complained of a burning pain in the stomach and was rolling about in agony. Chalk and water was immediately given to her and she recovered. Woodman reports recovery after taking 1/2 ounce of oxalic acid.

Salicylic acid in medicinal doses frequently causes untoward symptoms, such as dizziness, transient delirium, diminution of vision, headache, and profuse perspiration; petechial eruptions and intense gastric symptoms have also been noticed.

Sulphuric acid causes death from its corrosive action, and when taken in excessive quantities it produces great gastric disturbance; however, there are persons addicted to taking oil of vitriol without any apparent untoward effect. There is mentioned a boot-maker who constantly took 1/2 ounce of the strong acid in a tumbler of water, saying that it relieved his dyspepsia and kept his bowels open.

Antimony.—It is recorded that 3/4 grain of tartar emetic has caused death in a child and two grains in an adult. Falot reports three cases in which after small doses of tartar emetic there occurred vomiting, delirium, spasms, and such depression of vitality that only the energetic use of stimulants saved life. Beau mentions death following the administration of two doses of 1 1/2 gr. of tartar emetic. Preparations of antimony in an ointment applied locally have caused necrosis, particularly of the cranium, and Hebra has long since denounced the use of tartar emetic ointment in affections of the scalp. Carpenter mentions recovery after ingestion of two drams of tartar emetic. Behrends describes a case of catalepsy with mania, in which a dose of 40 gr. of tartar emetic was tolerated, and Morgagni speaks of a man who swallowed two drams, immediately vomited, and recovered. Instances like the last, in which an excessive amount of a poison by its sudden emetic action induces vomiting before there is absorption of a sufficient quantity to cause death, are sometimes noticed. McCreery mentions a case of accidental poisoning with half an ounce of tartar emetic successfully treated with green tea and tannin. Mason reports recovery after taking 80 gr. of tartar emetic.

Arsenic.—The sources of arsenical poisoning are so curious as to deserve mention. Confectionery, wall-paper, dyes, and the like are examples. In other cases we note money-counting, the colored candles of a Christmas tree, paper collars, ball-wreaths of artificial flowers, ball-dresses made of green tarlatan, playing cards, hat-lining, and fly-papers.

Bazin has reported a case in which erythematous pustules appeared after the exhibition during fifteen days of the 5/6 gr. of arsenic. Macnal speaks of an eruption similar to that of measles in a patient to whom he had given but three drops of Fowler's solution for the short period of three days. Pareira says that in a gouty patient for whom he prescribed 1/6 gr. of potassium arseniate daily, on the third day there appeared a bright red eruption of the face, neck, upper part of the trunk and flexor surfaces of the joints, and an edematous condition of the eyelids. The symptoms were preceded by restlessness, headache, and heat of the skin, and subsided gradually after the second or third day, desquamation continuing for nearly two months. After they had subsided entirely, the exhibition of arsenic again aroused them, and this time they were accompanied by salivation. Charcot and other French authors have noticed the frequent occurrence of suspension of the sexual instinct during the administration of Fowler's solution. Jackson speaks of recovery after the ingestion of two ounces of arsenic by the early employment of an emetic. Walsh reports a case in which 600 gr. of arsenic were taken without injury. The remarkable tolerance of arsenic eaters is well known. Taylor asserts that the smallest lethal dose of arsenic has been two gr., but Tardieu mentions an instance in which ten cgm. (1 1/2 gr.) has caused death. Mackenzie speaks of a man who swallowed a large quantity of arsenic in lumps, and received no treatment for sixteen hours, but recovered. It is added that from two masses passed by the anus 105 gr. of arsenic were obtained.

In speaking of the tolerance of belladonna, in 1859 Fuller mentioned a child of fourteen who in eighteen days took 37 grains of atropin; a child of ten who took seven grains of extract of belladonna daily, or more than two ounces in twenty-six days; and a man who took 64 grains of the extract of belladonna daily, and from whose urine enough atropin was extracted to kill two white mice and to narcotize two others. Bader has observed grave symptoms following the employment of a vaginal suppository containing three grains of the extract of belladonna. The dermal manifestations, such as urticaria and eruptions resembling the exanthem of scarlatina, are too well known to need mention here. An enema containing 80 grains of belladonna root has been followed in five hours by death, and Taylor has mentioned recovery after the ingestion of three drams of belladonna. In 1864 Chambers reported to the Lancet the recovery of a child of four years who took a solution containing 1/2 grain of the alkaloid. In some cases the idiosyncrasy to belladonna is so marked that violent symptoms follow the application of the ordinary belladonna plaster. Maddox describes a ease of poisoning in a music teacher by the belladonna plaster of a reputable maker. She had obscure eye-symptoms, and her color-sensations were abnormal. Locomotor equilibration was also affected. Golden mentions two cases in which the application of belladonna ointment to the breasts caused suppression of the secretion of milk. Goodwin relates the history of a case in which an infant was poisoned by a belladonna plaster applied to its mother's breast and died within twenty-four hours after the first application of the plaster. In 1881 Betancourt spoke of an instance of inherited susceptibility to belladonna, in which the external application of the ointment produced all the symptoms of belladonna poisoning. Cooper mentions the symptoms of poisoning following the application of extract of belladonna to the scrotum. Davison reports poisoning by the application of belladonna liniment. Jenner and Lyman also record belladonna poisoning from external applications.

Rosenthal reports a rare case of poisoning in a child eighteen months old who had swallowed about a teaspoonful of benzin. Fifteen minutes later the child became unconscious. The stomach-contents, which were promptly removed, contained flakes of bloody mucus. At the end of an hour the radial pulse was scarcely perceptible, respiration was somewhat increased in frequency and accompanied with a rasping sound. The breath smelt of benzin. The child lay in quiet narcosis, occasionally throwing itself about as if in pain. The pulse gradually improved, profuse perspiration occurred, and normal sleep intervened. Six hours after the poisoning the child was still stupefied. The urine was free from albumin and sugar, and the next morning the little one had perfectly recovered.

There is an instance mentioned of a robust youth of twenty who by a mistake took a half ounce of cantharides. He was almost immediately seized with violent heat in the throat and stomach, pain in the head, and intense burning on urination. These symptoms progressively increased, were followed by intense sickness and almost continual vomiting. In the evening he passed great quantities of blood from the urethra with excessive pain in the urinary tract. On the third day all the symptoms were less violent and the vomiting had ceased. Recovery was complete on the fifteenth day.

Digitalis has been frequently observed to produce dizziness, fainting, disturbances of vision, vomiting, diarrhea, weakness of the pulse, and depression of temperature. These phenomena, however, are generally noticed after continued administration in repeated doses, the result being doubtless due to cumulative action caused by abnormally slow elimination by the kidneys. Traube observed the presence of skin-affection after the use of digitalis in a case of pericarditis. Tardieu has seen a fluid-dram of the tincture of digitalis cause alarming symptoms in a young woman who was pregnant. He also quotes cases of death on the tenth day from ingestion of 20 grains of the extract, and on the fifth day from 21 grams of the infusion. Kohuhorn mentions a death from what might be called chronic digitalis poisoning.

There is a deleterious practice of some of the Irish peasantry connected with their belief in fairies, which consists of giving a cachetic or rachitic child large doses of a preparation of fox-glove (Irish—luss-more, or great herb), to drive out or kill the fairy in the child. It was supposed to kill an unhallowed child and cure a hallowed one. In the Hebrides, likewise, there were many cases of similar poisoning.

Epidemics of ergotism have been recorded from time to time since the days of Galen, and were due to poverty, wretchedness, and famine, resulting in the feeding upon ergotized bread. According to Wood, gangrenous ergotism, or "Ignis

Sacer" of the Middle Ages, killed 40,000 persons in Southwestern France in 922 A. D., and in 1128-29, in Paris alone, 14,000 persons perished from this malady. It is described as commencing with itchings and formications in the feet, severe pain in the back, contractions in the muscles, nausea, giddiness, apathy, with abortion in pregnant women, in suckling women drying of milk, and in maidens with amenorrhea. After some time, deep, heavy aching in the limbs, intense feeling of coldness, with real coldness of the surfaces, profound apathy, and a sense of utter weariness develop; then a dark spot appears on the nose or one of the extremities, all sensibility is lost in the affected part, the skin assumes a livid red hue, and adynamic symptoms in severe cases deepen as the gangrene spreads, until finally death ensues. Very generally the appetite and digestion are preserved to the last, and not rarely there is a most ferocious hunger. Wood also mentions a species of ergotism characterized by epileptic paroxysms, which he calls "spasmodic ergotism." Prentiss mentions a brunette of forty-two, under the influence of ergot, who exhibited a peculiar depression of spirits with hysteric phenomena, although deriving much benefit from the administration of the drug from the hemorrhage caused by uterine fibroids. After taking ergot for three days she felt like crying all the time, became irritable, and stayed in bed, being all day in tears. The natural disposition of the patient was entirely opposed to these manifestations, as she was even- tempered and exceptionally pleasant.

In addition to the instance of the fatal ingestion of a dose of Epsom salts already quoted, Lang mentions a woman of thirty-five who took four ounces of this purge. She experienced burning pain in the stomach and bowels, together with a sense of asphyxiation. There was no purging or vomiting, but she became paralyzed and entered a state of coma, dying fifteen minutes after ingestion.

Iodin Preparations.—The eruptions following the administration of small doses of potassium iodid are frequently noticed, and at the same time large quantities of albumin have been seen in the urine. Potassium iodid, although generally spoken of as a poisonous drug, by gradually increasing the dose can be given in such enormous quantities as to be almost beyond the bounds of credence, several drams being given at a dose. On the other hand, eight grains have produced alarming symptoms. In the extensive use of iodoform as a dressing instances of untoward effects, and even fatal ones, have been noticed, the majority of them being due to careless and injudicious application. In a French journal there is mentioned the history of a man of twenty-five, suspected of urethral ulceration, who submitted to the local application of one gram of iodoform. Deep narcosis and anesthesia were induced, and two hours after awakening his breath smelled strongly of iodoform. There are two similar instances recorded in England.

Pope mentions two fatal cases of lead-poisoning from diachylon plaster, self-administered for the purpose of producing abortion. Lead water-pipes, the use of cosmetics and hair-dyes, coloring matter in confectionery and in pastry, habitual biting of silk threads, imperfectly burnt pottery, and cooking bread with painted wood have been mentioned as causes of chronic lead-poisoning.

Mercury.—Armstrong mentions recovery after ingestion of 1 1/2 drams of corrosive sublimate, and Lodge speaks of recovery after a dose containing 100 grains of the salt. It is said that a man swallowed 80 grains of mercuric chlorid in whiskey and water, and vomited violently about ten minutes afterward. A mixture of albumin and milk was given to him, and in about twenty-five minutes a bolus of gold-leaf and reduced iron; in eight days he perfectly recovered. Severe and even fatal poisoning may result from the external application of mercury. Meeres mentions a case in which a solution (two grains to the fluid-ounce) applied to the head of a child of nine for the relief of tinea tonsurans caused diarrhea, profuse salivation, marked prostration, and finally death. Washing out the vagina with a solution of corrosive sublimate, 1:2000, has caused severe and even fatal poisoning. Bonet mentions death after the inunction of a mercurial ointment, and instances of distressing salivation from such medication are quite common. There are various dermal affections which sometimes follow the exhibition of mercury and assume an erythematous type. The susceptibility of some persons to calomel, the slightest dose causing profuse salivation and painful oral symptoms, is so common that few physicians administer mercury to their patients without some knowledge of their susceptibility to this drug. Blundel relates a curious case occurring in the times when mercury was given in great quantities, in which to relieve obstinate constipation a half ounce of crude mercury was administered and repeated in twelve hours. Scores of globules of mercury soon appeared over a vesicated surface, the result of a previous blister applied to the epigastric region. Blundel, not satisfied with the actuality of the phenomena, submitted his case to Dr. Lister, who, after careful examination, pronounced the globules metallic.

Oils.—Mauvezin tells of the ingestion of three drams of croton oil by a child of six, followed by vomiting and rapid recovery. There was no diarrhea in this case. Wood quotes Cowan in mentioning the case of a child of four, who in two days recovered from a teaspoonful of croton oil taken on a full stomach. Adams saw recovery in an adult after ingestion of the same amount. There is recorded an instance of a woman who took about an ounce, and, emesis being produced three-quarters of an hour afterward by mustard, she finally recovered. There is a record in which so small a dose as three minims is supposed to have killed a child of thirteen months." According to Wood, Giacomini mentions a case in which 24 grains of the drug proved fatal in as many hours.

Castor oil is usually considered a harmless drug, but the castor bean, from which it is derived, contains a poisonous acrid principle, three such beans having sufficed to produce death in a man. Doubtless some of the instances in which castor oil has produced symptoms similar to cholera are the results of the administration of contaminated oil.

The untoward effects of opium and its derivatives are quite numerous Gaubius treated an old woman in whom, after three days, a single grain of opium produced a general desquamation of the epidermis; this peculiarity was not accidental, as it was verified on several other occasions. Hargens speaks of a woman in whom the slightest bit of opium in any form produced considerable salivation. Gastric disturbances are quite common, severe vomiting being produced by minimum doses; not infrequently, intense mental confusion, vertigo, and headache, lasting hours and even days, sometimes referable to the frontal region and sometimes to the occipital, are seen in certain nervous individuals after a dose of from 1/4 to 5/6 gr. of opium. These symptoms were familiar to the ancient physicians, and, according to Lewin, Tralles reports an observation with reference to this in a man, and says regarding it in rather unclassical Latin: " . . . per multos dies ponderosissimum caput circumgestasse." Convulsions are said to be observed after medicinal doses of opium. Albers states that twitching in the tendons tremors of the hands, and even paralysis, have been noticed after the ingestion of opium in even ordinary doses. The "pruritus opii," so familiar to physicians, is spoken of in the older writings. Dioscorides, Paulus Aegineta, and nearly all the writers of the last century describe this symptom as an annoying and unbearable affection. In some instances the ingestion of opium provokes an eruption in the form of small, isolated red spots, which, in their general character, resemble roseola. Rieken remarks that when these spots spread over all the body they present a scarlatiniform appearance, and he adds that even the mucous membranes of the mouth and throat may be attacked with erethematous inflammation. Behrend observed an opium exanthem, which was attended by intolerable itching, after the exhibition of a quarter of a grain. It was seen on the chest, on the inner surfaces of the arms, on the flexor surfaces of the forearms and wrists, on the thighs, and posterior and inner surfaces of the legs, terminating at the ankles in a stripe-like discoloration about the breadth of three fingers. It consisted of closely disposed papules of the size of a pin-head, and several days after the disappearance of the eruption a fine, bran-like desquamation of the epidermis ensued. Brand has also seen an eruption on the trunk and flexor surfaces, accompanied with fever, from the ingestion of opium. Billroth mentions the case of a lady in whom appeared a feeling of anxiety, nausea, and vomiting after ingestion of a small fraction of a grain of opium; she would rather endure her intense pain than suffer the untoward action of the drug. According to Lewin, Brochin reported a case in which the idiosyncrasy to morphin was so great that 1/25 of a grain of the drug administered hypodermically caused irregularity of the respiration, suspension of the heart-beat, and profound narcosis. According to the same authority, Wernich has called attention to paresthesia of the sense of taste after the employment of morphin, which, according to his observation, is particularly prone to supervene in patients who are much reduced and in persons otherwise healthy who have suffered from prolonged inanition. These effects are probably due to a central excitation of a similar nature to that produced by santonin. Persons thus attacked complain, shortly after the injection, of an intensely sour or bitter taste, which for the most part ceases after elimination of the morphin. Von Graefe and Sommerfrodt speak of a spasm of accommodation occurring after ingestion of medicinal doses of morphin. There are several cases on record in which death has been produced in an adult by the use of 1/2 to 1/6 grain of morphin. According to Wood, the maximum doses from which recovery has occurred without emesis are 55 grains of solid opium, and six ounces of laudanum. According to the same authority, in 1854 there was a case in which a babe one day old was killed by one minim of laudanum, and in another case a few drops of paregoric proved fatal to a child of nine months. Doubtful instances of death from opium are given, one in an adult female after 30 grains of Dover's powder given in divided doses, and another after a dose of 1/4 grain of morphin. Yavorski cites a rather remarkable instance of morphin-poisoning with recovery: a female took 30 grains of acetate of morphin, and as it did not act quickly enough she took an additional dose of 1/2 ounce of laudanum. After this she slept a few hours, and awoke complaining of being ill. Yavorski saw her about an hour later, and by producing emesis, and giving coffee, atropin, and tincture of musk, he saved her life. Pyle describes a pugilist of twenty-two who, in a fit of despondency after a debauch (in which he had taken repeated doses of morphin sulphate), took with suicidal intent three teaspoonfuls of morphin; after rigorous treatment he revived and was discharged on the next day perfectly well. Potassium permanganate was used in this case. Chaffee speaks of recovery after the ingestion of 18 grains of morphin without vomiting.

In chronic opium eating the amount of this drug which can be ingested with safety assumes astounding proportions. In his "Confessions" De Quincey remarks: "Strange as it may sound, I had a little before this time descended suddenly and without considerable effort from 320 grains of opium (8000 drops of laudanum) per day to 40 grains, or 1/8 part. Instantaneously, and as if by magic, the cloud of profoundest melancholy which rested on my brain, like some black vapors that I have seen roll away from the summits of the mountains, drew off in one day,— passed off with its murky banners as simultaneously as a ship that has been stranded and is floated off by a spring-tide—

'That moveth altogether if it move at all.'

Now, then, I was again happy; I took only a thousand drops of Laudanum per day, and what was that? A latter spring had come to close up the season of youth; my brain performed its functions as healthily as ever before; I read Kant again, and again I understood him, or fancied that I did." There have been many authors who, in condemning De Quincey for unjustly throwing about the opium habit a halo of literary beauty which has tempted many to destruction, absolutely deny the truth of his statements. No one has any stable reason on which to found denial of De Quincey's statements as to the magnitude of the doses he was able to take; and his frankness and truthfulness is equal to that of any of his detractors. William Rosse Cobbe, in a volume entitled "Dr. Judas, or Portrayal of the Opium Habit," gives with great frankness of confession and considerable purity of diction a record of his own experiences with the drug. One entire chapter of Mr. Cobb's book and several portions of other chapters are devoted to showing that De Quincey was wrong in some of his statements, but notwithstanding his criticism of De Quincey, Mr. Cobbe seems to have experienced the same adventures in his dreams, showing, after all, that De Quincey knew the effects of opium even if he seemed to idealize it. According to Mr. Cobbe, there are in the United States upward of two millions of victims of enslaving drugs entirely exclusive of alcohol. Cobbe mentions several instances in which De Quincey's dose of 320 grains of opium daily has been surpassed. One man, a resident of Southern Illinois, consumed 1072 grains a day; another in the same State contented himself with 1685 grains daily; and still another is given whose daily consumption amounted to 2345 grains per day. In all cases of laudanum-takers it is probable that analysis of the commercial laudanum taken would show the amount of opium to be greatly below that of the official proportion, and little faith can be put in the records of large amounts of opium taken when the deduction has been made from the laudanum used. Dealers soon begin to know opium victims, and find them ready dupes for adulteration. According to Lewin, Samter mentions a case of morphin-habit which was continued for three years, during which, in a period of about three, hundred and twenty-three days, upward of 2 1/2 ounces of morphin was taken daily. According to the same authority, Eder reports still larger doses. In the case observed by him the patient took laudanum for six years in increasing doses up to one ounce per day; for eighteen months, pure opium, commencing with 15 grains and increasing to 2 1/4 drams daily; and for eighteen months morphin, in commencing quantities of six grains, which were later increased to 40 grains a day. When deprived of their accustomed dose of morphin the sufferings which these patients experience are terrific, and they pursue all sorts of deceptions to enable them to get their enslaving drug. Patients have been known to conceal tubes in their mouths, and even swallow them, and the authors know of a fatal instance in which a tube of hypodermic tablets of the drug was found concealed in the rectum.

The administration of such an inert substance as the infusion of orange-peel has been sufficient to invariably produce nervous excitement in a patient afflicted with carcinoma.

Sonnenschein refers to a case of an infant of five weeks who died from the effects of one phosphorous match head containing only 1/100 grain of phosphorus. There are certain people who by reason of a special susceptibility cannot tolerate phosphorus, and the exhibition of it causes in them nausea, oppression, and a feeling of pain in the epigastric region, tormina and tenesmus, accompanied with diarrhea, and in rare cases jaundice, sometimes lasting several months. In such persons 1/30 grain is capable of causing the foregoing symptoms. In 1882 a man was admitted to Guy's Hospital, London, after he had taken half of a sixpenny pot of phosphorous paste in whiskey, and was subsequently discharged completely recovered.

A peculiar feature of phosphorus-poisoning is necrosis of the jaw. This affection was first noticed in 1838, soon after the introduction of the manufacture of phosphorous matches. In late years, owing to the introduction of precautions in their manufacture, the disease has become much less common. The tipping of the match sticks is accomplished by dipping their ends in a warm solution of a composition of phosphorus, chlorate of potassium, with particles of ground flint to assist friction, some coloring agent, and Irish glue. From the contents of the dipping-pans fumes constantly arise into the faces of the workmen and dippers, and in cutting the sticks and packing the matches the hands are constantly in contact with phosphorus. The region chiefly affected in this poisoning is the jaw-bone, but the inflammation may spread to the adjoining bones and involve the vomer, the zygoma, the body of the sphenoid bone, and the basilar process of the occipital bone. It is supposed that conditions in which the periosteum is exposed are favorable to the progress of the disease, and, according to Hirt, workmen with diseased teeth are affected three times as readily as those with healthy teeth, and are therefore carefully excluded from some of the factories in America.

Prentiss of Washington, D.C., in 1881 reported a remarkable case of pilocarpin idiosyncrasy in a blonde of twenty-five. He was consulted by the patient for constipation. Later on symptoms of cystitis developed, and an ultimate diagnosis of pyelitis of the right kidney was made. Uremic symptoms were avoided by the constant use of pilocarpin. Between December 16, 1880, and February 22, 1881, the patient had 22 sweats from pilocarpin. The action usually lasted from two to six hours, and quite a large dose was at length necessary. The idiosyncrasy noted was found in the hair, which at first was quite light, afterward chestnut-brown, and May 1, 1881, almost pure black. The growth of the hair became more vigorous and thicker than formerly, and as its color darkened it became coarser in proportion. In March, 1889, Prentiss saw his patient, and at that time her hair was dark brown, having returned to that color from black. Prentiss also reported the following case a as adding another to the evidence that jaborandi will produce the effect mentioned under favorable circumstances: Mrs. L., aged seventy-two years, was suffering from Bright's disease (contracted kidney). Her hair and eyebrows had been snow-white for twenty years. She suffered greatly from itching of the skin, due to the uremia of the kidney-disease; the skin was harsh and dry. For this symptom fluid extract of jaborandi was prescribed with the effect of relieving the itching. It was taken in doses of 20 or 30 drops several times a day, from October, 1886, to February, 1888. During the fall of 1887 it was noticed by the nurse that the eyebrows were growing darker, and that the hair of the head was darker in patches. These patches and the eyebrows continued to become darker, until at the time of her death they were quite black, the black tufts on the head presenting a very curious appearance among the silver-white hairs surrounding them.

Quinin being such a universally used drug, numerous instances of idiosyncrasy and intolerance have been recorded. Chevalier mentions that through contact of the drug workmen in the manufacture of quinin are liable to an affection of the skin which manifests itself in a vesicular, papular, or pustular eruption on different parts of the body. Vepan mentions a lady who took 1 1/2 grains and afterward 2 1/2 grains of quinin for neuralgia, and two days afterward her body was covered with purpuric spots, which disappeared in the course of nine days but reappeared after the administration of the drug was resumed. Lewin says that in this case the severity of the eruption was in accordance with the size of the dose, and during its existence there was bleeding at the gums; he adds that Gouchet also noticed an eruption of this kind in a lady who after taking quinin expectorated blood. The petechiae were profusely spread over the entire body, and they disappeared after the suspension of the drug. Dauboeuf, Garraway, Hemming, Skinner, and Cobner mention roseola and scarlatiniform erythema after minute doses of quinin. In nearly all these cases the accompanying symptoms were different. Heusinger speaks of a lady who, after taking 1/2 grain of quinin, experienced headache, nausea, intense burning, and edema, together with nodular erythema on the eyelids, cheeks, and portion of the forehead. At another time 1 1/2 grains of the drug gave rise to herpetic vesicles on the cheeks, followed by branny desquamation on elimination of the drug. In other patients intense itching is experienced after the ingestion of quinin. Peters cites an instance of a woman of sixty-five who, after taking one grain of quinin, invariably exhibited after an hour a temperature of from 104 degrees to 105 degrees F., accelerated pulse, rigors, slight delirium, thirst, and all the appearances of ill-defined fever, which would pass off in from twelve to twenty-four hours. Peters witnessed this idiosyncrasy several times and believed it to be permanent. The most unpleasant of the untoward symptoms of quinin exhibition are the disturbances of the organs of special sense. Photophobia, and even transient amblyopia, have been observed to follow small doses. In the examination of cases of the untoward effects of quinin upon the eye, Knapp of New York found the power of sight diminished in various degrees, and rarely amaurosis and immobility of the pupils. According to Lewin, the perceptions of color and light are always diminished, and although the disorder may last for some time the prognosis is favorable. The varieties of the disturbances of the functions of the ear range from tinnitus aurium to congestion causing complete deafness. The gastro-intestinal and genito-urinary tracts are especially disposed to untoward action by quinin. There is a case recorded in which, after the slightest dose of quinin, tingling and burning at the meatus urinarius were experienced. According to Lewin, there is mentioned in the case reported by Gauchet a symptom quite unique in the literature of quinin, viz., hemoptysis. Simon de Ronchard first noted the occurrence of several cases of hemoptysis following the administration of doses of eight grains daily. In the persons thus attacked the lungs and heart were healthy. Hemoptysis promptly ceased with the suspension of the drug. When it was renewed, blood again appeared in the sputa. Taussig mentions a curious mistake, in which an ounce of quinin sulphate was administered to a patient at one dose; the only symptoms noticed were a stuporous condition and complete deafness. No antidote was given, and the patient perfectly recovered in a week. In malarious countries, and particularly in the malarial fevers of the late war, enormous quantities of quinin were frequently given. In fact, at the present day in some parts of the South quinin is constantly kept on the table as a prophylactic constituent of the diet.

Skinner noticed the occurrence of a scarlatiniform eruption in a woman after the dose of 1/165 grain of strychnin, which, however, disappeared with the discontinuance of the drug. There was a man in London in 1865 who died in twenty minute's after the ingestion of 1/2 grain of strychnin. Wood speaks of a case in which the administration of 1/100 grain killed a child three and one-half months old. Gray speaks of a man who took 22 grains and was not seen for about an hour. He had vomited some of it immediately after taking the dose, and was successfully treated with chloral hydrate. A curious case is mentioned in which three mustard plasters, one on the throat, one on the back of the neck, and another on the left shoulder of a woman, produced symptoms similar to strychnin poisoning. They remained in position for about thirty minutes, and about thirty hours afterward a painful stinging sensation commenced in the back of the neck, followed by violent twitching of the muscles of the face, arms, and legs, which continued in regular succession through the whole of the night, but after twelve hours yielded to hot fomentations of poppy-heads applied to the back of the neck. It could not be ascertained whether any medicine containing strychnin had been taken, but surely, from the symptoms, such must have been the case.

Tobacco.—O'Neill a gives the history of a farmer's wife, aged forty, who wounded her leg against a sewing-machine, and by lay advice applied a handful of chopped wet tobacco to it, from which procedure, strange to say, serious nicotin-poisoning ensued. The pupils were dilated, there were dimness of vision, confusion of thought, and extreme prostration. The pulse was scarcely apparent, the skin was white and wet with clammy perspiration. Happily, strychnin was given in time to effect recovery, and without early medical assistance she would undoubtedly have succumbed. There are several similar cases on record.

Although not immediately related to the subject of idiosyncrasy, the following case may be mentioned here: Ramadge speaks of a young Frenchman, suffering from an obstinate case of gonorrhea, who was said to have been completely cured by living in a newly painted house in which he inhaled the odors or vapors of turpentine.

White speaks of a case of exanthematous eruption similar to that of ivy-poison in mother and child, which was apparently caused by playing with and burning the toy called "Pharaoh's serpent egg."

The idiosyncrasies noticed in some persons during coitus are quite interesting. The Ephemerides mentions a person in whom coitus habitually caused vomiting, and another in whom excessive sexual indulgence provoked singultus. Sometimes exaggerated tremors or convulsions, particularly at the moment of orgasm, are noticed. Females especially are subject to this phenomenon, and it is seen sometimes in birds.

Winn reports the case of a man who, when prompted to indulge in sexual intercourse, was immediately prior to the act seized with a fit of sneezing. Even the thought of sexual pleasure with a female was sufficient to provoke this peculiar idiosyncrasy.

Sullivan mentions a bride of four weeks, who called at the doctor's office, saying that in coitus her partner had no difficulty until the point of culmination or orgasm, when he was seized with complete numbness and lost all pleasurable sensation in the penis. The numbness was followed by a sensation of pain, which was intensified on the slightest motion, and which was at times so excruciating as to forbid separation for upward of an hour, or until the penis had become flaccid. The woman asked for advice for her unfortunate husband's relief, and the case was reported as a means of obtaining suggestions from the physicians over the country. In response, one theory was advanced that this man had been in the habit of masturbating and had a stricture of the membranous portion of the urethra, associated with an ulcer of the prostate involving the ejaculatory ducts, or an inflammatory condition of all the tissues compressed by the ejaculatory muscles.

Hendrichsen quotes a case in which a spasmodic contraction of the levator ani occurred during coitus, and the penis could not be withdrawn while this condition lasted; and in support of this circumstance Hendrichsen mentions that Marion Sims, Beigel, and Budin describe spasmodic contractions of the levator and, constricting the vagina; he also cites an instance under his personal observation in which this spasm was excited by both vaginal and rectal examination, although on the following day no such condition could be produced. In this connection, among the older writers, Borellus gives the history of a man who before coitus rubbed his virile member with musk, and, similar to the connection of a dog and bitch, was held fast in his wife's vagina; it was only after the injection of great quantities of water to soften the parts that separation was obtained. Diemerbroeck confirms this singular property of musk by an analogous observation, in which the ludicrous method of throwing cold water on the persons was practised. Schurig also relates the history of a similar instance.

Among the peculiar effects of coitus is its deteriorating effect on the healing process of wounds. Boerhaave, Pare, and Fabricius Hildanus all speak of this untoward effect of venery, and in modern times Poncet has made observations at a hospital in Lyons which prove that during the process of healing wounds are unduly and harmfully influenced by coitus, and cites confirmatory instances. Poncet also remarks that he found on nine occasions, by placing a thermometer in the rectum, that the temperature was about 1 degrees F. lower just before than after coitus, and that during the act the temperature gradually rose above normal.

There are many associate conditions which, under the exciting influence of coitus, provoke harmful effects and even a fatal issue. Deguise mentions a man who had coitus 18 times in ten hours with most disastrous effects. Cabrolius speaks of a man who took a potion of aphrodisiac properties, in which, among other things, he put an enormous dose of cantharides. The anticipation of the effect of his dose, that is, the mental influence, in addition to the actual therapeutic effect, greatly distressed and excited him. Almost beyond belief, it is said that he approached his wife eighty-seven times during the night, spilling much sperm on the sleeping-bed. Cabrolius was called to see this man in the morning, and found him in a most exhausted condition, but still having the supposed consecutive ejaculations. Exhaustion progressed rapidly, and death soon terminated this erotic crisis. Lawson is accredited with saying that among the Marquesan tribe he knew of a woman who during a single night had intercourse with 103 men.

Among the older writers there are instances reported in which erection and ejaculation took place without the slightest pleasurable sensation. Claudius exemplifies this fact in his report of a Venetian merchant who had vigorous erections and ejaculations of thick and abundant semen without either tingling or pleasure.

Attila, King of the Huns, and one of the most celebrated leaders of the German hosts which overran the Roman Empire in its decline, and whose enormous army and name inspired such terror that he was called the "Scourge of God," was supposed to have died in coitus. Apoplexy, organic heart disorders, aneurysms, and other like disorders are in such cases generally the direct cause of death, coitus causing the death indirectly by the excitement and exertion accompanying the act.

Bartholinus, Benedictus, Borellus, Pliny, Morgagni, Plater, a Castro, Forestus, Marcellus Donatus, Schurig, Sinibaldus, Schenck, the Ephemerides, and many others mention death during coitus; the older writers in some cases attributed the fatal issue to excessive sexual indulgence, not considering the possibility of the associate direct cause, which most likely would have been found in case of a necropsy.

Suspended Animation.—Various opinions have been expressed as to the length of time compatible with life during which a person can stay under water. Recoveries from drowning furnish interesting examples of the suspension of animation for a protracted period, but are hardly ever reliable, as the subject at short intervals almost invariably rises to the surface of the water, allowing occasional respiration. Taylor mentions a child of two who recovered after ten minutes' submersion; in another case a man recovered after fourteen minutes' submersion. There is a case reported in this country of a woman who was said to have been submerged twenty minutes. Guerard quotes a case happening in 1774, in which there was submersion for an hour with subsequent recovery; but there hardly seems sufficient evidence of this.

Green mentions submersion for fifteen minutes; Douglass, for fourteen minutes; Laub, for fifteen minutes; Povall gives a description of three persons who recovered after a submersion of twenty-five minutes. There is a case in French literature, apparently well authenticated, in which submersion for six minutes was followed by subsequent recovery.

There have been individuals who gave exhibitions of prolonged submersion in large glass aquariums, placed in full view of the audience. Taylor remarks that the person known some years ago in London as "Lurline" could stay under water for three minutes. There have been several exhibitionists of this sort. Some of the more enterprising seat themselves on an artificial coral, and surrounded by fishes of divers hues complacently eat a meal while thus submerged. It is said that quite recently in Detroit there was a performer who accomplished the feat of remaining under water four minutes and eight seconds in full view of the audience. Miss Lurline swam about in her aquarium, which was brilliantly illuminated, ate, reclined, and appeared to be taking a short nap during her short immersion. In Paris, some years since, there was exhibited a creature called "l'homme-poisson," who performed feats similar to Lurline, including the smoking of a cigarette held entirely in his mouth. In all these exhibitions all sorts of artificial means are used to make the submersion appear long. Great ceremony, music, and the counting of the seconds in a loud voice from the stage, all tend to make the time appear much longer than it really is. However, James Finney in London, April 7, 1886, stayed under water four minutes, twenty-nine and one-fourth seconds, and one of his feats was to pick up 70 or 80 gold-plated half-pennies with his mouth, his hands being securely tied behind his back, and never emerging from his tank until his feat was fully accomplished. In company with his sister he played a game of "nap" under water, using porcelain cards and turning them to the view of the audience. "Professor Enochs" recently stayed under water at Lowell, Mass., for four minutes, forty-six and one-fifth seconds. The best previous record was four minutes, thirty-five seconds, made by "Professor Beaumont" at Melbourne on December 16, 1893.

For the most satisfactory examples of prolonged submersion we must look to the divers, particularly the natives who trade in coral, and the pearl fishers. Diving is an ancient custom, and even legendary exploits of this nature are recorded. Homer compares the fall of Hector's chariot to the action of a diver; and specially trained men were employed at the Siege of Syracuse, their mission being to laboriously scuttle the enemy's vessels. Many of the old historians mention diving, and Herodotus speaks of a diver by the name of Scyllias who was engaged by Xerxes to recover some articles of value which had been sunk on some Persian vessels in a tempest. Egyptian divers are mentioned by Plutarch, who says that Anthony was deceived by Cleopatra in a fishing contest by securing expert divers to place the fish upon the hooks. There was a historical or rather legendary character by the name of Didion, who was noted for his exploits in the river Meuse. He had the ability to stay under water a considerable length of time, and even to catch fish while submerged.

There was a famous diver in Sicily at the end of the fifteenth century whose feats are recorded in the writings of Alexander ab Alexandro, Pontanus, and Father Kircher, the Jesuit savant. This man's name was Nicolas, born of poor parents at Catania. From his infancy he showed an extraordinary power of diving and swimming, and from his compatriots soon acquired various names indicative of his capacity. He became very well known throughout Sicily, and for his patron had Frederick, King of Naples. In the present day, the sponge-fishers and pearl-fishers in the West Indies, the Mediterranean, the Indian Seas, and the Gulf of Mexico invite the attention of those interested in the anomalies of suspended animation. There are many marvelous tales of their ability to remain under water for long periods. It is probable that none remain submerged over two minutes, but, what is more remarkable, they are supposed to dive to extraordinary depths, some as much as 150 to 200 feet. Ordinarily they remain under water from a minute to one and a half minutes. Remaining longer, the face becomes congested, the eyes injected; the sputum bloody, due to rupture of some of the minute vessels in the lung. It is said by those who have observed them carefully that few of these divers live to an advanced age. Many of them suffer apoplectic attacks, and some of them become blind from congestion of the ocular vessels. The Syrian divers are supposed to carry weights of considerable size in their hands in order to facilitate the depth and duration of submersion. It is also said that the divers of Oceanica use heavy stones. According to Guyot-Daubes, in the Philippine Isles the native pearl-fishers teach their children to dive to the depth of 25 meters. The Tahitians, who excited the admiration of Cook, are noted for their extraordinary diving. Speaking of the inhabitants of the island of Fakaraya, near Tahiti, de la Quesnerie says that the pearl-fishers do not hesitate to dive to the depth even of 100 feet after their coveted prizes. On the Ceylon coast the mother-of-pearl fishers are under the direction of the English Government, which limits the duration and the practice of this occupation. These divers are generally Cingalese, who practice the exercise from infancy. As many as 500 small boats can be seen about the field of operation, each equipped with divers. A single diver makes about ten voyages under the water, and then rests in the bottom of the boat, when his comrade takes his place. Among other native divers are the Arabs of Algeria and some of the inhabitants of the Mexican coast.

It might be well to mention here the divers who work by means of apparatus. The ancients had knowledge of contrivances whereby they could stay under water some time. Aristotle speaks of an instrument by which divers could rest under water in communication with the air, and compares it with the trunk of an elephant wading a stream deeper than his height. In the presence of Charles V diving bells were used by the Greeks in 1540. In 1660 some of the cannon of the sunken ships of the Spanish Armada were raised by divers in diving bells. Since then various improvements in submarine armor have been made, gradually evolving into the present perfected diving apparatus of to-day, by which men work in the holds of vessels sunk in from 120 to 200 feet of water. The enormous pressure of the water at these great depths makes it necessary to have suits strong enough to resist it. Lambert, a celebrated English diver, recovered L90,000 in specie from the steamer Alphonso XII, a Spanish mail boat belonging to the Lopez line, which sank off Point Gando, Grand Canary, in 26 1/2 fathoms of water. For nearly six months the salvage party, despatched by the underwriters in May, 1885, persevered in the operations; two divers lost their lives, the golden bait being in the treasure-room beneath the three decks, but Lambert finished the task successfully.

Deep-sea divers only acquire proficiency after long training. It is said that as a rule divers are indisposed to taking apprentices, as they are afraid of their vocation being crowded and their present ample remuneration diminished. At present there are several schools. At Chatham, England, there is a school of submarine mining, in which men are trained to lay torpedoes and complete harbor defense. Most of these divers can work six hours at a time in from 35 to 50 feet of water. Divers for the Royal Navy are trained at Sheerness. When sufficiently trained to work at the depth of 150 feet seamen-divers are fully qualified, and are drafted to the various ships. They are connected with an air-pump in charge of trustworthy men; they signal for their tools and material, as well as air, by means of a special line for this purpose. At some distance below the water the extraordinary weight of the suits cannot be felt, and the divers work as well in armor as in ordinary laboring clothes. One famous diver says that the only unpleasant experience he ever had in his career as a diver, not excepting the occasion of his first dive, was a drumming in the ears, as a consequence of which, after remaining under water at a certain work for nine hours, he completely lost the use of one ear for three months, during which time he suffered agony with the earache. These men exhibit absolute indifference to the dangers attached to their calling, and some have been known to sleep many fathoms beneath the surface. Both by means of their signal lines and by writing on a slate they keep their associates informed of the progress of their work.

Suspension of the Pulse.—In some cases the pulse is not apparent for many days before actual death, and there have been instances in which, although the pulse ceased for an extended period, the patient made an ultimate recovery. In reviewing the older literature we find that Ballonius mentions an instance in which the pulse was not apparent for fourteen days before complete asphyxia. Ramazzini describes a case of cessation of the pulse four days before death. Schenck details the history of a case in which the pulse ceased for three days and asphyxia was almost total, but the patient eventually recovered. There is a noteworthy observation. in which there was cessation of the pulse for nine days without a fatal issue.

Some persons seem to have a preternatural control over their circulatory system, apparently enabling them to produce suspension of cardiac movement at will. Cheyne speaks of a Colonel Townshend who appeared to possess the power of dying, as it were, at will,—that is, so suspending the heart's action that no pulsation could be detected. After lying in this state of lifelessness for a short period, life would become slowly established without any consciousness or volition on the man's part. The longest period in which he remained in this death-like condition was about thirty minutes. A postmortem examination of this person was awaited with great interest; but after his death nothing was found to explain the power he possessed over his heart.

Saint Augustin knew of a priest named Rutilut who had the power of voluntarily simulating death. Both the pulsation and respiration was apparently abolished when he was in his lifeless condition. Burning and pricking left visible effects on the skin after his recovery, but had no apparent effect on his lethargy. Chaille reports an instance of voluntary suspension of the pulse.

Relative to hibernation, it is well-known that mice, snakes, and some reptiles, as well as bees, sometimes seem to entirely suspend animation for an extended period, and especially in the cold weather. In Russia fish are transported frozen stiff, but return to life after being plunged into cold water. A curious tale is told by Harley, from Sir John Lubbock, of a snail brought from Egypt and thought to be dead. It was placed on a card and put in position on a shelf in the British Museum in March, 1845. In March, 1850 after having been gummed to a label for five years, it was noticed to have an apparent growth on its mouth and was taken out and placed in water, when it soon showed signs of life and ate cabbage leaves offered to it. It has been said, we think with credible evidence, that cereal seeds found in the tombs with mummies have grown when planted, and Harley quotes an instance of a gentleman who took some berries, possibly the remnants of Pharaoh's daughter's last meal, coming as they did from her mummified stomach after lying dormant in an Egyptian tomb many centuries, and planted them in his garden, where they soon grew, and he shortly had a bush as flourishing as any of those emanating from fresh seeds.

Human hibernation is an extremely rare anomaly. Only the fakirs of India seem to have developed this power, and even the gifted ones there are seldom seen. Many theories have been advanced to explain this ability of the fakirs, and many persons have discredited all the stories relative to their powers; on the other hand, all who have witnessed their exhibitions are convinced of their genuineness. Furthermore, these persons are extremely scarce and are indifferent to money; none has been enticed out of his own country to give exhibitions. When one dies in a community, his place is never filled—proving that he had no accomplices who knew any fraudulent secret practices, otherwise the accomplice would soon step out to take his place. These men have undoubtedly some extraordinary mode of sending themselves into a long trance, during which the functions of life are almost entirely suspended. We can readily believe in their ability to fast during their periods of burial, as we have already related authentic instances of fasting for a great length of time, during which the individual exercised his normal functions.

To the fakir, who neither visibly breathes nor shows circulatory movements, and who never moves from his place of confinement, fasting should be comparatively easy, when we consider the number of men whose minds were actively at work during their fasts, and who also exercised much physical power.

Harley says that the fakirs begin their performances by taking a large dose of the powerfully stupefying "bang," thus becoming narcotized. In this state they are lowered into a cool, quiet tomb, which still further favors the prolongation of the artificially induced vital lethargy; in this condition they rest for from six to eight weeks. When resurrected they are only by degrees restored to life, and present a wan, haggard, debilitated, and wasted appearance. Braid is credited, on the authority of Sir Claude Wade, with stating that a fakir was buried in an unconscious state at Lahore in 1837, and when dug up, six weeks later, he presented all the appearances of a dead person. The legs and arms were shrunken and stiff, and the head reclined on the shoulder in a manner frequently seen in a corpse. There was no pulsation of the heart or arteries of the arm or temple—in fact, no really visible signs of life. By degrees this person was restored to life. Every precaution had been taken in this case to prevent the possibility of fraud, and during the period of interment the grave was guarded night and day by soldiers of the regiment stationed at Lahore.

Honigberger, a German physician in the employ of Runjeet Singh, has an account of a fakir of Punjaub who allowed himself to be buried in a well-secured vault for such a long time that grain sown in the soil above the vault sprouted into leaf before he was exhumed. Honigberger affirms that the time of burial was over 40 days, and that on being submitted to certain processes the man recovered and lived many years after. Sir Henry Lawrence verified the foregoing statements. The chest in which the fakir was buried was sealed with the Runjeet stamp on it, and when the man was brought up he was cold and apparently lifeless. Honigberger also states that this man, whose name was Haridas, was four months in a grave in the mountains; to prove the absolute suspension of animation, the chin was shaved before burial, and at exhumation this part was as smooth as on the day of interment. This latter statement naturally calls forth comment when we consider the instances that are on record of the growth of beard and hair after death.

There is another account of a person of the same class who had the power of suspending animation, and who would not allow his coffin to touch the earth for fear of worms and insects, from which he is said to have suffered at a previous burial.

It has been stated that the fakirs are either eunuchs or hermaphrodites, social outcasts, having nothing in common with the women or men of their neighborhood; but Honigberger mentions one who disproved this ridiculous theory by eloping to the mountains with his neighbor's wife.

Instances of recovery after asphyxia from hanging are to be found, particularly among the older references of a time when hanging was more common than it is to-day. Bartholinus, Blegny, Camerarius, Morgagni, Pechlin, Schenck, Stoll, and Wepfer all mention recovery after hanging. Forestus describes a case in which a man was rescued by provoking vomiting with vinegar, pepper, and mustard seed. There is a case on record in which a person was saved after hanging nineteen minutes. There was a case of a man brought into the Hopital Saint-Louis asphyxiated by strangulation, having been hung for some time. His rectal temperature was only 93.3 degrees F., but six hours after it rose to 101.6 degrees F., and he subsequently recovered. Taylor cites the instance of a stout woman of forty-four who recovered from hanging. When the woman was found by her husband she was hanging from the top of a door, having been driven to suicide on account of his abuse and intemperance. When first seen by Taylor she was comatose, her mouth was surrounded by white froth, and the swollen tongue protruded from it. Her face was bloated, her lips of a darkened hue, and her neck of a brown parchment-color. About the level of the larynx, the epidermis was distinctly abraded, indicating where the rope had been. The conjunctiva was insensible and there was no contractile response of the pupil to the light of a candle. The reflexes of the soles of the feet were tested, but were quite in abeyance. There was no respiratory movement and only slight cardiac pulsation. After vigorous measures the woman ultimately recovered. Recovery is quite rare when the asphyxiation has gone so far, the patients generally succumbing shortly after being cut down or on the following day. Chevers mentions a most curious case, in which cerebral congestion from the asphyxiation of strangling was accidentally relieved by an additional cut across the throat. The patient was a man who was set upon by a band of Thugs in India. who, pursuant to their usual custom, strangled him and his fellow-traveler. Not being satisfied that he was quite dead, one of the band returned and made several gashes across his throat. This latter action effectually relieved the congestion caused by the strangulation and undoubtedly saved his life, while his unmutilated companion was found dead. After the wounds in his throat had healed this victim of the Thugs gave such a good description of the murderous band that their apprehension and execution soon followed.

Premature Burial.—In some instances simulation of death has been so exact that it has led to premature interment. There are many such cases on record, and it is a popular superstition of the laity that all the gruesome tales are true of persons buried alive and returning to life, only to find themselves hopelessly lost in a narrow coffin many feet below the surface of the earth. Among the lower classes the dread of being buried before life is extinct is quite generally felt, and for generations the medical profession have been denounced for their inability to discover an infallible sign of death. Most of the instances on record, and particularly those from lay journals, are vivid exaggerations, drawn from possibly such a trivial sign as a corpse found with the fist tightly clenched or the face distorted, which are the inspiration of the horrible details of the dying struggles of the person in the coffin. In the works of Fontenelle there are 46 cases recorded of the premature interment of the living, in which apparent has been mistaken for real death. None of these cases, however, are sufficiently authentic to be reliable. Moreover, in all modern methods of burial, even if life were not extinct, there could be no possibility of consciousness or of struggling. Absolute asphyxiation would soon follow the closing of the coffin lid.

We must admit, however, that the mistake has been made, particularly in instances of catalepsy or trance, and during epidemics of malignant fevers or plagues, in which there is an absolute necessity of hasty burial for the prevention of contagion. In a few instances on the battle-field sudden syncope, or apparent death, has possibly led to premature interment; but in the present day this is surely a very rare occurrence. There is also a danger of mistake from cases of asphyxiation, drowning, and similar sudden suspensions of the vital functions.

It is said that in the eighty-fourth Olympiad, Empedocles restored to life a woman who was about to be buried, and that this circumstance induced the Greeks, for the future protection of the supposed dead, to establish laws which enacted that no person should be interred until the sixth or seventh day. But even this extension of time did not give satisfaction, and we read that when Hephestion, at whose funeral obsequies Alexander the Great was present, was to be buried his funeral was delayed until the tenth day. There is also a legend that when Acilius Aviola fell a victim to disease he was burned alive, and although he cried out, it was too late to save him, as the fire had become so widespread before life returned.

While returning to his country house Asclepiades, a physician denominated the "God of Physic," and said to have been a descendant of aesculapius, saw during the time of Pompey the Great a crowd of mourners about to start a fire on a funeral pile. It is said that by his superior knowledge he perceived indications of life in the corpse and ordered the pile destroyed, subsequently restoring the supposed deceased to life. These examples and several others of a similar nature induced the Romans to delay their funeral rites, and laws were enacted to prevent haste in burning, as well as in interment. It was not until the eighth day that the final rites were performed, the days immediately subsequent to death having their own special ceremonies. The Turks were also fearful of premature interment and subjected the defunct to every test; among others, one was to examine the contractility of the sphincter and, which shows their keen observation of a well-known modern medical fact.

According to the Memoirs of Amelot de la Houssaye, Cardinal Espinola, Prime Minister to Philip II, put his hand to the embalmer's knife with which he was about to be opened; It is said that Vesalius, sometimes called the "Father of Anatomy," having been sent for to perform an autopsy on a woman subject to hysteric convulsions, and who was supposed to be dead, on making the first incision perceived by her motion and cries that she was still alive. This circumstance, becoming known, rendered him so odious that he had to leave the community in which he practiced, and it is believed that he never entirely recovered from the shock it gave him. The Abbe Prevost, so well known by his works and the singularities of his life, was seized by apoplexy in the Forest of Chantilly on October 23, 1763. His body was carried to the nearest village, and the officers of justice proceeded to open it, when a cry he sent forth frightened all the assistants and convinced the surgeon in charge that the Abbe was not dead; but it was too late to save him, as he had already received a mortal wound.

Massien speaks of a woman living in Cologne in 1571 who was interred living, but was not awakened from her lethargy until a grave-digger opened her grave to steal a valuable ring which she wore. This instance has been cited in nearly every language. There is another more recent instance, coming from Poitiers, of the wife of a goldsmith named Mernache who was buried with all her jewels. During the night a beggar attempted to steal her jewelry, and made such exertion in extracting one ring that the woman recovered and was saved. After this resurrection she is said to have had several children. This case is also often quoted. Zacchias mentions an instance which, from all appearances, is authentic. It was that of a young man, pest-stricken and thought to be dead, who was placed with the other dead for burial. He exhibited signs of life, and was taken back to the pest-hospital. Two days later he entered a lethargic condition simulating death, and was again on his way to the sepulcher, when he once more recovered.

It is said that when the body of William, Earl of Pembroke, who died April 10, 1630, was opened to be embalmed, the hand raised when the first incision was made. There is a story of an occurrence which happened on a return voyage from India. The wife of one of the passengers, an officer in the army, to all appearances died. They were about to resort to sea-burial, when, through the interposition of the husband, who was anxious to take her home, the ship-carpenters started to construct a coffin suitable for a long voyage, a process which took several days, during which time she lay in her berth, swathed in robes and ready for interment. When the coffin was at last ready the husband went to take his last farewell, and removed the wedding-ring, which was quite tightly on her finger. In the effort to do this she was aroused, recovered, and arrived in England perfectly well.

It is said that when a daughter of Henry Laurens, the first President of the American Congress, died of small-pox, she was laid out as dead, and the windows of the room were opened for ventilation. While left alone in this manner she recovered. This circumstance so impressed her illustrious father that he left explicit directions that in case of his death he should be burned. The same journal also contains the case of a maid-servant who recovered thrice on her way to the grave, and who, when really dead, was kept a preposterous length of time before burial.

The literature on this subject is very exhaustive, volumes having been written on the uncertainty of the signs of death, with hundreds of examples cited illustrative of the danger of premature interment. The foregoing instances have been given as indicative of the general style of narration; for further information the reader is referred to the plethora of material on this subject.

Postmortem Anomalies.—Among the older writers startling movements of a corpse have given rise to much discussion, and possibly often led to suspicion of premature burial. Bartholinus describes motion in a cadaver. Barlow says that movements were noticed after death in the victims of Asiatic cholera. The bodies were cold and expressions were death-like, but there were movements simulating natural life. The most common was flexion of the right leg, which would also be drawn up toward the body and resting on the left leg. In some cases the hand was moved, and in one or two instances a substance was grasped as if by reflex action. Some observers have stated that reflex movements of the face were quite noticeable. These movements continued sometimes for upward of an hour, occurring mostly in muscular subjects who died very suddenly, and in whom the muscular irritability or nervous stimulus or both had not become exhausted at the moment of dissolution. Richardson doubts the existence of postmortem movements of respiration.

Snow is accredited with having seen a girl in Soho who, dying of scarlet fever, turned dark at the moment of death, but in a few hours presented such a life-line appearance and color as to almost denote the return of life. The center of the cheeks became colored in a natural fashion, and the rest of the body resumed the natural flesh color. The parents refused to believe that death had ensued. Richardson remarks that he had seen two similar cases, and states that he believes the change is due to oxidation of the blood surcharged with carbon dioxid. The moist tissues suffuse carbonized blood, and there occurs an osmotic interchange between the carbon dioxid and the oxygen of the air resulting in an oxygenation of the blood, and modification of the color from dark venous to arterial red.

A peculiar postmortem anomaly is erection of the penis. The Ephemerides and Morgagni discuss postmortem erection, and Guyon mentions that on one occasion he saw 14 negroes hanged, and states that at the moment of suspension erection of the penis occurred in each; in nine of these blacks traces of this erectile state were perceived an hour after death.

Cadaveric perspiration has been observed and described by several authors, and Paullini has stated that he has seen tears flow from the eyes of a corpse.

The retardation of putrefaction of the body after death sometimes presents interesting changes. Petrifaction or mummification of the body are quite well known, and not being in the province of this work, will be referred to collateral books on this subject; but sometimes an unaccountable preservation takes place. In a tomb recently opened at Canterbury Cathedral, a for the purpose of discovering what Archbishop's body it contained, the corpse was of an extremely offensive and sickening odor, unmistakably that of putrefaction. The body was that of Hubert Walter, who died in 1204 A.D., and the decomposition had been retarded, and was actually still in progress, several hundred years after burial.

Retardation of the putrefactive process has been noticed in bodies some years under water. Konig of Hermannstadt mentions a man who, forty years previous to the time of report, had fallen under the waters of Echoschacht, and who was found in a complete state of preservation.

Postmortem Growth of Hair and Nails.—The hair and beard may grow after death, and even change color. Bartholinus recalls a case of a man who had short, black hair and beard at the time of interment, but who, some time after death, was found to possess long and yellowish hair. Aristotle discusses postmortem growth of the hair, and Garmanus cites an instance in which the beard and hair were cut several times from the cadaver. We occasionally see evidences of this in the dissecting-rooms. Caldwell mentions a body buried four years, the hair from which protruded at the points where the joints of the coffin had given away. The hair of the head measured 18 inches, that of the beard eight inches, and that on the breast from four to six inches. Rosse of Washington mentions an instance in which after burial the hair turned from dark brown to red, and also cites a case in a Washington cemetery of a girl, twelve or thirteen years old, who when exhumed was found to have a new growth of hair all over her body. The Ephemerides contains an account of hair suddenly turning gray after death.

Nails sometimes grow several inches after death, and there is on record the account of an idiot who had an idiosyncrasy for long nails, and after death the nails were found to have grown to such an extent that they curled up under the palms and soles.

The untoward effects of the emotions on the vital functions are quite well exemplified in medical literature. There is an abundance of cases reported in which joy, fear, pride, and grief have produced a fatal issue. In history we have the old story of the Lacedemonian woman who for some time had believed her son was dead, and who from the sudden joy occasioned by seeing him alive, herself fell lifeless. There is a similar instance in Roman history. Aristotle, Pliny, Livy, Cicero, and others cite instances of death from sudden or excessive joy. Fouquet died of excessive joy on being released from prison. A niece of the celebrated Leibnitz immediately fell dead on seeing a casket of gold left to her by her deceased uncle.

Galen mentions death from joy, and in comment upon it he says that the emotion of joy is much more dangerous than that of anger. In discussing this subject, Haller says that the blood is probably sent with such violence to the brain as to cause apoplexy. There is one case on record in which after a death from sudden joy the pericardium was found full of blood. The Ephemerides, Marcellus Donatus, Martini, and Struthius all mention death from joy.

Death from violent laughter has been recorded, but in this instance it is very probable that death was not due to the emotion itself, but to the extreme convulsion and exertion used in the laughter. The Ephemerides mentions a death from laughter, and also describes the death of a pregnant woman from violent mirth. Roy, Swinger, and Camerarius have recorded instances of death from laughter. Strange as it may seem, Saint-Foix says that the Moravian brothers, a sect of Anabaptists having great horror of bloodshed, executed their condemned brethren by tickling them to death.

Powerfully depressing emotions, which are called by Kant "asthenic," such as great and sudden sorrow, grief, or fright, have a pronounced effect on the vital functions, at times even causing death. Throughout literature and history we have examples of this anomaly. In Shakespeare's "Pericles," Thaisa, the daughter to Simonides and wife of Pericles, frightened when pregnant by a threatened shipwreck, dies in premature childbirth.

In Scott's "Guy Mannering," Mrs. Bertram, on suddenly learning of the death of her little boy, is thrown into premature labor, followed by death. Various theories are advanced in explanation of this anomaly. A very plausible one is, that the cardiac palsy is caused by energetic and persistent excitement of the inhibitory cardiac nerves. Strand is accredited with saying that agony of the mind produces rupture of the heart. It is quite common to hear the expression, "Died of a broken heart;" and, strange to say, in some cases postmortem examination has proved the actual truth of the saying. Bartholinus, Fabricius Hildanus, Pliny, Rhodius, Schenck, Marcellus Donatus, Riedlin, and Garengeot speak of death from fright and fear, and the Ephemerides describes a death the direct cause of which was intense shame. Deleau, a celebrated doctor of Paris, while embracing his favorite daughter, who was in the last throes of consumption, was so overcome by intense grief that he fell over her corpse and died, and both were buried together.

The fear of child-birth has been frequently cited as a cause of death McClintock quotes a case from Travers of a young lady, happily married; who entertained a fear of death in child-birth; although she had been safely delivered, she suddenly and without apparent cause died in six hours. Every region of the body was examined with minutest care by an eminent physician, but no signs indicative of the cause of death were found. Mordret cites a similar instance of death from fear of labor. Morgagni mentions a woman who died from the disappointment of bearing a girl baby when she was extremely desirous of a boy.

The following case, quoted from Lauder Brunton, shows the extent of shock which may be produced by fear: Many years ago a janitor of a college had rendered himself obnoxious to the students, and they determined to punish him. Accordingly they prepared a block and an axe, which they conveyed to a lonely place, and having appropriately dressed themselves, some of them prepared to act as judges, and sent others of their company to bring him before them. He first affected to treat the whole affair as a joke, but was solemnly assured by the students that they meant it in real earnest. He was told to prepare for immediate death. The trembling janitor looked all around in the vain hope of seeing some indication that nothing was really meant, but stern looks met him everywhere. He was blindfolded, and made to kneel before the block. The executioner's axe was raised, but, instead of the sharp edge, a wet towel was brought sharply down on the back of the neck. The bandage was now removed from the culprit's eyes, but to the horror and astonishment of the students they found that he was dead. Such a case may be due to heart-failure from fear or excitement.

It is not uncommon that death ensues from the shock alone following blows that cause no visible injury, but administered to vital parts. This is particularly true of blows about the external genital region, or epigastrium, where the solar plexus is an active factor in inhibition. Ivanhoff of Bulgaria in 1886 speaks of a man of forty-five who was dealt a blow on the testicle in a violent street fight, and staggering, he fell insensible. Despite vigorous medical efforts he never regained consciousness and died in forty-five minutes. Postmortem examination revealed everything normal, and death must have been caused by syncope following violent pain. Watkins cites an instance occurring in South Africa. A native shearing sheep for a farmer provoked his master's ire by calling him by some nickname. While the man was in a squatting posture the farmer struck him in the epigastrium. He followed this up by a kick in the side and a blow on the head, neither of which, however, was as severe as the first blow. The man fell unconscious and died. At the autopsy there were no signs indicative of death, which must have been due to the shock following the blow on the epigastrium.

As illustrative of the sensitiveness of the epigastric region, Vincent relates the following case: "A man received a blow by a stick upon the epigastrium. He had an anxious expression and suffered from oppression. Irregular heart-action and shivering were symptoms that gradually disappeared during the day. In the evening his appetite returned and he felt well; during the night he died without a struggle, and at the autopsy there was absolutely nothing abnormal to be found." Blows upon the neck often produce sudden collapse. Prize-fighters are well aware of the effects of a blow on the jugular vein. Maschka, quoted by Warren, reports the case of a boy of twelve, who was struck on the anterior portion of the larynx by a stone. He fell lifeless to the ground, and at autopsy no local lesion was found nor any lesion elsewhere. The sudden death may be attributed in this case partly to shock and partly to cerebral anemia.

Soldiers have been seen to drop lifeless on the battle-field without apparent injury or organic derangement; in the olden times this death was attributed to fear and fright, and later was supposed to be caused by what is called "the wind of a cannon-ball." Tolifree has written an article on this cause of sudden death and others have discussed it. By some it is maintained that the momentum acquired by a cannon-ball generates enough force in the neighboring air to prostrate a person in the immediate vicinity of its path of flight.

Printed in Great Britain
by Amazon